Old Paint

Old Paint

A Medical History of Childhood Lead-Paint Poisoning in the United States to 1980

PETER C. ENGLISH

RUTGERS UNIVERSITY PRESS
New Brunswick, New Jersey, and London

Library of Congress Cataloging-in-Publication Data

English, Peter C.
  Old paint : a medical history of childhood lead-paint poisoning in the United States
to 1980 / Peter C. English.
    p. cm.
  Includes bibliographical references and index.
  ISBN 0-8135-2987-5 (alk. paper)
  1. Lead poisoning in children—United States—History—20th century. 2. Lead
based paint—Toxicology—United States—History—20th century. 3. Poisoning,
Accidents, in children—United States—History—20th century. I. Title.

RA1231.L4 E546 2001
615.9'25688'0830973—dc21

                                                                    2001019287

British Cataloging-in-Publication data for this book is available from the British Library.

Manufactured in the United States of America

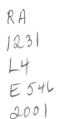

For Shirley Osterhout,
who taught hundreds of Duke medical students and pediatric house
officers about the dangers of accidental poisoning in children's lives

Contents

Illustrations

Preface

W<small>HEN</small> I <small>ENTERED</small> Duke Medical School in 1969, childhood lead-paint poisoning weighed heavily on the minds of northern child health professionals, public health officials, politicians, and parents. There was a broad national consensus about this health menace: at risk were toddlers, eating paint chips from peeling and flaking walls and ceilings of urban tenements that had fallen into decay and neglect.[1] Lead-paint poisoning thus merged into the larger issue of the crumbling inner city. Public health officials in Baltimore had initially described this household hazard twenty years earlier.[2] After Baltimore's initial portrait, one city after another, in what some public health officers termed the "lead belt," discovered the consequences of deteriorating paint in slum housing.[3] By 1969 lead poisoning was a disease clearly visible to parents and physicians. Lead-poisoned children had symptoms, often quite distressing and life-threatening, which prompted parents to seek medical attention. Severe abdominal pain; numbness and paralysis of hands, feet, arms, or legs; anemia; seizures; or coma prompted parents to pick up their sickened children and deliver them to community emergency rooms.

The lead poisoning about which I learned in medical school was largely gone by the time I joined the faculty in 1978. Worries about lead, of course, had not receded from view. Instead, medical technology, biochemical tests, and epidemiological surveys combined forces to redefine lead poisoning into a different disease.

Except in desperate cases, lead's visible symptoms disappeared, because children no longer ingested sufficient lead from peeling and flaking paint. But new worries arose. Biochemical blood tests indicated that lead interfered with the normal formation of heme, a constituent of hemoglobin. Later, psychological testing would reveal that amounts of lead that did not produce visible symptoms nonetheless interfered with brain function in more subtle ways. The older, highly visible lead poisoning evolved into the "silent epidemic," imperceptible without laboratory or psychological tests.

In part, technology helped to define the new lead poisoning. Until the mid-sixties, confirming the presence of lead required obtaining 5–10 cc of blood—no small task in a toddler—and much effort by a chemist. Health departments in Chicago and New York City pioneered with methods that needed less blood and less chemist time. These innovations set the stage for mass screening. The results, first published in the late sixties, indicated that many urban children had enough lead in their bodies to inhibit heme formation. What resulted was the birth of a new disease, which was termed "undue lead absorption." This new disease did not call attention to itself: parents did not know that their children suffered from it, nor did their pediatricians. Instead of seizures or coma, a child had only an elevated level of lead in the blood. Mass screening revealed that the new lead poisoning was as common as the old disease was rare.

The redefinition of lead poisoning in the late 1960s and early 1970s was just one of several transformations that this disease has undergone in the past century. These metamorphoses are grist for the historian's mill. I believe that most diseases change with time. Today's physician, who diagnoses tuberculosis with a skin test and an X-ray, would hardly recognize a nineteenth-century invalid with consumption. Rheumatic fever injured one million American hearts in 1940; at the end of the twentieth century it has virtually disappeared from the United States; what few cases appear in children's clinics are a pale reflection of the nineteenth-century form of the illness.[4] Heart attacks peaked in the 1950s; lung cancer may have peaked in the early 1990s. In 1900, neither heart attacks nor lung cancer were "blips" on the epidemiological radar screen.

The comings and goings of diseases are complicated, poorly understood processes. The effort of physicians and public health officials to combat illness is only one part of an intricate puzzle. To be sure, most diseases have biological components. But physicians and patients have to "see" the disease before they can study and understand it. In a medical sense, "seeing" is the interaction of what a patient complains about, what a physician finds on examination or in laboratory studies, and how the physician interprets the complaints and exam findings in terms of evolving medical theory. For example, a physician could not understand the common cold as a "viral disease" before viruses had been discovered. And after antibiotics flooded clinical practice, "viral" took on the specific meaning of "not bacterial," which patients and doctors often relegated to "untreatable" or, mistakenly, less important. Medicine and disease both change.[5]

Equally important to physicians' understanding of disease is the social context of the illness. It may seem illogical that a disease as concrete as pneumonia can be viewed quite differently by different cultures. For example, in 1900 American physicians believed that pneumonia was a problem of the elderly and almost never occurred in epidemics. Halfway around the world in South Africa, miners, working underground, died in droves from pneumonia at young ages. To combat the disease, South African doctors developed vaccines that greatly reduced its incidence among miners. American physicians dismissed the findings because they believed that the social setting of pneumonia in South Africa simply did not apply to pneumonia in the United States. Almost a century later, a new pneumococcal vaccine has been approved for practice. Only time will tell if American pediatricians and parents take advantage of it.[6]

Geography and social setting have greatly influenced the history of childhood lead poisoning in the United States. Although I was aware as a medical student in North Carolina that childhood lead-paint poisoning was an emerging public health concern, I did not see a single case. In my fourth year, I took a course in childhood poisoning with Shirley Osterhout, who was the director of the Duke Poison Control Center, where I learned about the dangers that peeling and flaking lead paint posed for toddlers. Having grown up in Elizabeth, New Jersey, in an older home that had many coats of lead paint and that was just a short distance from both the Garden State Parkway and the New Jersey Turnpike where cars and trucks spewed lead into the atmosphere, I found lead poisoning a disease that came distressingly close to home. I once asked Jay Arena, a pioneer in the poison control movement and a member of the Home Hazard Committee of the American Academy of Pediatrics that had first studied this problem in the 1950s, why we were not seeing the epidemic that was engulfing northern cities. Arena offered his opinion that deteriorating housing in the South had never been covered with lead paint. If decorated at all, these houses had been white-washed.

Trends in home decoration greatly influenced the history of childhood lead poisoning in northern cities as well. In the first years of the twentieth century—as one response to an intensified awareness of germs—public health reformers urged home owners to switch from wallpaper to glossy paint so that offending germs could be washed away. Concerned with the health of patients and schoolchildren, hospital administrators and school officials touted paint for sanitary reasons. Paints with lead pigments and driers could be scrubbed over and again.[7] Their vivid colors pleased home decorators; their ease of application made them the favorite of master painters. When a painted surface wore out, home owners and hospital and school officials asked painters to sand roughened surfaces and to paint over old coats. In wealthier neighborhoods, repainting might occur every five years, so that by mid-century these rooms had many layers of lead paint.

After World War II the character of many of the older, well-to-do neighborhoods changed. Families moved to the suburbs; large apartments in the cities were subdivided and rented to people who flocked there after the war. For the most part the new occupants, many of whom were southern African Americans, were transient tenants. In this new environment, landlords did not maintain painted walls when they aged. Peeling and flaking paint—which once would have been sanded and repainted—deteriorated. Paint flakes, containing a half century of lead paint, fell from ceilings and walls onto the hands and into the mouths of toddlers. Their parents—emigrants from the South who had previously lived in dwellings that had never been painted—were unaware of the dangers of eating lead paint, a health concern that northern public health officials had identified in the 1920s in connection with infants' chewing on cribs and toys that were then painted with lead paints.

When I moved to New York Hospital for residency, the contrast between the rural South and the urban North could not have been more marked. Childhood lead poisoning was the subject of intense media scrutiny. Jack Newfield's series of detailed articles in the *Village Voice* had alerted the city to the perils facing children as a result of crumbling paint in decaying apartments.[8] I had read this series in North Carolina, drawn to it more because I had met Newfield when he came to Duke in 1967 than because of its relevance to the care I was then providing to children at Duke Hospital. At New York Hospital there were always two or three children admitted for chelation therapy, a method of removing lead from their bodies. It was a routine procedure, so common that we had standard protocols for treating poisoned toddlers.

When I returned to North Carolina after residency, I left this daily familiarity with the treatment of lead poisoning. In the South symptomatic cases were virtually nonexistent; asymptomatic cases were more likely from pottery glazes than from paint. The few paint cases came from urban redevelopers who were fixing up older homes in affluent neighborhoods.

The lead worries so prevalent in the North did not cease with the demise of symptoms. Most distressing to parents and public health officials were subtle neurological, behavioral, and intellectual injuries. As these injuries became known, public health officials progressively scaled back the exposure to lead that was considered "safe." One indication of this dramatic shift in opinion is expressed in the amount of lead in the body considered toxic, measured in micrograms of lead in 100 ml of whole blood (micrograms/deciliter). From experience in the 1930s and 1940s—when blood lead measurements first became available—pediatricians learned that seizures and coma occurred at blood levels between 100 and 300 micrograms/dl. By 1991 the Centers for Disease Control had lowered the level of concern to 10 micrograms/dl. The Committee on Environmental Health of the American Academy of Pediatrics explained to members in 1993:

> During the last 30 years the Centers for Disease Control and Prevention (CDC) has revised downward the definition of the blood level at which lead poisoning occurs from 60 micrograms/dl whole blood in the early

1960s, to 30 micrograms/dl in 1975, and 25 micrograms/dl in 1985. The 1991 CDC Statement "Preventing Lead Poisoning in Young Children" recommended lowering the community intervention level to 10 micrograms/dl. . . . In 1987 the American Academy of Pediatrics stated that lead levels greater than 25 micrograms/dl were unacceptable for children. The Academy now recognizes that impairment of cognitive function begins to occur at levels greater than 10 micrograms/dl, even though clinical symptoms are not seen.[9]

In this heightened concern over levels of lead once considered normal, even house dust licked from sticky fingers—containing lead from air pollution and small bits of pulverized paint—emerged as a new hazard. I therefore screened all my patients for lead, no matter where they lived. The decaying inner city no longer provided a convenient boundary for the disease.

Three people deserve special thanks. First is Shirley Osterhout, whom I first met as an inspirational teacher of childhood poisoning and who later became a wonderful colleague and pediatrician for our son, David. Second is Betsy Adams, whose careful attention to details brought this manuscript to readiness. The third is my wife, Sarah, for her careful reading, criticism, and copyediting.

I would like to acknowledge that I began my research on childhood lead poisoning in preparation of an affidavit submitted on behalf of defendants in *The City of New York, the New York City Housing Authority, and the New York City Health and Hospitals Corporation* v. *The Lead Industries Association, Inc., et al.*

I also want to thank the Mary Duke Biddle Foundation for awarding me a publication grant for this book.

Old Paint

Prologue

IT IS HARD TO appreciate how far lead has receded from our everyday environment. At the beginning of the twentieth century, the widespread use of lead-containing insecticides resulted in lead in virtually every foodstuff, including breast milk. Over the course of the century, the amount of dietary lead decreased remarkably. When Robert Kehoe, a leader in industrial medicine, measured the amount of lead in the average American diet in the 1930s, he estimated that it ranged between 160 and 280 micrograms/day.[1] Forty years later, the lead content of food was unchanged.[2] After tetraethyl lead was removed from gasoline and lead solder from cans in the late 1970s, dietary lead fell to 85 micrograms/day. By 1990, it was 10 micrograms/day.[3] A year later dietary lead for toddlers averaged 5 micrograms/day.[4]

Lead pipes and solder added lead to water. At the turn of the century, estimates of the lead content of water flowing through lead pipes were 100 micrograms/liter or higher.[5] In the 1930s, when Kehoe measured lead in water flowing through pipes joined with lead solder, he found that the water contained 30 micrograms/liter.[6] By 1972 the value had fallen to 10 micrograms/liter;[7] by the early 1990s, lead in water was 1–2 micrograms/liter.[8]

Tetraethyl lead, added to gasoline in the 1920s to improve engine efficiency and counteract engine "knock," steadily added lead to the atmosphere over the next half century. In 1933 the U.S. Public Health Service determined that the average urban street corner had 9 micrograms of lead/cubic meter of air.[9] When Kehoe's laboratory measured atmospheric lead in the 1950s, investigators discovered that the air in Philadelphia contained 2.3 micrograms/cubic meter; in Los Angeles, 5.2 micrograms/cubic meter; in New York City, 2.8 micrograms/cubic meter; in Cincinnati, 1.6 micrograms/cubic meter.[10] Ten years later, when concern erupted over environmental pollution, the lead content of air remained at the same level, but public health officials and environmentalists now interpreted these amounts as health risks.[11] In the 1970s, the lead content of air breathed by urban dwellers had fallen to 1–3 micrograms/cubic meter, although it could be higher depending on traffic congestion.[12]

One measure of the elimination of lead from the environment has been the dramatic decline of blood lead levels in the general population. In 1942 officials at the Baltimore Health Department calculated that the average blood lead level for persons—who had no increased lead exposure—was 30 micrograms/dl.[13] In 1976–1980 the average blood lead level, based on a far larger national sample, had fallen to 12.8 micrograms/dl. Two decades later, it was 2.0 micrograms/dl.[14]

This progressive lowering has had a paradoxical effect on public health officials. On the one hand, less lead has been interpreted as a story of wonderful environmental and public health achievement. On the other hand, the acceptable limit of 10 micrograms/dl—set by the Centers for Disease Control in 1991—is so low that many more children are considered at risk. By some estimates, 3 million tons of lead paint remain on the walls of 57 million dwellings. Of these, 14 million—housing 3.8 million children—are considered in disrepair. Perhaps 4–5 million tons of lead from gasoline have fallen from the atmosphere and remain in the soil.[15]

I see the history of childhood lead poisoning as a dynamic epidemiological evolution. It is fair to say that a children's doctor in 1900 would scarcely perceive the worries of a pediatrician a century later. The nature of the disease has radically changed—for victims, parents, and public health officials. Lead in the child's domestic environment has greatly lessened and the sources altered. Medical understanding of the lead hazard has evolved and with it have come changes in public health responses. Policy over the past century has been forged through interactions among child health officials, public health communities on the local, state, and national levels, the lead-paint industry, and researchers.

This history focuses on lead-paint poisoning in the United States to 1980 and on the responses of public health officials and the lead-paint industry to this changing hazard. To cut off the story at 1980 is somewhat arbitrary, in that ideas and responses to childhood lead poisoning continue to change. History, however, requires some distance from events. The end point of 1980 comes just after the federal ban on tetraethyl lead in gasoline and the reduction of the lead content of paint to less than 0.06 percent, or essentially the elimination of lead from paint. While the focus is on children in the United States, the story also includes the health of lead workers and painters in the United States and Europe, and children exposed to lead in Britain, Europe, and Australia. I have restricted this history largely to lead-paint poisoning. Although the story cannot be told without some understanding of the intersections with tetraethyl lead,

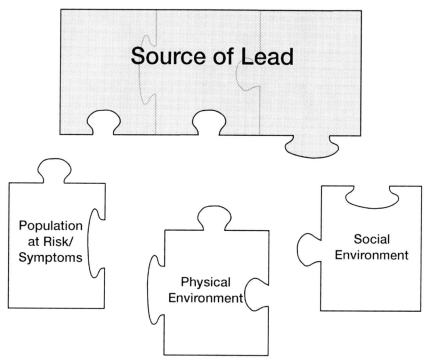

Figure 1. Historical Epidemics

the history of air pollution is far too complicated for detailed inclusion here. The removal of lead from paint was a complex story that involved paint technology, manufacturers, the industrial hygiene movement, the poison control movement of the American Academy of Pediatrics, urban public health departments, pediatricians, researchers, and governments at state, city, and federal levels.

With its focus on the health and safety of the home, the history of childhood lead-paint poisoning is important to both pediatricians and public health officials. It is also important to historians of disease, raising issues of the social construction of disease, technology and the definition of disease, therapy, and the effect of various public health measures: education, voluntary industry bans, labels, local bans, and federal laws.

Until recently, there have been relatively few histories of childhood lead poisoning. Some thought-provoking analyses have been written by pediatricians and public health officials who have made lead poisoning a focal point of their careers.[16] Historians, sociologists, and public policy scholars have also examined childhood lead poisoning.[17] These accounts are insightful, and I have profited from each. My history differs in two key respects. First, I see the history of childhood lead poisoning as a dynamic process, one that requires the historian to place the epidemic into constantly changing social and medical contexts. I believe it imperative to keep the perceived understanding of the nature of the domestic lead hazard and the medical concerns for children firmly rooted in the social context of the period. In the 1930s, for example, pediatricians worried about children who developed seizures and coma and therefore directed their recommendations to household situations that might expose a child to this amount of lead. In contrast, pediatricians a half century later were alarmed over subtle neurological injuries caused by far smaller amounts of lead than those required to provoke seizures and coma, and correspondingly their public health recommendations were far different. Second, I see the lead-paint industry as adjusting to the changing nature of the hazard and working collaboratively with the public health community as the nature of the domestic hazard evolved. This judgment is controversial. Recent publications by Christian Warren and especially by David Rosner and Gerald Markowitz have severely criticized the industry for impeding public health efforts.[18]

I have found it useful to employ an ecological model when considering complex epidemics. This model seeks to identify the agent causing the epidemic; the population at risk and their experience of illness; the social environment in which the epidemic occurred; and the physical environment. (See figure 1.) Childhood lead-paint poisoning provides an excellent example of this ecological model, which helps to conceptualize this dynamic epidemic.

Part I

Lead Poisoning before 1920

Chapter 1

Children and Lead
before 1920

On August 17, 1913, a five-year-old child in Baltimore's Home of the Friendless complained about a pain in his face and head. He slept poorly and appeared ill. The following morning his condition worsened, and he developed a stiff neck and seizures before lapsing into coma. These distressing symptoms prompted his transfer to Johns Hopkins's children's hospital, the Harriet Lane Home. There his doctors, Henry M. Thomas and Kenneth D. Blackfan, initially believed that he suffered from a severe infection of the central nervous system. To their surprise, tests for meningitis—bacterial and tubercular—and neuro-syphilis were repeatedly unrewarding. As Thomas and Blackfan observed their young patient over the next few days, they noted additional distressing problems. His left eye turned inward, his right optic nerve was swollen, and his retinas displayed hemorrhages. Despite these troubling symptoms and the frustration of not having a diagnosis, the boy improved so that a week later he was "nearly well." Able to speak, he complained of a stomachache and headache. After a month in the Harriet Lane Home, he returned to the Home of the Friendless, restored to health but still an enigma.

He remained healthy for six months, until March 1914. Then he suddenly complained of headache and vomiting, developed seizures, and once again lapsed into coma. The boy was quickly transferred to the Harriet Lane Home, where the same doctors once more suspected an infection of the central nervous system and once more were unable to prove it. A diagnostic dilemma brought the boy's condition into sharp scrutiny. On one exam, a doctor noted that there was a faint bluish discoloration in the gum around one tooth. This unlocked the puzzle, because physicians were accustomed to seeing similar markings in factory workers who inhaled or swallowed too much lead on the job. Physicians at Johns Hopkins had not considered lead poisoning in the boy because it was not reckoned a problem for children, unless they worked as a painter's apprentice or in a lead-manufacturing plant.

Once the diagnosis was suspected, Thomas and Blackfan puzzled over the source of lead, because this boy was neither an apprentice nor a child laborer. During the course of his hospitalization, they found his mouth filled with paint flakes that he had gnawed off his hospital crib. On visiting his bed at the Home of the Friendless, they noted that he had also chewed paint from his furniture there. Alerted to his habit, nurses noted that "he would gnaw any painted object unless he was most carefully watched."

The boy recovered and returned to the Home of the Friendless in early May. Three weeks later he developed seizures once more. He died before he could be sent back to the Harriet Lane Home.[1]

One year later, a two-year-old boy with seizures came to the Harriet Lane Home. Blackfan, schooled from the earlier case, looked closely at the toddler's gums and found a similar blue line. He still checked for infection, for in 1915 this was by far the most common cause of seizures in a young child. In this two-year-old, Blackfan also noted an abnormality in the red blood cells—stippling—a diagnostic aid used in factory workers suspected of lead poisoning. The boy was discharged after two weeks. Unfortunately, just one day later, he seized again, and died shortly after being rushed back to the Harriet Lane Home. Blackfan asked the boy's father about a source of lead and learned "that the child would gnaw any painted article, and that he and his brother had recently ruined a set of parlor furniture by eating paint from it."[2] Six months later, his fraternal co-conspirator, now just two years old, also developed seizures. Of note, Blackfan found that around the time of his brother's death the boy had suffered from abdominal pains so severe that a surgeon operated for suspected appendicitis. At surgery, the appendix was not inflamed, and the surgeon was perplexed about the cause of the abdominal distress. Blackfan surmised that unsuspected lead poisoning had been the culprit. Blackfan attempted to control the boy's seizures; despite enormous efforts, this toddler also died.

At the end of July 1915 another boy, three years of age, came to the Harriet Lane Home with seizures and coma. He had a blue line on his gums. The boy improved in the hospital, but once he awoke from his coma, he displayed a paralysis of his facial muscles. Fortunately, this child survived. Blackfan was unable to determine his source of lead.

Not only were these four boys the first children that Blackfan had encountered with lead poisoning, but the three who died were the first reported American cases of toddlers poisoned from gnawing paint from cribs or other furniture at home. Lead poisoning was not a new disease in the second decade of the twentieth century, but when it occurred it did so in environments very different from the surroundings of these infants. Lead poisoning was a disease of workers employed in one of the many lead trades. Physicians therefore normally thought of lead poisoning as a disease of adults.

Over the course of the nineteenth century, physicians and workers came to appreciate the large number of telltale signs and symptoms of lead poisoning or "plumbism" on the job. Most common were abdominal cramps, or colic, which could incapacitate workers. Particularly distressing was numbness or even paralysis of fingers, hands, wrists, toes, feet, and ankles, complaints that went by the terms foot-drop, wrist-drop, or peripheral neuropathy (because the symptoms demonstrated injury to peripheral nerves). Lead in greater amounts damaged the brain or central nervous system, resulting in seizures, coma, and even death. Many lead workers had a light blue line on the gums above the teeth, which was the product of lead and poor oral hygiene. Many were pale from anemia.[3]

In addition to adults, a few children in the nineteenth century, and to a lesser extent in the twentieth century, also worked in lead industries, thus providing physicians with some information about how children experienced lead poisoning. Industrial hygiene was thus a logical place for Blackfan to turn in search of insights. What he found was an occupational disease so different from the one his young patients suffered that it offered few helpful guides. For example, Blackfan recognized that most lead workers were poisoned through inhaling the clouds of dust that swirled around the workplace. This environment did not occur in the homes of Baltimore's infants. In contrast, Blackfan's patients chewed and swallowed far smaller amounts of lead.[4]

At the time that Thomas and Blackfan observed their cases, there were foreign examples of children who had developed lead poisoning at home. Children in Queensland, a remote and tropical region of northern Australia, had suffered from household lead poisoning, and Thomas and Blackfan's published papers give evidence that they explored the outlines of this Australian epidemic. What Thomas and Blackfan discovered was a disease that differed in symptoms, in age of victims, and in contexts from the disease that their patients experienced in Baltimore.

In addition, Blackfan knew that there were a few cases of American children lead-poisoned in their homes. These afflicted children also provided limited insights, because they had ingested the metal in ways and in circumstances considerably different from those of the children whom Blackfan and Thomas treated at the Harriet Lane Home. Consequently pediatricians in the United States had to develop an entirely new way to conceptualize the domestic hazard of lead. This view shaped public health efforts until the late 1940s.

Domestic Lead Poisoning in Children

For information about household lead poisoning, American pediatricians could read about the experiences of a small number of children which revealed that lead paint was an uncommon source of lead at the time that Blackfan encountered his cases in 1914–1917. In particular, Blackfan turned to an epidemic of lead poisoning suffered by children and adults in Philadelphia following the ingestion of pastry buns that had been dyed with a food coloring made from lead chromate. This epidemic was recent and numerically significant. Even more important to Blackfan, the victims of bun poisoning had seizures, the symptom he was seeing in Baltimore's children after gnawing paint from cribs. In 1887 David Stewart investigated the home of a Philadelphian family of nine who had been struck—sequentially—with vomiting, headaches, and seizures. Four children died. Dr. Stewart suspected lead poisoning from the blue gum lines that several victims had. Stewart made a home visit, investigating the usual sources of lead: water pipes, pottery glazes, linings of "iron" pots. None contained lead. On questioning the family about possible food contamination, Dr. Stewart learned that they shopped at a new bakery. A visit to the bakery revealed that a member of the baker's family had also died of convulsions. On questioning the baker, Dr. Stewart determined that the baker had used chromium yellow (lead chromate) as a substitute for egg yolk to produce more enticing yellow pastries.[5] Two years later a physician in Baltimore, William Glenn, reviewed the medical literature and found over one hundred cases of lead poisoning caused by the use of lead pigments as food colorings. Following Stewart's example, Glenn investigated Baltimore bakeries, but he discovered none using the dangerous substitutes. He did, however, find lead chromate in candies sold at street fairs.[6] In 1895 Stewart reported sixteen additional cases with seizures in Philadelphia. Once again, several cases occurred in the home of a baker.[7] Two features made these patients noteworthy: the source of lead and the seizures. Stewart informed his readers that L. Tanquerel des Planches, a renowned French industrial hygienist of the mid-nineteenth century, had claimed that lead encephalopathy was the rarest problem he encountered in a career devoted to industrial lead poisoning. For Stewart, seizures were the most common complaint.

In the nineteenth century childhood lead poisoning was rare in England and the United States, but when it occurred contaminated food was often the source. A family tragedy in London in 1810 set the stage: a mother and several children died of seizures after eating sugar that had been stored in a container that had once held white lead.[8] Stewed pears stored in a lead-glazed earthen pot were the source of a poisoning case in Boston;[9] cider ladled from a tub newly painted with white lead and linseed oil sickened three or four children in Cortlandville, New York, in 1843;[10] adulterated flour led to an 1849 epidemic in Stourbridge, England;[11] tea brewed in a kettle that had once melted lead sickened a family in New Brunswick, Canada;[12] food packaged in a can with lead soldering resulted in a case of paralysis in Maryland;[13] and at least one death in Horselydown, England,[14] in 1888, one year after Dr. Stewart first reported lead chromate in Philadelphia's pastries. In 1904 Henry M. Thomas, who would later publish with Kenneth Blackfan the case of the boy who died from paint chewed from his crib, reported on a five-year-old girl poisoned from canned foods whom he treated in the neurology clinic at Johns Hopkins.[15] The danger of lead poisoning from canned fruits and vegetables was a major concern of Harvey Wiley, a government chemist who was instrumental in the passage of the Federal Food and Drug Act of 1906.[16]

Other outbreaks of poisonings were caused by lead in the water supply coursing through the lead pipes and aqueducts used in many of the new waterworks in the middle decades of the nineteenth century. One report about lead pipes came from Addlestone, near Stratford-upon-Avon, in 1848;[17] New Orleans experienced a widespread epidemic in 1850 that raised the question of lead in the city's water;[18] a year later lead lining a cistern at a girls' school in England sent many to the infirmary;[19] Boston investigated reports of contaminated water in its waterworks in 1852,[20] as did Bacup in England.[21]

Infants were poisoned when suckling on mothers' cracked nipples that had been treated with ointments containing lead.[22] They could also be poisoned from lead in powder, used directly on the baby[23] or on mothers' faces. Lead powder resulted in considerable poisoning in Asian countries, where white powder was in vogue,[24] but it also poisoned infants in the United States.[25]

American Lead-Paint Poisoning Cases

When Thomas and Blackfan published their first case in 1914, there were about ten prior domestic lead-paint poisoning cases in children in the United States. Three or four involved children poisoned from drinking cider from a tub painted with white lead paint in 1843.[26] These cases should fall under the category of contaminated foods.

The first case of a child poisoned by childhood domestic lead paint that I have found in the American medical literature occurred in New York City in 1883. Henry D. Chapin, a prominent pediatrician, described two brothers who developed stomachaches, nearly complete paralysis, and blue gum lines. Chapin explained:

> On examining the premises in which these children lived, I found their father was a painter, and that for two years some remains of paint had been kept in a closet immediately adjoining the sleeping-room of the children. There was some white lead and turpentine, and a few bottles with coloring matter. At Christmas the father painted the rooms in

which the children spent most of the day with two coats of white paint, after which they were stained and grained. About a week after this the first symptoms of lead-poisoning manifested themselves.[27]

These cases were similar to painters' apprentice cases that industrial hygienists described in connection to worries about children in the workplace. The boys were present when their father prepared and painted their room; shortly afterward they developed symptoms. And it was conceivable that the boys played in the closet where their father kept his painting clothes.

Playing among their father-painter's paints and utensils was the source of lead in three children described by Wharton Sinkler in Philadelphia in 1894. Sinkler had been alerted to domestic lead poisoning by discussing the yellow bun cases with David Stewart. (Stewart wrote to Sinkler that there were now seventy-nine pastry cases.) The children Sinkler treated were ten, six, and three years of age. He described his search for the cause of their symptoms: "On inquiring into the history of the children I found that their father was a painter, but the mother strenuously denied that they had been exposed to contact with the paints. When the third case was brought to me I asked my friend, Dr. J. H. Rhein, to visit the home of the children; and he discovered the fact that there was a great deal of white lead lying about, and that the children had frequently played in the paint-room, and were often daubed with paint."[28] Sinkler also mentioned a six-year-old girl who developed lead palsy in Boston "after having been exposed to a freshly-painted house." This child had been under the care of James J. Putnam.[29] This case appears also to have been acquired under circumstances similar to those of an "occupational" exposure, since it occurred during the process of painting.

After reviewing the medical literature available to him, Sinkler concluded that the rarity of lead poisoning in children stemmed from young people's lack of susceptibility to the effects of lead.[30] But he recognized the ubiquitous sources of lead in the domestic environment: "The sources of lead-poisoning are so numerous that it is remarkable that more cases do not occur. Drinking-water in cities, from passing through lead pipes, frequently becomes charged with lead. Lead is to be found in cooking utensils, in red rubber, which is sometimes used for making nipples for nursing-bottles, in the solder used in cans, coverings of sweetmeats, and in lead chromate, which is used in coloring toys, cloths, and other articles."[31]

A year later a physician from San Francisco, Leo Newmark, reported the case of an eight-year-old girl with lead palsy. He claimed that the source of lead was undried, tacky paint on the child's bed.[32]

In 1896 a physician at Mt. Sinai Hospital in New York City, R. Abrahams, investigated a case of an infant who had been poisoned while playing with solid "lead soldiers and sailors, lead horses, ship, and utensils, and many other accouterments of military and naval life."[33] Abrahams raised the additional possibility that "*painted* wooden toys" might pose a risk, although he himself had not encountered such a case.

W. F. Hamilton, a physician at Montreal's Royal Victoria Hospital, added in 1905 another poisoned painter's child. Hamilton also reported the sad tale of an impoverished family who kept warm by burning "barrel staves gathered from a neighboring paint factory,"[34] anticipating the epidemics of lead poisoning during the Depression when many poor families burned wooden battery cases that were saturated with lead. In 1909 H. W. Wright, a physician-in-training at the New York State Hospital for Crippled Children, reported the case of an eight-year-old girl who suddenly developed seizures, "drop wrist," and "drop foot." He suspected lead poisoning and identified paint as a possible culprit. Wright did not state whether the girl had been present when her room had been painted or whether any member of the staff had seen the girl actually consume paint.[35]

This was the sum of domestic lead-poisoning cases in the United States when Thomas and Blackfan treated their first patient in 1914. From this context, it is easy to see why that five-year-old boy who died from seizures stood out so starkly in their minds. In America, most children were poisoned by adulterated foods, contaminated water, cosmetics, and nipple creams. Of the cases attributed to paint, three or four were more accurately instances of contaminated food (Shipman, 1843), two children were poisoned from burning painted barrel staves (Hamilton, 1905), and six were painters' children who played in their fathers' work materials and should be thought of as workplace exposures (Chapin, 1884; Sinkler, 1885; Hamilton, 1905). Two children apparently acquired lead during the process of painting their homes and should also be grouped as workplace exposures (Putnam, Wright, 1909). Only one child acquired lead from housepaint long after it had been applied (Newmark, 1895), and even in this case there was some doubt whether the paint had ever completely dried. Before 1914 there was no reported case of childhood lead poisoning from paint—dried on an object or a surface—in the American medical literature.

Chapter 2

The Queensland Epidemic

Between 1890 and 1930 Queensland parents and physicians were confronted with many children with symptoms of foot-drop, wrist-drop, and eye palsies. Queensland doctors speculated that the epidemic, which was occurring nowhere else in Australia, was caused by lead acquired from the accidental ingestion of decaying household lead paint. This idea was unique. When physicians in the 1890s thought about household childhood epidemics of lead poisoning—a rare event—they did so in terms of contaminated water supplies or food.[1]

In the first half of the twentieth century, American public health officials knew only the outlines of this epidemic in northern Australia. Most of the detailed reports were published in minor, regional medical journals. The *Australasian Medical Gazette*, *Transactions of the Intercolonial Medical Congress of Australia*, and *Transactions of the Australasian Medical Congress* did not have wide American readership. The *Union List of Serials* (the librarians' tool for identifying periodical holdings in U.S. libraries) identifies only a few American libraries with runs of these journals. It is probable that only the occasional American physician would have read the details of the epidemic in the original reports; most American physicians almost certainly relied on summaries that were published by Queensland doctors in the *British Medical Journal* or on brief discussions of the Queensland epidemic that appeared in the few American articles on childhood lead-paint poisoning that were published before 1930.[2]

What is more significant is that the information that American physicians culled from these summaries seemed not to apply to the handful of cases that American physicians were beginning to identify in a child's home. The ecological setting of tropical Queensland was so exotic and the symptoms bringing most victims to Australian doctors so peculiar that American physicians—noting the differences—relegated the Queensland observations to the uniqueness of the tropics, the way that American physicians viewed pneumonia among young South African miners in a different category than pneumonia in elderly Americans.

Queensland seemed remote and tropical. It extends from a latitude of approximately fifteen to thirty degrees south, or to place it in northern hemispheric terms, a distance that would span from Miami to Nicaragua. It is removed from the major Australian population centers of Sydney and Melbourne, and in 1900 had only a rudimentary road and rail system. Brisbane, with a population of about 120,000 in 1900, was by far the largest city. It was plagued by poor sanitation and ill health.[3]

Queensland was hot. Monthly high temperatures in Brisbane ranged from a winter "low" of 83 degrees in July to a summer high of 108.9 in January. It was also bright, with tropical sun beaming down steadily throughout the year. Only in June was it even partially overcast.[4] At the turn of the twentieth century American physicians often looked to foreign examples for knowledge, but their gaze was decidedly toward Britain, France, and Germany, not toward the South Pacific.[5]

Queensland Cases

In 1892 John Lockhart Gibson, a native of Queensland who had received his general medical education in Edinburgh and his specialty training (eyes, ears, nose, and throat) in Vienna, Berlin, and London before returning to practice in Brisbane in 1885, published what he believed were the first cases of lead poisoning among children in Queensland.[6] One coauthor was A. Jefferis Turner, who later published case studies of additional patients. Gibson described ten children with paralysis of some of the muscles in the arms and hands (wrist-drop) and legs and feet (foot-drop). Two of the ten children had suffered seizures. Other signs of possible lead poisoning such as blue gum lines and lead colic were absent. Most of the children were anemic. In part, he arrived at the diagnosis by exclusion: the slow onset distinguished these children from polio victims; their youth distinguished them from alcoholics. Attempts to find lead in the urine of two patients failed. He considered but rejected sucking on "tin foil" as the source of lead.[7]

Gibson and Turner had seen sixty-six cases by 1897, enough to analyze the common elements. The average age was six; girls outnumbered boys by almost three to one. Turner divided cases into four groups: foot/wrist-drop (the most numerous), abdominal pain, seizures (uncommon but serious), and a peculiar

cluster of children with what Gibson called "ocular neuritis," in which the optic nerve and the oculomotor nerves were damaged. This hampered the children's
ability to see and to move their eyes.

Significantly, ocular neuritis became for Gibson, the region's only eye specialist, the hallmark of the Queensland cases. Gibson believed these eye complaints were unique to Queensland, and this was the aspect of the epidemic that
he chose to inform the international community about.

By 1897 Gibson and Turner were able to detect lead in the urine of many
of the children. The patients came from several towns in Queensland. The children improved in the hospital but sickened upon returning home. Turner termed
this tendency to relapse at home "toxicity of habitation." He suspected that
drinking water—which was gathered from roofs and stored in tanks—was the
source of the lead. When he sampled the water in a number of cases, he discovered lead in three.[8] That same year T. E. Green, a resident medical officer at
Brisbane's Hospital for Sick Children who was working with Gibson, described
three additional children—all of whom died—with peripheral neuritis.[9]

In 1904 Gibson reported four new cases of children with ocular neuritis.
Once again he attributed this eye condition, which he had first described and
named, to lead poisoning. Of note, he abandoned water as the possible source
of lead and in its place proposed lead paint. He investigated the homes of the
children and discovered that they were indeed painted. He rubbed the surfaces
with cloths, and the government analyst detected lead in many of the powdery
samples. Gibson also described the setting: "oppressive heat," where most of the
lead was found in white powder from decaying paint on the outside floors, walls,
and railings of the verandas where children played. The government analyst did
not detect lead from cloths rubbed "on the ceiling [inside the house] whose paint
was very glossy and showed no signs of wear and tear."[10] What troubled Gibson
was that normally only one member of a family had symptoms while all lived in
the same chalky environment. On questioning parents he found that the children with symptoms were nail-biters or thumb-suckers.

Here we need a brief discussion of the nature of the lead chalk that these
children ate. For comparison, it is instructive to contrast it with the lead found
in household dust seventy years later, when American public health officials
turned their attention to dust. The powder that Gibson and Turner described
was quite different from the dust that concerned pediatricians in the 1970s.
Gibson identified seemingly pure white lead powder, like the chalk dust that
covers hands and erasers in a schoolroom. Queensland physicians measured the
lead that saliva-moistened fingers attracted in some of these sun-burnt houses.
L. J. Jarvis Nye calculated that three adult fingertips collected 1.4 *milligrams* of
lead.[11] Elliott Murray measured up to 7.0 *milligrams* on just two saliva-moistened
fingertips.[12] In the 1970s physicians worried about brown house dust—of which

lead paint was only one constituent—in quantities that contained far less lead. For example, when James W. Sayre measured the lead from both hands of urban children in 1974, he found that the median had 20 micrograms.[13] In other words, just two fingertips in Queensland might contain as much as seven hundred hands in Rochester a half century later. To put this difference into perspective, the relative exposure in Rochester compared with Queensland was the disparity between one baby aspirin and a 150-pill bottle of adult aspirin.

In 1907 J. Macdonald Gill reported three cases of peripheral neuritis in children from Sydney. In contrast to the prevalence of the disease in Queensland, Gill stated, "there is no doubt but that it is a rare disease in Sydney."[14]

One year later Gibson described ocular neuritis to an international audience in the *British Medical Journal*:

> I am anxious that an account of the cases should have wide circulation,
> not only because I think they throw more light on the special clinical
> manifestations of lead on the ocular nerves than has been recorded by
> others, but because they appear to constitute a type of ocular disease
> unknown in the medical literature of Europe. [two paragraphs later] I am
> satisfied also that cases cannot be very infrequent in warm climates,
> other than Queensland, where sources of the poison similar to those
> pointed out in this paper are available.[15]

Gibson then explained that the hot climate in Queensland turned outside paint on railings and verandas to powder.

For Gibson, the purpose of the article was to describe an ocular syndrome that he and colleagues were seeing in the tropics. Although he mentioned that Brisbane physicians had treated 262 cases of lead poisoning, his article focused on what he considered to be the singular aspects in Queensland: the 68 children with eye disease. Gibson attributed the epidemic of lead poisoning in Queensland to the architectural style of houses with elevated, painted verandas.

Turner's address to the Australasian Medical Congress (also published for an international audience in the *British Medical Journal*) analyzed the same 262 cases. He elaborated on the particular setting for childhood lead poisoning in Queensland:

> Nearly all the dwellings in Queensland are built of wood, and in the
> towns the wood is covered by paint consisting largely of white lead.
> Exposed to our hot summer sun this paint rapidly withers and becomes
> reduced to a powdery condition. This is particularly noticeable on ve-
> randah railings. The verandahs are favourite playgrounds for young
> children, who clasp the railings with their moist hands, which become
> covered with poison. Thence it finds its way to the child's mouth, espe-
> cially in children who suck their fingers or bite their nails.[16]

Turner then analyzed the Brisbane cases. Many children had abdominal complaints, but he explained that they were less well defined than in adults. Foot-drop was common (wrist-drop was more common in adults). Some children stopped breathing from paralysis of the diaphragm. Some had kidney findings. Only "now and again [did] children suffering from chronic plumbism develop eclamptic seizures." Turner claimed credit for first recognizing "the most insidious and most damaging" effect of these cases: "acute optic neuritis associated with oculo-motor paresis" (what Gibson, who also claimed priority, called ocular neuritis).

Turner concluded his remarks to his Australian audience with a plea to restrict lead paint in Brisbane:

> Paint containing lead should never be employed on outside surfaces,
> such as fences, walls, and particularly verandah railings, in places where
> children, especially young children, are accustomed to play. Zinc-white,
> or some other paint free from lead, should be substituted. Unfortunately
> we in Brisbane still from ignorance no longer excusable, allow our
> houses to be poisoned traps for children's fingers, and every year fur-
> nishes its quota of ill-health and suffering, crippling, hopeless and per-
> manent blindness, and occasionally death as the consequence. This is
> certainly a matter which calls for legislative interference.[17]

What both papers emphasized to their international audiences was that the Queensland epidemic of childhood lead-paint poisoning resulted from a unique climatic and social setting, producing a unique constellation of symptoms, one of which had been described only in Queensland.

In the next decade Gibson published additional papers. Two called for Australian physicians to drain cerebral spinal fluid in order to prevent blindness and improve the squint caused by ocular neuritis.[18]

In 1914 A. Breinl and W. J. Young added twenty-two cases from Townsville, a community located on the coast in northern Queensland. In some respects these children were similar to the ones in Brisbane: foot- and wrist-drop were common, as were vague abdominal complaints. "Brain symptoms are common, ranging from obstreperousness and fretfulness to a state resembling mania." Although Breinl and Young mentioned that "not rarely convulsions are the outcome of chronic lead poisoning in children," they described only one of their patients with a lengthy seizure. Of note, the Townsville patients differed significantly from the Brisbane patients in that only one had eye symptoms. Lead was found in the urine of eighteen of the children. Breinl and Young ended their study with a query: "It is striking that cases similar to those described above should not have been recorded from other parts of the tropics where lead paint is employed. Whether this be due to local conditions prevalent in Queensland only, to the difficulty of diagnosis, or to the lack of a definite clue associating such symptoms with lead, remains to be seen."[19]

E. S. Littlejohn, a physician from Camperdown, a small town in New South Wales west of Melbourne, answered this query in terms of Queensland's climate, child care, and housing:

> In Queensland it is mostly too hot for young children to play out in the sun; they spend much of their time on the verandahs, where they can play protected from the heat of the sun. In New South Wales, on the other hand, the children play for the most part in the garden or yards or streets and only exceptionally on the verandahs.
>
> Furthermore, in Queensland towns the homes are almost always built of wood and are raised on piles, the verandahs being therefore railed in, nearly always with painted railings and it is interesting to note in this connexion that in the country, where the houses are not raised off the ground, the verandahs are low and unrailed or the railings unpainted, cases of lead poisoning do not occur. In New South Wales the houses are mostly of brick, are mostly low on the ground and the verandahs are very often unrailed altogether or protected with brick or cement walls. Hence the circumstances of daily life of the children in New South Wales are totally different from those of the children in Queensland as regards their liability to lead poisoning from this cause.[20]

The American Understanding of the Epidemic

The Queensland epidemic differed sharply from the experience of childhood lead poisoning in the United States in the first decade of the twentieth century. The first report of the epidemic in the American medical literature came in a textbook chapter written by David Edsall in 1907. Edsall was a pioneer in industrial medicine in the United States and later became dean of the Harvard Medical School and dean of the Harvard School of Public Health. In this capacity, he assembled the first university faculty to study the effects of lead poisoning.

Edsall referred to the Queensland epidemic in three places. The most detailed comment came in the section "Lead Poisoning in Children." Edsall noted the prevalence of foot-drop in the Queensland epidemic. What caught his attention were the eye ailments.[21] These distinctive ocular findings implied to Edsall that children might have a greater susceptibility to lead, because similar findings were quite rare in adults.[22] Edsall also noted Gibson's description of paint powder in Queensland housing.[23] Significantly, Edsall did not generalize the tropical findings to the American context.

Readers of child health literature first learned of the Queensland epidemic in 1914, when encountering Henry M. Thomas and Kenneth D. Blackfan's case report. Their patient suffered eye symptoms, so Thomas and Blackfan reviewed the published literature about ocular neuritis, noted the scarcity of prior papers, and properly detailed Gibson's description of ocular neuritis in Queensland. Thomas and Blackfan also noted Gibson's view that the source of lead was "dried paint from the railings of long-painted verandas or garden fences."[24] In 1917 Blackfan added three additional cases from Johns Hopkins. From this study, it is possible to see an emerging difference in the American focus on childhood lead poisoning. Blackfan's attention centered on seizures and coma, which pediatricians often grouped together under the category of encephalopathy. He noted Gibson, Turner, Breinl, and Young—citing their papers in some detail— but pointed out that "in the cases reported from Australia, convulsions were observed very infrequently, though mild cerebral disturbances were frequently present."[25] Blackfan picked up on differences between the Australian and the American cases that became even more evident later. One analysis of 259 children admitted with a diagnosis of lead poisoning in Brisbane's Hospital for Sick Children between 1914 and 1932 recorded that only 8 children had encephalopathy.[26] In the United States, virtually all of the children who were admitted to hospitals with the diagnosis of lead poisoning had experienced poorly controlled seizures or were in coma. Blackfan also noted the source of lead from the Queensland cases: "Gibson considers the ingestion of lead as the most likely source of infection, although he appreciates that it may occur from the inhalation of dust containing lead. He points out that children who bite their fingernails and suck their fingers are much more frequently affected, and believes that their hands became contaminated with dried paint from porch railings and houses."[27]

Of particular import, Blackfan's patients obtained lead from entirely different sources than lead-poisoned children in Queensland. Case I (the boy described in the 1914 paper) "had nibbled from the railings of his crib." Cases II and III (brothers) "would gnaw any painted article, and . . . he and his brother had recently ruined a set of parlor furniture by eating the paint from it." In Case IV Blackfan did not determine the source of lead. From these cases, he concluded: "I would urge that energetic prophylactic measures be taken with children who habitually eat painted articles in order to guard against the development of lead poisoning. Since my attention has been directed to lead poisoning, I have found a number of children who nibble the white paint from enameled cribs."[28]

Blackfan signaled a marked contrast in the way in which physicians in Queensland and the United States viewed lead poisoning. In Queensland, doctors focused on ocular neuritis and peripheral neuropathy (foot-drop and wrist-drop) and identified the primary source of lead from outside lead-paint powder created by the desiccating tropical sun. (See figure 2.) In America, physicians focused on seizures and coma and identified the primary source of lead as lead-

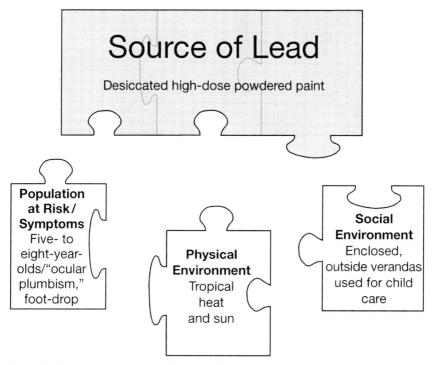

Figure 2. Queensland Lead-Paint Poisoning Epidemic, 1904

painted cribs and articles from inside the house. (See figure 3.) In the American scene there was no mention of desiccated lead powder or climate.

Some Queensland children did suffer seizures and coma, but to learn about this required reading the detailed reports in the Australian literature. Gibson, an eye specialist, elected to emphasize the eye findings, and this is what American physicians noted. Turner addressed the question that many Australian physicians were raising: why was childhood lead poisoning seemingly limited to Queensland? His answer—which stressed climate, housing, and child care—was duly noted by American physicians.

In 1923 L. Emmett Holt, Jr., one of America's most prominent pediatricians, further distanced the Queensland epidemic from the American experience. First, Holt noted that many patients in the United States were younger than those in Queensland.[29] The case that Holt reported obtained lead from an ointment placed on the mother's nipples. Holt then reviewed the sources of lead in childhood cases as reported in the published medical literature. Reflecting the American and European experience, Holt—placing Queensland in its proper context—concluded that domestic childhood lead poisoning occurring outside of Australia did not for the most part involve paint.[30]

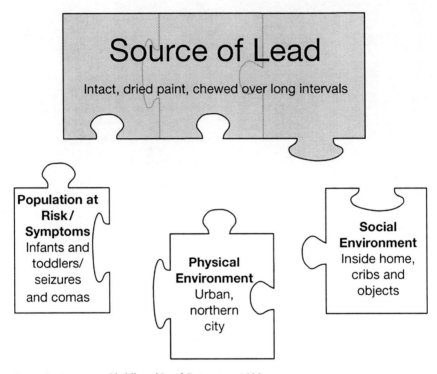

Figure 3. American Childhood Lead Poisoning, 1920

In his general pediatric textbook, first published in 1926, the one paragraph Holt devoted to lead poisoning reflected his concern for encephalopathy and his identification of the source of lead. By then, Holt was more concerned about paint than he had been in the earlier paper: "An infrequent cause of convulsions in young children is an encephalopathy due to lead poisoning. We have seen thirty or more such cases. The condition is a serious and often fatal one. The poisoning was usually caused by the child's nibbling and swallowing the paint from his crib or furniture."[31]

There are only four additional American references to the Queensland epidemic before 1930, and all refer to Gibson's eye findings. In 1924 John Ruddock mentioned that "Gibson reported a group of eye symptoms, which he referred to as 'plumbic ocular neuritis.' "[32] In 1926 Charles McKhann included the Queensland epidemic in a footnote; his only direct reference to Australia was about lead amblyopia.[33] Also in 1926, Joseph Aub, in what became the standard work in the United States on lead poisoning, mentioned Gibson's "ocular neuritis."[34] Carl Vernon Weller, a pathologist at the University of Michigan, noted the unique source of lead and climate.[35] What these opinions demonstrated was that American physicians were aware of the Queensland epidemic—at least in outline form—and that they took away from it precisely those elements that the Australian physicians emphasized: peculiar ocular findings and lead obtained from powder produced by outside paint desiccated from the severe tropical heat and sun.

This epidemic may have alerted American pediatricians to the danger of lead-paint powder, but the evidence suggests that they considered the environmental context of tropical Queensland so exotic that it did not apply to American children. In no American account were children found covered with high-concentration lead powder. There were additional contrasts. In the United States, much younger children suffered lead poisoning; the symptoms that most concerned American pediatricians were coma, seizures, and encephalopathy; and the social setting was urban infants and toddlers, inside the house, resting in cribs, chewing paint on crib railings or on objects. Lead was a facet of disease in both countries, but the circumstances could not have been more different.

Queensland's Unique Mark: Nephritis

In 1920 the Australasian Medical Congress met in Brisbane and adopted a measure asking the government of Queensland to prohibit "the use of lead paint on verandah railings and outside surfaces within reach of children's fingers." This met with some opposition from "powerful moneyed interests" and some physicians.[36] Despite these reservations, the Parliament of Queensland in 1922 passed a Health Act that reflected the particular circumstances of housing and climate in Queensland: "No paint containing more than five per centum of soluble lead shall be used or put within four feet from the floor or ground on the outside of any residence, hall, school, or other building to which children under the age of fourteen years have access, or on any veranda railing, gate, or fence."[37]

By focusing on outside paint, the legislators clearly understood that the danger resulted from the damaging effects of the harsh climate on outside painted surfaces. As Gibson explained to a British audience: "Such paint inside our houses or unexposed to the sun and outside atmosphere, does not powder at all appreciably."[38] This legislation was unique and quite different from laws restricting the use of lead paint that had been passed in a few European countries. In Queensland, the law aimed at protecting children; in Europe all laws restricting the use of lead paint aimed at protecting painters at the time of applying paint or preparing a wall (sanding) prior to painting. Of note, other Australian states did not pass legislation similar to Queensland's, reflecting the common understanding that childhood lead-paint poisoning was a problem restricted to tropical Queensland.[39] Because lead-paint poisoning, especially the Queensland variant of ocular neuritis, did not occur elsewhere in Australia, Gibson offered an explanation to British ophthalmologists: "It has been difficult for those practising in other parts of Australia to recognize the special conditions under which our children live, and the special facilities they have for ingesting lead."[40]

In the early 1920s the Queensland cases peaked, and by the early 1930s lead poisoning had almost disappeared. Some attributed this remarkable decline to the legislation, although in the opinion of one physician: "it is quite true that this Act has not been rigidly enforced, and has been entirely ignored by many painters." Nevertheless, he adds, "there have been instances in which painters who have used lead paint on veranda railing have been compelled to burn off and repaint the work with non-poisonous paints."[41] Other reasons given for the decline in childhood lead-paint poisoning were effective public health education, postwar prosperity (houses were painted more often), smaller families (greater parental supervision of children), earlier recognition of lead poisoning by physicians, better hygiene (more baths), a change in the style of housing that was less confining for children, decreasing the lead content of pigment by mixing zinc-based pigments with lead pigments, and the work of the Crèche and Kindergarten Society that provided day care for poor children.[42] The disappearance of childhood lead-paint poisoning from Brisbane was welcome if not fully understood.

New cases of lead poisoning had vanished from Brisbane, but that happy fact did not signal the end of concern in Queensland. Beginning in the early 1920s, young adults began dying from kidney disease. The numbers were few, but the population was sparse to begin with. Statisticians believed that deaths from chronic nephritis in Queensland were several times higher than expected when compared with kidney deaths in other Australian states. Local physicians, among them L. J. Jarvis Nye, were puzzled by this greater incidence of nephritis, and they sought possible explanations by questioning patients and by examining hospital records. What they found was that many adults with kidney disease had been diagnosed with lead poisoning as children. In one calculation, 33 of 186 kidney patients (18 percent) had a history of prior lead poisoning. Another series found 30 percent with "definite plumbism" and 16 percent with "indefinite plumbism."[43] Nye concluded that the epidemic of Queensland nephritis was a late effect of childhood lead-paint poisoning.

Nye's hypothesis resulted in a governmental investigation and in an Interim Report published by the Commonwealth Department of Health in 1932. This panel noted Nye's numbers but was generally more skeptical about the causal connection between childhood lead-paint poisoning in Queensland and excess kidney deaths in adults because lead paint was so common and kidney disease so rare.[44] What the Commonwealth Health Department proposed was that lead-paint poisoning in childhood accelerated the deaths of people destined to die of kidney disease.[45] This lukewarm endorsement irked Nye, who gathered his

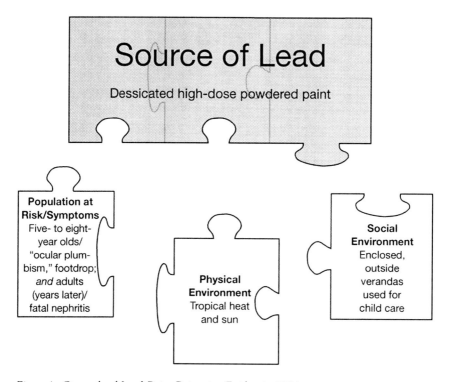

Figure 4. Queensland Lead-Paint Poisoning Epidemic, 1934

cases and sharpened his argument in a book, *Chronic Nephritis and Lead Poisoning* (1933).[46] By the mid-1930s, the ecology of childhood lead poisoning in Australia had changed. (See figure 4.) Keith Fairley[47] in 1934 and R. Elliott Murray in 1939 reviewed the evidence and supported Nye's contention. Murray added a second significant source of lead in Queensland: lead arsenate insecticide. He reported that cabbages in Brisbane markets in 1931 had between 100 and 600 mg of lead arsenate per cabbage.[48]

The American Understanding of Queensland Nephritis

Queensland nephritis appears to have been another unique and isolated phenomenon of lead poisoning in the tropics. Although debate over nephritis occupied Australian physicians for much of the 1930s, epidemics of kidney failure following lead poisoning simply did not occur outside of the Queensland context. Physicians had long known that lead could produce transient renal abnormalities, such as sugar in the urine, but chronic nephritis leading to death was completely unknown to American physicians.

American physicians did learn about Queensland nephritis. In the "Foreign Letters" section of the *Journal of the American Medical Association* in October 1939, the Australian correspondent presented a two-paragraph summary of Murray's 119-page book.[49] The following year the *Journal* carried an editorial on the subject. It was curious that the editorial writers summarized Nye's 1933 book and not Murray's more recent volume. What American readers gleaned from the editorial was that lead-poisoned children in Queensland often died from chronic kidney disease. Once again, American physicians and public health workers learned of the specific environment that resulted in childhood lead-paint poisoning in Queensland: "The characteristic feature of a house of the poor folk in Queensland is a large veranda the function of which is to afford protection from the rays of the tropical sun to the infants and children while the mother is away at work. The railings are painted with white paint. The siccative action of the tropical sun dries up the linseed oil and leaves the pigment, which in this case is the very toxic lead carbonate, in the form of a chalky powder."[50]

The unpublished correspondence of Robert Kehoe, the leading American authority on industrial lead poisoning from 1930 to 1965, sheds additional light on the American reception of the Queensland story. In 1946 and 1947, Kehoe and Nye exchanged letters about lead poisoning, nephritis, and the Queensland climate. In their correspondence it is possible to see how an American well versed in lead poisoning viewed the Australian experience. What the letters show is that Nye believed that the Queensland climate, housing style, and child care arrangements (which he termed a pen) were responsible for the Australian cases. In his response, Kehoe focused on Nye's nephritis theory and flatly explained to Nye that he simply had seen nothing similar in the United States. Furthermore, Kehoe doubted whether lead could cause serious kidney disease at all.[51]

The Queensland childhood lead-poisoning epidemic and nephritis may have indirectly influenced the history of lead poisoning in the United States in the late 1940s. After the publication of a provocative study in 1943 linking lead poisoning to later school failure, Felix Wormser and the Lead Industries Association (LIA), a trade organization for the lead industry about which we will learn more in Chapter 5, directed greater attention to childhood cases. For background reading, Kehoe, who advised LIA officials, sent Wormser a copy of Nye's book and several references from Australia (he mentions only Fairley's paper specifically). Wormser reached Kehoe's conclusion about lead and nephritis; but the Queensland epidemic may have nudged Wormser to look beyond the nephritis and to examine more closely the home environment.[52]

The unique Queensland complication of serious kidney disease has continued to perplex researchers. There is little doubt that nephritis occurred in Australia in children lead-poisoned in the first years of the twentieth century, but it is equally certain that this did not occur elsewhere.[53] Julian Chisholm, a Baltimore pediatrician who was at the forefront of lead research, concluded in 1969, "The observation that late lead nephropathy has been found as a sequel of plumbism during early childhood in Queensland, but not elsewhere, remains a mystery. . . . I can only say that we have not found it in a group of adolescents studied in Baltimore."[54]

Analysis in the 1950s

Australians have continued to study the Queensland epidemic. In the 1950s D. A. Henderson examined the records of 401 children admitted to Brisbane's Hospital for Sick Children between 1915 and 1935 with a diagnosis of lead poisoning. These would include some of Gibson and Turner's patients and most of Nye's (among other patients admitted by physicians who did not publish papers). What was striking was that 108 died of nephritis, a finding unique in the world. What was equally startling was that Henderson concluded that only 125 children appeared on his chart review to have suffered from lead poisoning.[55] What may have happened in Brisbane was that physicians incorrectly labeled with "lead poisoning" children who suffered similar symptoms, an understandable occurrence in the midst of any epidemic. When compared with cases from the United States, the Brisbane children were older, suffered more peripheral neuropathy and blue gum lines, had less encephalopathy, and, of course, far more nephritis.[56]

With the benefit of a century's hindsight, Jane Lin-Fu, a U.S. Children's Bureau pediatrician, expressed disappointment and frustration that American physicians and public health officials had not immediately accepted the Queensland notion that dust from decomposing lead paint presented health risks to children: "In the U.S., the early Australian papers were initially viewed with indifference; some considered childhood lead poisoning to be unique to Australia."[57] Even at home, "the Queensland experience had little impact elsewhere in Australia."[58] As Lin-Fu explained, "These important observations were promptly forgotten, to be rediscovered only in the early 1970s."[59] Considering the same epidemic and its failure to galvanize American medical opinion, Julian Chisholm suggested in 1989: "For seventy years, Gibson's observations lay fallow. Indeed, for many years, the epidemic of lead poisoning in Queensland children was not believed by physicians elsewhere who apparently considered the Queensland physicians primitive and perhaps addlepated by the heat."[60]

Lin-Fu and Chisholm were correct that American physicians in the first half of the twentieth century did not view this epidemic in the same fashion that a pediatrician or a public health worker might at the end of the century. Lin-Fu and Chisholm were not correct in concluding that the lessons to be learned from Queensland were precisely the same ones that American pediatricians gained from Rochester, New York, household dust in the 1970s. Rather, Thomas, Blackfan, and others viewed Queensland's chalky exposures in the same light that they also viewed workplace "clouds of dust": both were thought so different as to not apply to toddlers who chewed paint from their cribs and toys.[61]

Chapter 3

The Scientific Study of The American Workplace

WHEN THOMAS AND BLACKFAN first identified lead-poisoned children in their homes, European industrial hygienists had been struggling for several decades to curb lead poisoning in the workplace. By most accounts, industry in the United States lagged far behind in recognizing the health hazards of lead and in taking steps to curb exposures. Virtually all public health measures concerning lead poisoning had industrial worries at their origin, and so it is here where the historian of household lead poisoning must begin. From the outset, it was clear that there were significant differences between workers on the job and toddlers at home. Nevertheless, industrial health was where child health professionals—out of necessity—needed to start.

Alice Hamilton (1869–1970) was a sensitive barometer for American ideas and practices on a wide variety of issues concerning the lead industry from 1908, when she first turned her attention to industrial safety, to 1936, when she published *Recent Changes in the Painters' Trade*.[1] Hamilton was familiar with the inner workings of the lead industry: mining, processing, manufacturing, and the use of various products, among them lead paint. She was widely admired for the depth of her understanding by labor, manufacturers, public health officials, industrial hygienists, academic scientists, and government officials on the urban, state, and federal levels.

Throughout much of her career, European countries provided the benchmark for safety in the lead industry. Alice Hamilton was familiar with European opinions and practices: she knew European industrial hygienists, attended their conferences, visited their production plants, admired their safety record, and made critical comparisons between practices in Europe and the United States. She also followed the European debate over the prohibition of lead-based paint for interiors, reporting to her American audience the differences in opinion among countries and among various factions within countries.

Alice Hamilton's career demonstrates the evolution of the American approach to lead hazards: surveys and personal persuasion, state regulations, federal government reports and monitoring, and the conferences sponsored by the surgeon-general—pioneered in the mid-1920s—that brought together scientists, industrial hygienists, public health officials, labor, and government officials. Hamilton believed that the workplace was dangerous. She also believed that the workplace could be made safe. In her view, dust from lead paint presented health risks to painters, but she believed that dust management was achievable.

Hamilton had a long and rich career that intersected with many exciting currents, including progressives' interest in health and well-being in the tenements, the development of industrial medicine, feminism, especially women in medicine, and industrial sponsorship of health-related research. Here I have elected to focus tightly on Hamilton's evolving views of the dangers of lead in the workplace and how child health professionals interpreted her work in assessing the dangers of lead paint for toddlers at home.

Alice Hamilton was born in 1869 into a privileged family in Fort Wayne, Indiana. As a child she experienced a protected life of home schooling, expansive grounds, a cordon of servants, and summers in West Virginia and Mackinac Island. While at Miss Porter's School in Farmington, Connecticut, she was stunned to learn that her father had squandered the family fortune: she would have to earn her own way. Marriage did not appeal, so she decided on medicine to maintain her independence and to perform a useful service.[2]

Because her education had not been directed toward a profession, Hamilton had to start at an undistinguished local medical school before moving on to the University of Michigan, which had an admirable tradition of educating women physicians. Her internship at a Boston dispensary brought her into close contact with the terrible health conditions of the urban poor. Then it was off to Europe in 1895 to learn bacteriology in the laboratories of German savants. On her return, Hamilton spent time at Johns Hopkins Medical School. On the whole, she was well educated by the standards of medical training of her time.

Alice Hamilton experienced the obstacles facing many women physicians. Most doors of professional advancement—a lucrative practice, hospital appointments, university professorships—were not open to her. She avoided the path toward pediatrics and obstetrics that many women physicians traveled. Hamilton did not wish to be a woman physician for women; rather, she wanted to find a place in the mainstream. As many outsiders discover, Alice had to create a niche of her own.[3]

At first her quest landed her at Hull House, the urban settlement project founded by Jane Addams in Chicago. Like other residents, Hamilton earned her way elsewhere by day; in off hours she participated in uplifting the neighborhood served by Hull House. In all, Alice Hamilton lived at Hull House for much of the next twenty-two years. She taught classes, offered medical advice, and even ran baby clinics, although she had disdained this career pathway. In this setting, Hamilton was exposed to a wide sweep of reformers who ranged from progressive to radical. She later recounted that she never accepted the notion that anarchy achieved much of value. She was, however, an advocate for a strong labor movement. At Hull House, she witnessed the oppressive life of urban immigrants: poverty, unhealthy food, unsafe and unsanitary tenements, prostitution, and cocaine addiction. These conditions occupied her time but did not excite her. Then she discovered illness in the workplace.[4]

In choosing to enter what the British called "industrial hygiene" and what Americans later termed "industrial medicine" and still later "occupational medicine," Alice Hamilton solved several personal and professional problems. Industrial hygiene was almost nonexistent in the United States, so it did not conform to a pattern that excluded women physicians. Of equal importance, industrial hygiene was not a designated "woman's track." Factory medicine permitted her to enter, work, and achieve in a man's world. Her Hull House experience gave her particular sensitivity to the plight of poor, immigrant workers.[5]

Her earlier studies of cocaine addiction, typhoid fever, prostitution, and tuberculosis caught the eye of progressive politicians in Illinois, and in 1908 Hamilton was one of five physicians appointed to make a state survey of industrial illness. The task was overwhelming, so the panel focused on industrial poisons, Alice selecting lead. Lead hygiene in the workplace became the center of her professional life for the next three decades.[6]

Preparing the "Report of the Illinois Commission on Occupational Diseases" (1911) both educated Hamilton and made her visible to the industrial hygiene movement.[7] She learned much from this introduction. For example, she realized that lead found its way into far more products and industries than the commission had ever contemplated: printers, potters, painters, battery makers, and dozens of other types of workers all came into contact with lead.[8] Lead was never an abstract notion to Hamilton. She visited plants and witnessed the conditions; later she would study them in great detail. She spoke to physicians, hospital attendants, and sickened workers to get a sense of occupational lead poisoning, its early signs, and its destructive course in workers' bodies. Painters caught her attention early because they were so numerous.[9]

One observation stood out: industrial plumbism depended on factory cleanliness, which varied widely in industrial settings.[10] "This means," she wrote, that "the care of the men depends entirely upon the good will of the man in charge."[11] From the start, she articulated a philosophy of convincing industrial leaders that it was in their best interests to improve the health conditions of their employees.[12]

The Illinois commission realized that it did not have sufficient expertise in industrial plumbism, so in 1910 it sent Hamilton to Brussels to attend the International Congress of Occupational Accidents and Diseases. This was her first contact with the leading European industrial hygienists whom she had previously encountered only through their published papers.

For over half a century, European industrial health reformers such as L. Tanquerel des Planches had correctly drawn attention to lead dust and powder in the workplace.[13] The British industrial hygienists Thomas Legge and Kenneth Goadby reiterated the concern over the dangers: "Aetiologically, therefore, the relationship of dust-contaminated air and poisoning is undeniable." Legge and Goadby worried about dust so thick that they could see it by flashing a light through it.[14]

Thomas Oliver, another noted British industrial hygienist, also worried about the workplace dangers for painters:

> Lead poisoning is more prevalent among house painters than it ought to be. Painters when at work are not always strictly observant of details of personal hygiene. The practice of holding the brush between the teeth, of holding putty, which is a lead product, in the palm of the hand, of not always having the opportunity for washing before eating, or of misusing the opportunity when it exists, predisposes them to plumbism. Inhalation of dust given off during the sand-papering of dried painted surfaces, also of the fumes given off during the burning off of old paint, are sources of lead poisoning.[15]

On this European visit, Alice Hamilton inspected many lead factories in Britain and two in Germany. French factories did not permit her inspection.

The congress and her visits to European factories brought home to Hamilton just how far ahead of the United States Europe was in industrial hygiene. America had no reliable statistics on workplace diseases, no health or safety regulations, no field of industrial hygiene, and no system of insurance to compensate workers sickened on the job. When she returned from Europe, she brought her observations to the attention of superintendents of the National Lead Company and to medical audiences in many publications.[16]

Also attending the congress was Charles O'Neill, U.S. commissioner of labor, who asked Hamilton to make a detailed survey of the lead industry in the United States.[17] The Bureau of Labor (which in 1912 became the U.S. Department of Labor) could not afford to offer her a salary, so she sold her finished reports to the department on completion. Nor could the United States government provide Hamilton with the authority to enter the factories she wished to inspect. Persuasion alone had to suffice.

Alice Hamilton wrote ten reports on the lead industry for the Department of Labor between 1910 and 1920. Each report was rich in its fieldwork. She inspected as many factories as she could; every report is impressively detailed with example piled upon example.[18] Hamilton did not rely on factory management to provide her with information. She consulted with factory physicians, physicians who had no employment connections, local hospital records, workers, their wives and priests, and local drug store proprietors. What set her reports apart was that Hamilton coupled her inspections with a thorough understanding of the manufacturing processes she was studying. This analysis permitted her to conclude that health risks were not equally distributed throughout an industry, a plant, or even an assembly line. In any given factory, there might be workers at great risk and others at no risk. The same job at different factories could have widely different health hazards depending on the enlightenment of those in charge. On the completion of her inspection, Hamilton presented her findings in person to the manager, praising what the factory was doing right, pointing out unhealthy areas, and suggesting how improvements might be made. She offered to return and document progress.

A reading of Hamilton's reports demonstrates the evolution of her thinking about lead safety in the workplace. Her first report, "The White Lead Industry in the United States" (1911), revealed much of what ailed the industry. American manufacturers employed the "Old Dutch" method to produce lead carbonate, a process that yielded far more dust than different processes used in European factories. Dust was responsible for disease; vigorous dust management was the key to health. This meant keeping dust down by wetting and washing the floors and by removing air-suspended dust with ventilation and exhaust fans. Workers needed separate work clothes that were frequently laundered, adequate washing facilities to remove dust, and lunch rooms that were free from dust and away from the production line.

Lead Dust in the Workplace

Hamilton was overwhelmed by the "clouds of dust" she encountered in all of the lead industries. One of the worst was the pottery, tile works, and porcelain industry.[19] This was a booming field in the first decades of the twentieth century as inside plumbing with sinks, bathtubs, and toilets reached most American homes and apartments. Hamilton's reports speak for themselves: "Vast clouds of dust which fill the air so that one can hardly see [27]. . . . there are piles of dust in the corners and on the stairways, and the windows and walls are coated with dust [30]. . . . women workers often go home in the skirts they have worn all day, covered with a long coat to hide the white dust [32]. . . . there is no dust-free place [39]. . . . there was so much dust in the air that she would almost choke; they had to wear some of their street clothes in the winter to work in because it was so cold, and when they got home they could always shake the dust out of their skirts [51]." Hamilton concluded, "One must, however, visit the factories personally to realize how much of this dust there is; in one of the cleaner enameling rooms the furnaces, which were built out into the room, were covered with a deposit of more than 2 inches of the finer enamel dust . . . in every plant visited walls, ceilings, and windows were white with dust, and in spite of the ventilators in the rooms, hoods, and open windows, the air is always cloudy when work is going on" [40].[20] Hamilton found similar "clouds of dust" in her inspection of the smelting industry[21] and the storage battery industry.[22] Her vivid descriptions conveyed the dusty work environment of lead factories. In no fashion did she or others think these extreme conditions occurred in homes.

Other industrial hygienists attempted to quantify the amount of lead that was required to poison a worker. Tanquerel did not calculate this directly, but at one point he did provide the amount of lead, given orally as a medicine, that resulted in the development of lead colic. He stated that patients could take between 1 grain and 130 grains before symptoms occurred, or between 64 milligrams and 1000 milligrams. By present-day understanding this was an enormous dose of lead.[23]

Several industrial hygienists measured the amount of dust in the work environment and then calculated how much lead a worker inhaled over the course of a ten-hour day. The numbers were astounding; a lead worker inhaled between 6 and 25 milligrams of lead per shift.[24]

Legge calculated that an atmosphere with less than 5 milligrams of lead per 10 cubic meters of air would not produce encephalopathy or paralysis in a lead worker. This calculation resulted in two figures that were used by industrial physicians for decades: (1) air that contained less than 0.5 milligrams per cubic meter (or 500 micrograms/cubic meter) was thought safe for workers; and (2) it was believed that a worker could inhale about 2 milligrams of lead a day without developing lead poisoning. Ludwig Teleky, a Viennese industrial hygienist, thought the daily dose was about 1 milligram over several months.[25]

From these numbers, it is possible to see why industrial hygienists were so worried. With the Teleky/Legge measure of 1–2 milligrams of lead per day considered a threshold to produce industrial plumbism, a worker in many dusty environments could be exposed to between three and twenty-five times the threshold dose in the course of a single workday.

The Teleky/Legge measure was the standard for two decades. Alice Hamilton used these numbers in 1914, and to them she added a threshold determination from a New York City rubber factory in 1912: 8 milligrams of lead per day.[26] In 1930 the American Public Health Association still relied on these same figures.

By 1940, Robert Kehoe solidified the safe threshold daily dose for lead workers with human experiments that showed that a lead worker could ingest up to 2 milligrams per day without developing symptoms.[27] Kehoe reduced this threshold dose to 0.3–0.6 milligrams per day in 1947.

The Legge air concentration of 0.5 mg/cubic meter was used as a standard until 1933, when a U.S. Public Health Service study recommended lowering it to 0.15 mg/cubic meter. The number was raised to 0.20 mg/cubic meter in 1957 and lowered again to 0.15 mg/cubic meter in 1972.[28]

Hamilton's prescription for all dusty workplaces was similar to that she had given to the white lead industry: at every phase of production, dust creation needed to be minimized. When dust was formed, it required prompt removal. Workers needed protective clothing, washing facilities, and separate eating places. Hamilton noted social conditions that worsened health on the job. Non-English-speaking immigrants held most of the dangerous jobs; no attempts were made to educate them. When they sickened, immigrants simply left the factory, thus making the full state of the danger invisible. Hamilton discovered this problem by leaving the factories and going into the neighborhoods. She observed that unionized laborers could often negotiate better working conditions, but that immigrants usually did not belong to unions. She compared these pottery conditions with those in Europe: "No British, German, or Austrian pottery was seen in which dust was tolerated in the dipping room, in which glaze scraping and brushing were carried on without any device for removing the dust, or which failed to provide a lunch room and wash rooms for the workpeople."[29]

Painters and Other Lead Workers

Lead dust was also a hazard in painting, where it was produced when painters sandpapered and scraped surfaces.[30] Hamilton's plan for safety extended her program for dust management to painters. She modified it to include wet sanding so that dust would not billow up into the atmosphere.

In *Hygiene of the Painters' Trade*, Hamilton expanded on her method in two ways. First, she added paint chemistry to her fieldwork. This addition allowed her to understand that both solvents *and* pigments had health risks. No paint was completely safe; each type of paint required different safety measures; all paints could be safely used if the appropriate measures were applied. Second, Hamilton turned to the human physiology of absorption in order to explain lead hazards. Here she entered the unsettled debate of how and where lead was absorbed. Some European authorities believed that most lead entered the human system through the intestinal tract; others thought that inhaled lead contributed to the problem; still others believed that inhaled lead was actually swallowed and that the lungs could not absorb lead. Hamilton also studied how the solvents of lead-free paints entered the human system through the lungs.

The next year Hamilton studied the smelting and refining and storage battery industries. Each extended her views of occupational safety. Her analysis of lead smelting convinced her that the main danger for lead workers came from lead in the air, the "clouds of dust" that she had first encountered in the white lead and pottery industries and which were compounded by lead fumes that the superheating of lead produced. Airborne dust and fumes were so overwhelming that she shifted her focus from workers' personal hygiene to reducing lead in the atmosphere of the workplace. What was needed was regular factory inspections and frequent medical inspections of all employees. Americans needed compulsory insurance to cover industrial diseases, and states needed to mandate companies to report all lead diseases to a central registry.[31] The automobile and the radio created an overwhelming demand for lead storage batteries, and Hamilton was particularly critical of the lead hazards in this growth industry.[32]

Just before the outbreak of World War I in 1914, Hamilton took stock of efforts to improve safety in the lead industries. Impressed with the progress to date, she reminded her readers that the history of industrial hygiene in the United States had been very short, just three years since the publication of her Illinois report. She observed: "The white lead industry in the United States is more dangerous than in England or Germany, because we use dry methods where they use wet, and therefore have a more serious dust problem. Owing partly to the evident risks, this industry has of late undergone great reforms, and in the majority of our plants there is a constant and intelligent effort to protect the men."[33]

During the war, Alice Hamilton turned her talents to the inspection of munitions plants. Some used lead, but this was not her major concern. What sickened workers, many of them women recently employed in the factory workforce, were fumes and dust created by the manufacture of TNT. This worry over volatile solvents underscored Hamilton's newly articulated concern over polluted air in the workplace and her long-standing concern over solvents in lead-free paints. She also revisited lead manufacturing plants and determined that enough progress had been made to permit women to work at many lead jobs.[34]

Hamilton saw the war as pivotal to the development of industrial medicine in the United States. Munitions and lead manufacturing brought widespread apprehension about industrial poisons. Employers now took greater note of these dangers and understood that toxins were forcing some workers to leave production lines, thus increasing the cost of training new workers. The U.S. Public Health Service added industrial hygiene to its agenda during the war, and in-

dustrial medicine was becoming a respectable field in some of the nation's leading medical schools.[35]

Lead Research at Harvard

Hamilton's efforts during the war brought her to the attention of David Edsall,
newly appointed dean of the Harvard Medical School, who was committed to
developing industrial medicine at Harvard. Edsall, whom we met earlier when
he discussed the Queensland epidemic in 1907, invited Hamilton to give the
Cutter Lectures at Harvard in 1919 and then offered her a faculty position, the
first for a woman on the Harvard medical faculty.[36] The most significant research on the scientific aspects of lead poisoning in the first third of the twentieth century occurred at Harvard University. Although the inspiration for the
research once again was industrial poisoning, insights about lead metabolism
served as the theoretical underpinning for pediatricians when thinking about
children poisoned at home. In addition, a strategy developed at Harvard in the
1920s became one of two standard treatments for the disease.

Hamilton, who was quite familiar with leaders in the lead industry, persuaded
the National Lead Institute to fund studies at Harvard.[37] After her initial field
investigations, she had been highly critical of the medical profession in the
United States for largely ignoring industrial health: "There is here a great ne-
glected field in American medicine and one of growing importance, for each
year the number of industrial establishments which employ physicians increases,
and the opportunity for expert hygienic control of our dangerous trades increases.
But there will have to be a more general understanding of the problems of industrial hygiene before the service rendered by the majority of company physicians becomes of much real value."[38] What concerned Hamilton was that
industrial physicians simply did not understand the scientific underpinnings of
the diseases they were asked to treat. By 1920 she was convinced that some leaders of the lead industry wanted to improve health conditions at their factories,
if for no other reason than to trim outlays for workman's compensation.[39] Ham-
pering reform, however, was a clear understanding of lead metabolism in the
human body.

Obviously Hamilton selected Harvard as the site for her new studies in part
because she had accepted Edsall's invitation to join the medical school faculty
there.[40] But more significantly, Harvard was the only American university with
a track record in industrial health.[41]

Before becoming dean, David Edsall had spent more than a decade studying industrial diseases, including those faced in the lead industry. In 1912 he
organized the Industrial Diseases Clinic at Harvard. After a slow start, the clinic

attracted an avalanche of patients—most suffering from industrial poisoning—that grew to nearly five thousand patients yearly, or 20 percent of the total number of patients seen in Harvard's outpatient clinics. Lead poisoning was the diagnosis of just under 10 percent of patients.[42] From the start, Edsall wanted to study industrial diseases in the laboratory. One of his interests was the absorption of poisons through the respiratory tract. This had great significance for many industries, including lead.

Funding research in the early twentieth century normally required support from industry or from a few recently organized foundations, many of which, of course, had been endowed by industrialists. Edsall had some success in persuading manufacturers in New England to fund his research. When he became dean of the medical school in 1916, Edsall made industrial hygiene one of the fields of study that he wished to nurture at Harvard. Along with Hamilton, Edsall hired Cecil Drinker, who, in addition to pioneering research, founded and edited the *Journal of Industrial Hygiene*. Edsall persuaded New England manufacturers to donate an additional $125,000 to fund research. Edsall soon expanded Harvard's program in industrial health by developing the School of Public Health, which opened its doors in 1921 with a large grant from the Rockefeller Foundation.[43]

This environment attracted leaders of the lead industry. George Shattuck, a prominent member of the Harvard faculty, remembered: "The members of the Lead Institute gave a total of over $60,000 to be used over a period of three years for the scientific study of lead poisoning, simply because they broad-mindedly thought a new fundamental study of lead poisoning ought to be made."[44]

The lead industry's offer to support research at Harvard was characteristic of a few manufacturers in the first decades of the century. To be sure, the funding was motivated by self-interest. Nevertheless, the research was noticeably independent of industry control.[45] Harvard hired the researchers—Joseph C. Aub, Lawrence T. Fairhall, A. S. Minot, and Paul Reznikoff—who selected the topics for study. There is some evidence that the lead industry would have preferred a different research agenda but bowed before the logic of allowing the Harvard scientists investigative freedom.[46] All findings were openly published in medical journals, including the *Journal of Industrial Hygiene, Journal of the American Medical Association, Journal of Biological Chemistry, Journal of Experimental Medicine, American Journal of Physiology, Archives of Neurology and Psychiatry, Quarterly Journal of Medicine, American Journal of Public Health,* and *Journal of the American Chemical Society*. Aub's laboratory instituted the first research program on lead in the United States.[47] Beginning with the initial publications, its findings became the core of contemporary understanding of lead poisoning.[48]

Some historians have raised the question whether any research funded by the lead industry in the 1920s was truly independent;[49] others attest to the intellectual character and independence of the research.[50] Aub was quite clear on the subject. In his "Third Report on the Investigation of Lead Poisoning," he declared: "The funds for the investigation were donated by the National Lead Institute. It is very gratifying that this organization has not at any time offered suggestions as to any policy or point of view, but has allowed the work to run its course and to demonstrate the truth without regard for a possible economic effect upon the lead industries."[51]

Edsall, Aub, and Hamilton wanted research that would investigate the basic metabolism of lead in living animals. They did not believe that the field was yet mature enough to study workers directly. Medical schools had recently been invigorated by close unions to research universities. The spirit of research, inspired by European examples, was sparked by the belief that the greatest chance of discovery resulted from allowing scientists freedom to roam in the laboratory.[52] To Joseph Aub, this meant starting with the basics.[53] He explained:

> The problem of lead poisoning has been studied [at Harvard] neither as an industrial hazard nor in the light of preventive medicine, but with the desire to understand more fully the chemistry, physiology, and clinical aspects of the disease itself. This point of view was taken because the other types of investigation have been carried out frequently in recent years, and do not permit careful scientific work. Any measures for preventing the deleterious effects of lead must be fundamentally dependent upon an understanding of its action in the organism if they are to be effective. We have, therefore, undertaken an investigation of the problems of the absorption, retention, and excretion of lead by the body, and we have been able in this way to obtain a far clearer conception of how and why lead produces the clinical signs characteristic of lead poisoning and also of the conditions which control its excretion.[54]

Aub's research group started with the fundamentals. Toward the end of the nineteenth century, some physicians had been able to detect the presence of lead in urine in living patients and in some bodily organs at autopsy.[55] The difficulty lay in determining the amount. Even in workers poisoned to death by lead, the concentration of lead in bodily tissues was measured in parts per million. In 1922 Lawrence Fairhall developed a technique that he believed could detect as little as 1 part lead in 10,000,000 parts urine,[56] which A. S. Minot confirmed was more accurate than her earlier technique, an innovation just three years earlier.[57] As Fairhall explained years later, when he was principal industrial toxicologist of the U.S. Public Health Service: "With respect to the heavy metals, investigations in industrial hygiene are concerned with quantities that are very small. Unfortunately these very small amounts are concealed in quantities of biological material which are enormously large in proportion. Thus, a significant amount of a metal in a day's output of urine of 1,500 cc. may be

30 or 40 micrograms. This represents a concentration of 3 or 4 parts in 150,000,000."[58]

From the start, Fairhall's technique won high marks. Carl Weller, a pathologist at the University of Michigan, in 1925 praised Fairhall's method:

> The work of the Harvard group on lead and of L. T. Fairhall in particular, has made it possible to do satisfactory qualitative tests for exceedingly small amounts of lead present in relatively large quantities of biologic material. Results of chemical research on the bodily fluids and organs of cases of lead poisoning have formerly been notoriously inconsistent and uncertain. There can be but little doubt that much of the older work is without value. Lead has escaped detection, and other substances have been confused with lead, so that errors in both directions have occurred. From both quantitative and qualitative standpoints the newer methods are much superior.[59]

Not all researchers were able to duplicate Fairhall's technique. Robert Kehoe, who would emerge as the recognized authority on human lead poisoning in the 1930s, was highly critical of Fairhall's method and developed his own procedure.[60] In an exchange of letters, each challenged the other to an on-site demonstration. This duel seems never to have taken place.

Physicians had known that workers absorbed lead from breathing in lead dust or from swallowing lead. What happened to the lead after it entered the body from either site was not known. Investigation required careful animal studies that employed Fairhall's method of determining lead in bodily fluids and organs. Minot found that most swallowed lead passed through the digestive tract unabsorbed. The small amount that was absorbed was filtered through the liver and biliary system before entering the bloodstream. In contrast, animals absorbed nearly all inhaled lead which entered the bloodstream in the lungs without the benefit of filtering. Once in the blood, lead traveled to bones, where it was stored. Minot's demonstration of lead metabolism had direct implications for lead workers and their employers. Inhaled lead was far more dangerous than swallowed lead. Minot and Aub confirmed Minot's ideas with human autopsy studies.[61]

Lead workers suffered from anemia. The Harvard group set out to determine whether anemia occurred because lead inhibited the making of red blood cells or because lead destroyed them. They determined that lead both disrupted production and caused red blood cells to break up.[62] The Harvard research team also investigated lead palsy.[63]

Toward the end of the 1920s and into the 1930s, Aub's group investigated how lead entered the bones and how—by manipulating calcium in the diet of lead-poisoned workers—lead could be eliminated from bones and ultimately from the body. In these studies, Aub's team made one of the first studies in humans of parathyroid hormone, which helps to regulate bodily calcium. Aub's "high-calcium" treatment was one of only two available therapies for lead poisoning until after World War II.[64]

Research of the Harvard group became the cornerstone of understanding the metabolism of lead poisoning in the United States. Virtually every article on childhood lead poisoning published after 1926 cited Aub and his colleagues. The historian Christopher Sellers has concluded that the work of Aub's industry-funded laboratory at Harvard provided "the foundation of our modern understanding of this ailment."[65]

Some of Aub's findings found quick appreciation in the lead industry. In 1923 Edward Cornish, president of the National Lead Company, wrote to Dean Edsall:

> I quite agree that it is already being demonstrated that scientific investigation of lead poisoning, even though commenced for the sole purpose of acquiring knowledge, is likely to result in great advantage to everyone whose business brings him into contact with lead. The statement that lead absorbed through the lungs is more injurious and dangerous than lead absorbed through the stomach is very interesting. . . . We have been influential in procuring a sandpaper which will not be unduly expensive and can be used wet. We hope that it will be adopted generally at an early date. Your finding that lead is relatively more dangerous when absorbed through the lungs will assist us in inducing painters to adopt wet sandpapering.[66]

Alice Hamilton's Years at Harvard

With Hamilton's move to Harvard, the character of her career changed. She did less fieldwork, although she continued to revisit factories that she had inspected over the past decade. She returned to the laboratory and pursued her interest in solvents and fumes, studying carbon monoxide, aniline dyes, and mercury poisoning. Only occasionally did she collaborate with Joseph Aub and his coworkers.

Hamilton served as a transition to the next generation of industrial medicine[67] as she turned her attention to writing her textbook,[68] serving on governmental commissions, and assessing safety in the lead industry.[69] In essence, she emerged as the recognized authority in the field.

During her first years at Harvard, Hamilton became involved in the controversy surrounding the introduction of the antiknock ingredient, tetraethyl lead, into gasoline. The story of gasoline and tetraethyl lead takes this history a bit away from its main focus, but part of the story has relevance. Soon after tetraethyl lead was first added to gasoline, several employees died at the manufacturing plant, and concern emerged from many quarters over its safety. A study by the U.S. Bureau of Mines cleared the new substance, but Hamilton and others raised objections about its safety.[70] The Ethyl Corporation temporarily removed tetraethyl lead from the marketplace. The surgeon general convened a conference of industrial hygienists, university scientists, manufacturers, labor leaders, public health officials, and government bureaucrats. Questions over safety emerged; the surgeon general appointed a committee of experts to study workplace issues. This committee conducted experiments and returned with conclusions about the safety of tetraethyl lead that were approved by the larger conference. This American approach to solving health issues in the workplace greatly appealed to Hamilton. She thought it superior to lawsuits or legislative action, because it placed the decision in the hands of experts who understood the issues better than politicians, lawyers, or judges.[71]

Hamilton raised a concern over the contamination of the atmosphere with tetraethyl lead. Her fears would resurface decades later. At this later point, the histories of air pollution and childhood lead paint merged.

In her last publications about lead hazards in the workplace, Hamilton detailed the "enormous improvement" that had been made in the white lead industry,[72] identified areas that still needed work, and outlined new hazards.[73] When she viewed the painting industry in the 1920s and 1930s, Hamilton thought that the lead hazard was essentially manageable because its dangers were so well known and because dust precautions were widely used. In addition, manufacturers had reduced the lead content in many interior paints and removed it altogether from paint intended for furniture. Unfortunately, not all aspects of painting were safer for painters. Spray painting with quick-drying paints increased the dangers to the painter by dispersing the solvents into enclosed rooms.[74] Masks could trap virtually all lead but were unable to filter solvent vapors.[75] Hamilton could thus end her career with the knowledge that her efforts had enhanced safety for lead workers, though challenges remained.

Chapter 4

Lead Hazards, Lead Safety, and Alice Hamilton

ALICE HAMILTON'S LONG experience with lead safety in the workplace placed her in an ideal position to survey many controversies that swirled through the industrial hygiene movement. In some cases Hamilton was an observer; in others she was an active participant. Hamilton never wrote directly on household childhood lead-paint poisoning. Nevertheless, her opinions about workplace safety informed pediatricians and influenced decisions that had direct bearing on the subject.

The Special Vulnerability of Women and Children to Lead

Some industrial hygienists worried that women and child workers were more vulnerable to the effects of lead than men. The question arises: Did American pediatricians, public health officials, and leaders of the lead industry believe that health concerns in the workplace translated precisely to home exposures? And if they did, what were the perceived lessons? The historian has to be careful here. No pediatrician, public health official, or industrial health leader addressed these questions directly. When they did speak of children, industrial physicians did so in terms of children in the workplace, assisting either factory workers or painters on the job. These young people were usually adolescents—children, to be sure, but older than the six- to eight-year-olds in Queensland and the infants and toddlers who worried Thomas, Blackfan, and Holt. It is noteworthy that there was virtually no articulated concern about dried lead paint—from physicians, public health workers, or industrial leaders—as applied to the wall, ceiling, or furniture.

For the most part, American physicians maintained firm boundaries between industrial health risks and home safety. When physicians did discuss the lessons from the workplace, the context of the discussion was usually whether children suffered from the same symptoms as adults following exposure to lead.[1] Physicians did make two connections between workplace and home. First, workers or painters—covered with powder and dust on the job—could bring this high-dose powder home on their clothing or skin. Two of the changes that occupied industrial health reformers and industry officials were special clothing at the workplace and showers to wash away lead powder.[2] Second, industrial officials worried about the effects of high-dose lead on pregnant workers.[3] Lead was a known abortifacient; it was the "active ingredient" of commonly used home remedies for inducing abortions, such as Diachylon pills, during the nineteenth and early twentieth centuries.[4] One of the reforms that both physicians and industry leaders urged was removing women from the lead paint-producing factories.[5] Of note, European laws that placed restrictions on the use of lead paint did so out of concern for the painter or others in the room at the time of painting and sanding. These laws were not aimed at the safety of the occupants of the home after the paint had dried.

Standard texts on industrial lead poisoning contain few comments about the effects of lead on child workers. At the turn of the twentieth century, most texts on industrial exposures of lead referred to the pioneering nineteenth-century *Lead Diseases: A Treatise* by the French physician L. Tanquerel des Planches.[6] Tanquerel believed that children developed symptoms similar to those of adults but that children were rarely exposed, except on the job.[7] In his experience, Tanquerel found that most victims of lead encephalopathy were men between twenty and fifty years of age. He had only encountered four workers under twenty with encephalopathy.[8]

The British industrial hygienists Thomas Legge and Kenneth Goadby were also concerned about the dangers of lead to children in the workplace. In *Lead Poisoning and Lead Absorption* (1912), they stated:

> Young persons are regarded as more liable to lead poisoning than adults, although it is difficult to obtain definite figures on the point, the duration of employment acting as a disturbing factor in estimating the susceptibility of young persons. They may have worked in a lead works for a year or more without showing any signs of poisoning, but develop them later in adult life, although it is very likely that absorption had taken place during an earlier period. . . . The general clinical conclusions of appointed surgeons and certifying surgeons in the various lead factories would be, we believe, that the susceptibility of young persons is at least twice that of adults, and there is some ground for supposing that the tissues of an adult when growth has ceased more readily adapt them-

selves to deal with absorption and elimination of poisonous doses of lead than do the tissues of a young person.[9]

Thomas Oliver, another British industrial hygienist, also worried about the health of adolescents in the lead industry:

> Lead exerts its malign influence with a rapidity and severity greater in young children than in old. Young adults especially are quickly brought under its sway.
>   On February 17, 1898, the Home Secretary [Sir M. White Ridley] announced in the House of Commons that there had been 37 cases of lead poisoning among boys under 18 years of age which had proved fatal. Work in a white lead factory is not an occupation for young persons of either sex.[10]

What these few references to children in the industrial literature demonstrated was a concern for teenagers in the workplace and a general notion that adolescent workers might be more vulnerable to lead than adults, the result of a natural recklessness or physiological susceptibility. In none of the texts was there any comment on infants or toddlers exposed to lead at home. As such these workplace experiences did not prove particularly relevant to American pediatricians.

   What worried industrial hygienists was the creation of pure lead-paint dust in the workplace—dust that would hang in the atmosphere, coat a painter's skin, hair, or clothing, and settle on the floor like chalk dust in a classroom. What did not worry the industrial hygienists in the first years of the twentieth century was the health risk sanding posed to infants, toddlers, or other members of the household once the painters had cleaned up after their work. To be fair, industrial reformers focused tightly on the health risks of workers. This is not to imply that Alice Hamilton and others were indifferent to householders or their children. It was simply that industrial hygienists honed their arguments sharply to the workplace.

   Hamilton, like all physicians, knew that lead was an effective abortifacient, used commonly by women after abortions became illegal in the 1880s. She was also aware that some European industrial hygienists worried about the high miscarriage rate among lead workers. In fact this was often the reason given for removing women from lead industries. In the United States, however, in contrast to Europe, Hamilton often observed that miscarriage was not a problem because women (and adolescents) were seldom employed in the lead industry prior to World War I.[11]

   During the war, women did enter the lead industry in great numbers, and it was then that Hamilton gave serious thought to women's vulnerability to lead.[12] The issue for Hamilton was whether the improvements in health conditions in the lead industry made it safe for women to work or whether conditions were so unsafe that women should be banned from the workplace.[13]

Hamilton concluded that most jobs in the lead industry were safe enough for women. Because so few American women had been employed as lead workers, Hamilton turned to European industrial hygienists for her understanding. There she found controversy. British physicians believed that women had a lower threshold for lead poisoning. In contrast, German physicians thought that women did not have any special vulnerability, but that factory women—when compared with German factory men—were more impoverished, more overworked, and more undernourished, thus setting them up for greater susceptibility to lead exposure.

Hamilton carved out an opinion between the British and the German positions. In most instances, women reacted to lead in the same fashion as men. She did think there were two areas where women were more susceptible: encephalopathy and risk to fetuses. She relied entirely upon European sources for the latter, because she could find no American studies. On the basis of the European findings, Hamilton concluded that pregnant women and married women of child-bearing age should not work in lead factories.[14]

Hamilton recognized that few women in 1919 were house painters. Nevertheless, she saw no reason why they could not paint as long as they followed the same precautions that she outlined for men: "In employing women in any branch of the painting trade it will be necessary to prohibit dry rubbing down of lead paint, mixing dry lead compounds with paint, using dirty drop cloths, and chipping off old lead paint. It will also be necessary to insist on the provision of hot water, nailbrushes, soap, and towels for their use."[15]

The European Debate over Interior Paint

From the perspective of the twenty-first century, it is tempting to speculate what might have happened to childhood lead poisoning if home decorators had chosen paint that did not contain lead pigment. In fact, there was a European debate over the removal of lead from paints for interiors both before and after World War I. This debate did not make a significant transatlantic jump, but it is instructive nonetheless.

After a number of decades of attempting to moderate lead poisoning among painters, several European nations in 1910 debated whether workplace safety was even possible. Those who concluded that it was not advocated banning lead paint from the insides of buildings. The concern was over inhaling lead-paint dust while preparing a wall for repainting. Outside painting was not a concern because the dust dissipated into the atmosphere. The first point to keep in mind is that this was a *European* debate. At no time until the 1950s was there any call to restrict the use of lead-based paint on walls and ceilings in the United

States. Second, the European debate was an enormously complicated affair. One study in 1923 published the legislation on lead safety in the workplace from a number of Europeans nations: it covered 135 small-print pages.[16] Third, there was never a single "point of view" coming from Europe. In every period, there were nations that favored a ban and those that opposed a ban; there were groups within each country who supported a ban and those who did not. Fourth, there was a general shift in European opinion from supporting a ban before the war to opposing a ban after the war, although again this was far from clear-cut. Fifth, the debate Hamilton watched took place in major industrialized nations. She was not indifferent to legislative proposals from less industrialized countries, but she took her cues from Britain, France, Germany, and Austria.

No one doubted that lead-based paint was hazardous. The issue was whether safety measures that controlled dust reduced the danger. If not, a ban made sense. Alice Hamilton first encountered this debate when she visited Europe in 1910. At that point most European nations had rigorous legislation to prevent dust in the workplace. For painters, this meant wet sandpapering, cleanliness, separate work clothes, and washing facilities. Hamilton admired these regulations, and on her return, she advocated them for the United States.

A ban was a far greater step. Here European nations divided. Many considered a ban for interior surfaces. Germany and Britain debated and rejected a ban before and after the war. Austria and France passed a ban. Even in France, Hamilton reported dissent from master painters: "The statistics on lead poisoning in the painter's trade in France have been the subject of bitter controversy between those who advocate the prohibition of white lead paint and the master painters. It is difficult to glean impartial statements from the mass of evidence on both sides."[17] In this early point in her career, Hamilton seemed open to considering a ban on lead paint for interior uses in Europe, but she concluded that any movement to ban lead paint from both interiors and exteriors as "radical and premature."[18]

After the war, Hamilton again surveyed the European scene.[19] In 1924 she described the postwar debate:

> The French argue that it is not possible to control conditions under which the painter works, now indoors, now outside, now for one contractor, now for another; that he cannot be given proper washing facilities in new buildings nor regular medical supervision. Therefore . . . they now refuse to take halfway measures with regard to lead paint, and white lead is no longer made in France and white lead paint is not supposed to be used. The British and the Germans have followed their usual method of trying to minimize the risks rather than revolutionize the industry. [Hamilton then went on to describe wet sandpapering and other dust precautions.][20]

Hamilton's most detailed analysis of the European debate—which she described as an "active controversy"—came in her 1925 textbook, *Industrial Poisons in the United States*. She reviewed the French position. Then she observed that the International Labour Organization's proposal to ban lead-based paints for interiors reopened the debate in Britain and Germany. In Britain, Hamilton noted a shift in the debate toward the dangers of solvents and away from the concern over lead pigments. Dust precautions took care of lead, but solvent vapors were harder to control. Hamilton reported that some German industrial hygienists believed that medical inspection of painters detected lead poisoning in the early stages. Hamilton next detailed several British committees that considered the subject in some depth at different points from 1911 to 1923.[21] In 1923 a parliamentary inquiry reviewed the issue of banning lead pigments for interior use, advances in dust control, and the ILO proposal. Committee members recommended to the government that Britain adopt laws that would implement the Geneva convention. The government was not persuaded that any change was needed; in fact it believed that wet sanding had rendered interior painting safer. The government decided not to accept the recommendation of the parliamentary committee. In 1926 Parliament passed the Lead Paint Protection against Poisoning Act, which did not include a ban.[22] The "Foreign Letters" correspondent for the *Journal of the American Medical Association* captured the shift in British opinion for an American audience.[23]

In *Exploring the Dangerous Trades* (1943), Alice Hamilton gave reasons why U.S. industry and labor both opposed the ILO proposal. She tied the American rejection to postwar isolationism and fear of European socialism.[24]

Ludwig Teleky, the Viennese industrial hygienist who favored the ban, reported to an American audience that German painters were divided over this issue. The Union of German Painters and Varnishers and the Social Democratic Guild of Painters favored the ban, but the Master Painters opposed it.[25]

On Restricting Lead Paint in the United States

Although it appears likely that Hamilton was at least open to the idea of a European ban early in her career, she refrained from endorsing a similar proposal for the United States because of her concern for the health risks posed by alternatives to lead paint. In addition, she believed that any restriction on lead pigments would be unacceptable to American painters. As her career progressed, she became convinced that safety was possible for painters on the job.[26]

On February 12, 1913, she wrote a letter to Charles H. Verrill, her superior at the Department of Labor. In it she responded in great detail to criticism leveled by a physician, Dr. Sutton, who was employed by the American Encaustic Tile Works of Zanesville, Ohio.[27] Sutton had gone over Hamilton's head to complain about her conclusions about his tile plant. Near the end of her letter to Verrill, Hamilton added:

> When I was in Denver I succeeded in speaking to the International
> Congress of Master Painters as an employee of the Bureau of Labor, not
> as a friend of the National Lead Company, and as I spoke against the use
> of white lead in interior work, I think no one connected me with them
> in any way. When I had finished, a master painter from Washington
> asked why the government did not begin at home, and went on to say
> that the interior work in the federal building is all done with lead paint
> and sandpapered. This is like the statement I wrote you before to the
> dangerous methods used in the naval yards. The White Lead people
> have been much agitated over that Cincinnati inquiry and I am hearing
> them on all sides. You will let me have the chemist's report when it is
> ready, will you not? I should like to write the thing up for the *Journal of
> the American Medical Association.*[28]

In this speech to the Master Painters, Hamilton explained her position on the proposed ban: "Now, when I say that this is an avoidable danger, I do not mean that it has to be avoided by prohibition of the use of lead paint for interior work. I am not going to advocate that because I think it would be utterly useless for me to do so, and I would not receive any backing from practical painters if I suggested such a thing. They would think that I was suggesting something that was perfectly preposterous."[29] Dry sandpapering of old lead paint was what Alice Hamilton was against. The master painter from Washington chided her on just this point. In her letter to Verrill, Hamilton amplified her conclusion by calling attention to a similar concern she had with painting in naval yards.[30]

Although Hamilton never advocated a ban on the use of lead paint for interiors, she did support legislative safeguards for painters: "This study of the painters' trade in the United States shows that there are many elements of danger, most of them avoidable, and it shows that if protective legislation is to be passed it should be directed toward the prevention of poisonous fumes and dust, and the provision of facilities for bodily cleanliness."[31]

The final sentence of Hamilton's report was curious, because it seemingly contradicted what she had argued throughout her narrative: "The total prohibition of lead paint for use in interior work would do more than anything else to improve conditions in the painting trade."[32] It is this sentence that has led other historians to conclude that Hamilton advocated a ban in the United States. Yet this comment does not fit with the rest of her report or with her speech to the Master Painters. She had argued persuasively that painters could manage the hazard of lead dust with wet sandpapering and strict personal cleanliness and that "no paint need be dangerous if it is used with sufficient caution."[33]

In 1913 only Austria had a ban (with many exceptions) in effect; France had passed one, but it had not yet been executed. The war would further delay implementation. Britain and Germany, whose industries Hamilton had closely studied and admired, rejected a ban both before the war and after. In 1913 Hamilton reported that no American state legislature was considering a ban.

The sentence concluding her report was an isolated one. Although Hamilton wrote extensively on painting and safety, she never again published a similar phrase.

The Dangers of Lead-Free Paint

There is another reason why this sentence does not fit with Hamilton's thinking. In *Hygiene of the Painters' Trade* (1913), Hamilton argued that no paint was completely safe. Using lead pigments had risks; using leadless paints posed different risks because of the solvents involved. In 1913 Hamilton considered the risks from lead-free paints to be considerable. Her comment in her letter to Charles Verrill about the Cincinnati study—the one that "agitated" the white lead people and provoked comments "on all sides"—underscored her concern about the use of lead-free paints. In *Hygiene of the Painters' Trade*, she reported on a study by Dr. John Landis, Cincinnati health officer, which detailed the serious illnesses that painters suffered after using quick-drying lead-free paint. In her analysis of these paints—which contained zinc-based pigments such as lithopone—she concluded: "This enormous proportion of benzine explains why the paint dries so rapidly and why currents of air must be excluded from the room which is being painted. It is clear that these painters were suffering from symptoms of acute benzine poisoning, complicated in one case at least with chronic turpentine poisoning."[34] She could not responsibly advocate a ban on lead-based paints because there was no alternative that was completely safe.

In her autobiography, Hamilton offered another slant on this period in the history of painting:

> In those days [1913] there were only two poisons which threatened the majority of painters, lead and turpentine, and painters were perfectly familiar with the effects of both. But since in the painter's eye the only good paint was lead paint with turpentine, and since he took pride in a good job, he never objected to the use of these two poisonous substances—indeed he preferred them. The new, cheap, quick-drying paints, with leadless pigment and naphtha, were beginning to come in, but the painter despised them and complained far more of the dopeyness and headache and nausea caused by naphtha fumes than he complained of lead poisoning.[35]

Hamilton's method of investigating health dangers in the workplace gave her an appreciation of the potential hazards of all paints, not just of those with lead pigment. She always informed her readers that pigment and solvent both involved health risks. Painters, of course, knew this. The toxicity of lead-free paints was quite evident to them; they found the solvents sickened them while the paint was applied. There were also long-range health effects. Hamilton devoted a long section of *Hygiene of the Painters' Trade* to the toxicity of solvents and in particular to the Cincinnati study already discussed.[36] She concluded: "The danger in the use of leadless paints and of paint removers comes from the liquid vehicle and is increased by lack of proper ventilation. If quickly drying, flat finish paints are used in close, ill-ventilated rooms, serious poisoning from the fumes of coal tar products and of turpentine may result."[37] So concerned was Hamilton about these solvents that she advocated legislation to "forbid the use in unventilated rooms of paints or paint removers containing volatile poisons."[38]

She also worried, of course, about lead pigments. But she carefully defined the risk, which was found in mixing dry pigments (which she did not believe occurred in the United States)[39] and in the dust created by sandpapering and scraping lead paint.[40] Her solution to lead dust was wet sandpapering, separate work clothes, clean drop cloths, washing facilities, and separate lunch rooms.[41] In other words, she believed in 1913 that all paints had health risks, but that with the proper precautions, all paints could be used safely.

Over the years, Hamilton grew less concerned about lead pigments and more worried about the solvents in lead-free paints. It is possible to see the evolution of her concern about solvents during World War I. She inspected munitions industries, and discovered that most illness came from volatile fumes.[42] The fumes that worried her came from TNT. At Harvard after the war, she continued her study of volatile solvents.[43] She was aware that the British industrial hygienists Oliver and Goadby also perceived the increased danger to painters from solvents.[44]

The new technology of spraying compounded the issue. Spraying quick-drying, lead-free paints permitted painters to cover more surfaces in less time. Unfortunately spraying also dispersed toxic solvents.[45] In contrast, Hamilton argued in 1925 that "the avoidance of danger from the use of lead pigments is a simpler problem."[46] The use of masks had no effect on reducing the danger to painters from volatile fumes.[47]

In *Recent Changes in the Painters' Trade* (1936), Hamilton still worried about both pigment and solvents. In general she thought that the dangers from lead were considerably less for painters, because all knew the necessary precautions and because there was less lead used in paints designed for interior use.[48] Spraying and new solvents concerned her far more than lead.[49]

At all points in her career, Hamilton believed that lead pigment, while presenting some risk to painters, was a manageable problem with proper precautions.

At no time did she think that lead-free paints carried no risk. At all times, Hamilton's concern was the painter and never the occupant of the house.

The discussions of the dangers of lead paint for the insides of homes—both in Europe and in the United States—thus focused on the health of painters, not of inhabitants. Hamilton and others believed that appropriate precautions offered adequate protection to painters to prevent lead poisoning. In only one instance have I found a possible contradiction to this generally held view. A paragraph from a 1914 speech delivered by Henry A. Gardner, director of the Scientific Section of the Paint Manufacturer's Association, appears to have raised a concern regarding inhabitants living in a painted room. To the master painters who formed Gardner's audience, virtually every aspect of his speech conformed with the standard views of industrial hygienists such as Alice Hamilton, whose *Hygiene of the Painters' Trade* he cited. For example, Gardner identified health problems of both pigments and solvents, paying special attention to dust production and paint removal. At one point, he mentions a danger to inhabitants from lead coming from painted surfaces. I suspect that Gardner was referring to the danger posed to inhabitants from lead dust created from sanding and scraping at the time of repainting, but his phrasing is imprecise. Even sixty years later, when physicians first identified house dust as a potential source of lead and when it was technologically possible to measure small amounts of lead in the atmosphere, no pediatrician or public health official worried about airborne lead in a painted room after the painter had finished painting, cleaned up, and the paint dried.

Fumes from Drying Paint: A Cause of Lead Poisoning?

Alice Hamilton also commented on a long debate, extending back to Tanquerel, concerning whether lead paint gave off lead-containing vapors while drying, thus potentially exposing inhabitants to a lead hazard when they simply sat, played, or slept in a recently painted room.

Tanquerel had warned painters and inhabitants of rooms being painted: "Everyone knows the pernicious effects of oil painting with a base of carbonate of lead, upon the workmen who apply it; also upon those who dwell in close places where this paint is newly used. Oil paint mixed with carbonate or white of zinc, has no deleterious influence upon the workmen, or upon the inhabitants of the newly painted apartments."[50] Tanquerel did not expressly mention whether his concern was for vapors from wet paint or for dust from sanding, but many industrial hygienists interpreted his comments as a warning about dangerous vapors. Other nineteenth-century physicians were adamant that no one could be lead-poisoned merely by sleeping in a room that had been freshly painted.[51]

Tanquerel was an influential leader, and his worry over drying vapors extended into the twentieth century. In 1904, for example, the French Chamber of Deputies heard from M. Breton on the dangers of fumes, a discussion that was later briefly summarized in *SWP*, a trade publication of the Sherwin-Williams Company. Breton, picking up Tanquerel's thread, tried to prove that drying lead paint gave off fumes containing lead. Tanquerel and Breton's error was certainly understandable. Illness from paint fumes and lead poisoning shared some symptoms, such as headache and abdominal distress. In the middle of the nineteenth century, most paints contained lead pigments. It seemed logical to Tanquerel that fumes must contain lead. In 1903 Breton tried to prove this false notion, and after conducting experiments, he believed that he had done so.

British industrial hygienists properly saw that Breton had made several errors in technique, and when they repeated Breton's experiments, they were unable to find any lead in the fumes. The British correctly attributed the sickness from fumes to the inhalation of turpentine, not to lead.

Why did Tanquerel and Breton believe that zinc paints did not cause this problem? Alice Hamilton explained the European scientific debate[52] and her understanding of the controversy to her readers in *Hygiene of the Painters' Trade*. Recent chemical experiments showed that the sickness from fumes came from aldehydes given off from drying paints. Turpentine and linseed oil—the liquid portion of lead paint—yielded aldehydes when drying. Hamilton knew that zinc-based paints also produced sickness when painters inhaled fumes in poorly ventilated work areas. In her report, she explained that zinc-based paints did not contain linseed oil, but they included benzene. This was the solvent that had so worried her from the reports of painters in Cincinnati in 1912.[53] Two years later, Henry Gardner discussed the same debate and scientists that Hamilton had considered and reached the same conclusion: "It is apparent that many other cases of lead poisoning have, without justice, been attributed to the vapors from white lead paints."[54] Gardner, in contrast to Hamilton, attributed the fume sickness to carbon monoxide.

The Honorable Marion Rhodes, 1910

This curious notion of the danger of lead vapors even reached a committee room in the U.S. Congress. In 1910 Marion Rhodes, a congressman from Missouri, wanted to extend the labeling provision of the Food and Drug Act to cans of lead paint. As Rhodes pointed out, when someone purchased lead carbonate as a medicine from a druggist, the box had a poison label.[55] Rhodes thought painters should have the same warning on cans of paint so that they would know to take the recognized precautions to prevent lead poisoning while painting.[56] Other committee members challenged the need: "Is there any painter so ignorant that he does not know that white lead is poisonous?" To this objection,

Representative Rhodes conceded: "I rather doubt that there are any painters but have some sort of conception that it is poisonous."[57] Rhodes explained—in a general way—that painters were at risk from inhaling lead dust while painting.

Then committee members questioned Rhodes on whether lead paint was dangerous to occupants once dried on the wall:

> MR. SIMS: For instance, suppose those doors are painted with white lead; does it become dangerous for us to occupy this room?
>
> MR. RHODES: Dr. Thomas Oliver, of London, an eminent scientist says it does.
>
> MR. SIMS: What do you say about it?
>
> MR. RHODES: I say it does, but perhaps not to any appreciable extent. It is not to that source that we are looking for the greatest danger. It is in the manufacturing of the article, and . . . in the use of other poisonous pigments.[58]

At several points Rhodes reassured fellow committee members: "In order that I may not be misunderstood, I desire to say this bill does not seek to prohibit the use of white lead in this country."[59] The congressional committee saw little need for a warning label and remained unconvinced about the dangers of lead poisoning from fumes coming from painted walls and ceilings. It rejected Marion Rhodes's bill.[60]

Rhodes was not correct in his statement that Oliver believed a person was in danger of becoming lead-poisoned simply by living in a room that had once been painted with lead paint. Like Gardner and Hamilton, Oliver believed that painters or inhabitants might suffer from fumes given off while the paint was drying. Oliver addressed this topic at length in *Lead Poisoning: From the Industrial, Medical, and Social Points of View* (1914). He reviewed the scientific evidence, adding his experience, and concluded that the symptoms suffered by inhabitants of newly painted rooms resulted from solvents such as benzene and turpentine, not lead. Of course, he would not have expressed any concern for the door in the congressional hearing room, with its paint long dried.[61]

Hamilton's Assessment of Industry Responsiveness

Another reason Alice Hamilton did not seek to ban lead paint from interiors was her conviction that the lead industry was responsive to her pleas for work safety. Even though she was appalled by the lack of precautions she encountered when she first entered the lead industry, she was equally struck by the openness of some industrial leaders to reform. In her speech to the superintendents of the National Lead Company, Hamilton praised the reform-minded spirit of National Lead and its officer, Edward Cornish: "I do not know when I have been more gratified by anything than by the information I received from Mr. Cornish that the National Lead Company intends to have medical inspection in all its plants."[62] In Cornish's response to Hamilton's reform program, it is possible to see why she held the National Lead leader in such high regard:

> Not a single suggestion that would work to the improvement of the
> sanitary conditions of any of our plants has ever been turned down by
> the Board of Directors, when presented in an intelligent manner that
> carried conviction that it was a real improvement. [Cornish then de-
> tailed several dust reduction measures.] We now have physicians in all of
> our plants, and we are feeling our way along toward the compulsory
> examination of all of the men. . . . I know that there can be no sugges-
> tion that you make that will not be considered. There is no suggestion
> that you can make that will not be followed unless we can persuade you
> that perhaps it is not a good one. Differing from many physicians, I have
> always found Dr. Hamilton willing to look at a thing from the practical
> as well as the theoretical side. I assure you, Doctor, that we appreciate
> very much your assistance, and we are trying to profit by it to the utter-
> most.[63]

Hamilton did not find avid listeners among the management of all lead companies, but her experiences with industry leaders convinced her that most acted
responsibly when confronted by the facts. She did not simply take the word of
those at the top; she returned to factories to witness the improvements firsthand. In *Exploring the Dangerous Trades*, she detailed one remarkable transformation, concluding:

> This was one of the many experiences which convinced me that the
> iniquitous conditions I so often found were not a proof of deliberate
> greed or even of actual indifference, but rather of ignorance and an
> indolent acceptance of things as they are. An alert and trained factory
> inspection service would have had little difficulty in righting these
> matters, for the employers were mostly very well-meaning, but through-
> out those early years I cannot remember ever seeing a single inspector or
> even hearing about one.[64]

Hamilton found instances, of course, of dusty workplaces and unsympathetic
managers. Even in these cases, she elected to continue her strategy of inspection, quiet confrontation, and specific suggestions of reform. Unlike some ac-
tivists of the Progressive Era, Hamilton chose not to become a muckraker: "That
was the era of the muckraking article. *McClure's Magazine* was in full activity,
and as I went back to my hotel I was strongly tempted to write an article [de-
scribing a particularly unhealthy situation]. But on soberer reflection I gave it
up. The result would be only a temporary flurry, no lasting reform, and it would

make any further work on my part impossible. A muckraking writer would not be permitted to visit other plants."[65] Hamilton was a pragmatic reformer.[66]

Hamilton reached her opinion on the openness of industrial leaders to reform on the basis of her appraisal of progress, which—she always reminded her readers—was occurring at a very quick clip. Her Illinois report not only convinced manufacturers to begin making changes but also led to the passage of a statute regulating the industry.[67] By 1914 Hamilton could see that company physicians were recognizing earlier the signs and symptoms of industrial plumbism and that the cases were becoming milder.[68] She praised the white lead industry for quick strides: "The white lead industry in the United States is more dangerous than in England or Germany, because we use dry methods where they use wet, and therefore have a more serious dust problem. Owing partly to the evident risks, this industry has of late undergone great reforms, and in the majority of our plants there is a constant and intelligent effort to protect the men. The same thing is true of all but a few of the red lead factories."[69] After the war, Hamilton again cited continuing progress: "It seldom happens nowadays that very acute or severe forms of lead poisoning are caused by exposure to lead during work. Some years ago men did at times develop severe symptoms of colic and even convulsions after only a few weeks' exposure to lead dust in the smelters or white-lead works, or in storage-battery plants, or in enameling sanitary ware. But improvements in factory hygiene that have been made of late years have caused such distressing occurrences to become almost a thing of the past."[70]

When Alice Hamilton delivered the Cutter Lectures at Harvard in 1919, she described the progress the lead industry was making: "Since 1910, when this industry was investigated, very far-reaching improvements have been made, especially in the white-lead branch."[71] In 1925 she repeated this observation in her textbook: "The white lead industry has undergone enormous improvement during the past ten years, not only with regard to construction and operation but also with regard to the personal care of the men."[72] The following year she amplified this assessment in the pioneering monograph authored by her colleagues in Joseph Aub's laboratory: "This industry has undergone very radical improvement in the last ten years and almost all white lead works are now equipped with excellent mechanical devices to prevent dust, with ample washing facilities, a clean lunch room and washable working clothes, provided and laundered by the management."[73] When Hamilton last surveyed the painting industry in 1936, she once again remarked on the exceptional changes she had witnessed in improved safety: "The changes in the last 20 years have affected both materials and methods of work. Changes in materials have resulted in the displacement of lead pigments in house painting to a certain extent, especially interior decoration."[74]

Other industrial hygienists shared her assessment of continuing progress in the health of lead workers. Frederick Hoffman, comparing statistics between the United States and European nations, concluded in 1933: "The foregoing international data reflect the conclusion that lead poisoning in this country is at the present time comparatively unimportant as a labor problem demanding, of course, eternal vigilance on the part of employers who are fully aware of the risk and its penalties under governmental compensation." Several pages later, Hoffman summarized: "A detailed analysis of the American experience, 1914–1933, reveals evidence that many occupations formerly subject to an excessive death rate from lead poisoning are now comparatively free therefrom. This is particularly true of painters, potters, rubber workers, glass workers, printers, and lead workers generally."[75] Industrial health worries for lead-paint safety in the United States thus focused entirely on the painter and not on the inhabitants living within painted homes.

Part II

Gnawing Toddlers

Chapter 5

Children and the Lead Industries Association, 1925–1935

W ITH NO EXAMPLE that completely fit babies lead-poisoned in their homes, U.S. pediatricians fashioned a new understanding suitable to the American scene. Between 1914 and 1923, Henry Thomas, Kenneth Blackfan, and L. Emmett Holt, Jr., added another five children to the country's experience with domestic lead poisoning.[1] The sources of lead in these cases were: one crib (Thomas and Blackfan, 1914), two painted articles and furniture (Blackfan, 1917), one nipple cream (Holt, 1923), and one unknown (Blackfan, 1917). In 1920 Robert Strong, a physician at Tulane University School of Medicine, described another crib case, a nineteen-month-old boy ("the child had been seen to bite paint from the rail of the bed").[2] In 1924 John Ruddock, a physician from Los Angeles, contributed two cases in which the children had gnawed paint from cribs and furniture. To these now familiar sources, Ruddock observed that the children also ingested lead by chewing on windowsills and railings: "Case 1. . . . every bit of paint on porch railings, window sills[,] crib, bureau, chairs and even white enameled door casings, as high as the child could reach, had been gnawed off. [C]ase 2. . . . the mother stated that the child gnawed the paint from the crib and the window sills, and had an uncontrollable desire to chew any painted object."[3] In 1925 Isaac Abt, in his textbook *Pediatrics, by Various Authors*, mentioned: "I recall two cases in which children ate the paint from the household furniture."[4]

In sum, there were only eight reported cases of lead poisoning in the United States through 1925 where the source of lead was thought to be paint dried on a crib or an object.[5] In contrast, American child health professionals in the first decades of the twentieth century were swamped with other pressing medical problems. High infant and childhood mortality rates from poor nutrition and infectious diseases were of paramount concern.[6] Pediatricians in the first decades of the century were not indifferent to lesser health problems, but out of necessity they focused on malnutrition, diarrhea, and respiratory illnesses.[7]

Pica

What struck Ruddock about his patients was their voracious compulsion to gnaw on nonfood objects, a behavior that physicians and child psychiatrists called *pica*. Ruddock was astonished that these children chewed "every bit of paint on porch railings, window sills, crib, bureau, chairs, and even white enameled door casings, as high as the child could reach." Ruddock's identification of pica was the first articulation of a cardinal pillar in medical thinking about domestic childhood lead poisoning that persisted for over half a century.

Ruddock explained to his readers that pediatricians had a variety of opinions about why some children aggressively sought out nonfood objects to chew. Some had wasting from serious illnesses or nutritional deficiencies, such as rickets or anemia, and the search for odd foods might be interpreted as a quest to balance the diet. Most, however, were not obviously sick from any disease. Ruddock insisted that children with pica differed from normal children:

> [In the opinion of John Thomson] the morbid craving develops in early
> infancy, as opportunity for its indulgence offers, apart from any very
> noticeable cachexia, and without anemia, passing off gradually in most
> cases, even if untreated, when the child is about 3 years old. [Two para-
> graphs later Ruddock discussed the views of Henry Koplik.] Koplik be-
> lieves that this peculiar condition in children is an exaggeration of the
> normal habit in young infants of invariably placing everything within
> reach in their mouths.[8]

This "morbid craving" got these children into trouble when the objects they chewed were covered in lead paint.

Ruddock's discussion mirrored the views of major pediatric texts. For example, Holt—who would later write on childhood lead poisoning—included a paragraph on pica for the first time in the sixth edition of his *Diseases of Infancy and Childhood* (1912): "Pica or perverted appetite is an inordinate desire to eat various substances, such as dirt, sand, mortar, or coal. It is most frequently seen in infants but may occur in older children. This habit is met with in those who are mentally defective, but not rarely in other children. These patients are usually highly neurotic and exhibit some of the other habits common to this class."[9] Another prominent pediatric text explained: "The normal infant soon learns by trial that only certain articles he picks up are good to eat. The child with pica, on the other hand, seems unable to acquire this knowledge, and even develops an unnatural craving for inedible articles, such as sand, wool from blankets, hair from his head, coal, ashes, plaster from the wall, etc."[10]

By far the longest discussion occurred in Abt's multivolume text, *Pediatrics* (1925). In the section on etiology Abt outlined a variety of reasons given for "unnatural appetite": debilitating health from a number of diseases, "nervous temperament," and mental deficiency. The text concluded that "despite these various views as to the cause of pica, nothing is definitely known as to the exact etiology."[11] For treatment, all three textbooks and Ruddock's article recommended that parents closely supervise children with pica and remove the objects of their craving from their reach.

It is important here to step ahead of our story to understand the significance of Ruddock's observation for the history of childhood lead poisoning. In 1924, or for that matter in 1970, lead poisoning was understood as a cluster of easily visible symptoms that included seizures, coma, and severe abdominal pain. In order to ingest sufficient lead to provoke these complaints, a child had to consume considerable lead. Only those children with pica were likely to persist in chewing cribs, toys, or woodwork to swallow enough lead. Pediatricians understood that pica differed from the normal tendency for toddlers to put things into their mouths. Normal "mouthing" behavior may have permitted many infants to consume small bits of lead, but almost certainly mouthing did not allow sufficient lead in the toddler's system to provoke visible symptoms. Fifty years after Ruddock, when "lead poisoning" was defined as an "invisible" disease measurable by psychological tests and biochemical analyses, pediatricians understood that tiny amounts of lead were harmful. In this heightened environment, normal mouthing of all infants became a worry.

In 1925, the outlines of what became—over the next decade—the American ecology of childhood lead-paint poisoning were present: toddlers with morbid appetites (pica), chewing paint inside the home from objects, furniture, cribs, and in two instances porch railings and windowsills, in northern cities.(See figure 5.)

America's First Epidemics

The mid-1920s witnessed the first American reports of lead poisoning that included more than just a few sporadic cases. Compared with the major health issues, such as pneumonia or tuberculosis, lead poisoning was still quite minor, but there was a growing concern that it was a greater worry than pediatricians had previously thought.

One issue was clear: lead poisoning produced life-threatening illness. As Thomas, Blackfan, Holt, and others had perceived earlier, lead poisoning could result in encephalopathy. This was what worried pediatricians.

A second issue was also clear: the location in the home where the child encountered the lead was important. The historian has to be careful in making

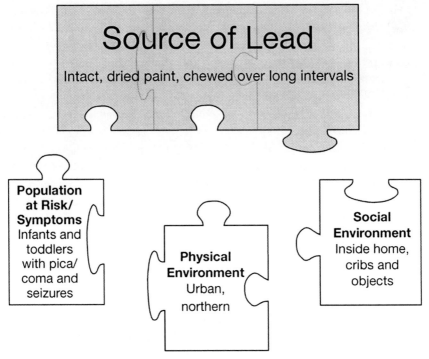

Figure 5. American Childhood Lead Poisoning, 1925

this assessment. Most studies contained lists of potential sources of lead that had been reported in various articles reaching back well into the nineteenth century. These lists were not meant to suggest that the author had actually seen cases in which an infant had become poisoned from sucking on a lead nipple shield or from licking his mother's make-up. Rather, these inventories indicated that the author was aware of what had come before him and the wide variety of potential sources.

To ascertain the perceived lead hazard requires an examination of the specific case histories. This is somewhat frustrating, because authors often included only a few specific cases in their published accounts. Nevertheless, it is essential to look closely at these in order to get a sense of the problem until 1940. By far the greatest concern was for objects and furniture within the grasp of infants or toddlers. The usually identified culprits were cribs and toys. As we shall see, when health departments in Boston and Baltimore raised the initial alarm regarding lead paint, they counseled parents about chewing paint from cribs and toys. Pediatricians were also aware that some children gnawed lead from windowsills, porch railings, or woodwork. As such, these locations were often listed as potential sources of lead. But case histories reveal only a few woodwork cases before 1940. There was only one report—an autopsy summary—that attributed a child's lead poisoning to flakes of lead paint crumbled off a wall.[12] As individual case histories revealed, the source of lead was normally *repainted* cribs, furniture, and toys. This led to public health efforts to alert parents to the danger of repainting furniture with unsuitable paints.

A third point of consensus was that a child had to "chew," "gnaw," or "nibble" the painted object for a long time. Observers stated that children chewed objects for months, even years. Virtually all studies confirmed Ruddock's observation that children at risk were ones who had aggressive eating behaviors, or pica. Cribs and toys were the constant environment of children; it was not mystifying why these were the major sources of lead.

A fourth point of agreement was that lead poisoning was a most visible illness. Although the condition shared symptoms with other diseases, any observer could see a child with seizures or coma. Peripheral neuropathy, abdominal pain, and anemia were less serious, but also very easily perceived problems. Before World War II, there were no concerns about subtle injuries, imperceptible to observers without sophisticated psychological tests, which would fill the medical literature a half century later. In this sense, pediatricians looked upon lead ingestion without symptoms similarly to the way they looked upon an infection that did not produce disease.

A fifth area of consensus was the children at risk. Every report identified toddlers, roughly one to three years of age. Only a few cases occurred in babies, fewer still in kindergarten children.

A sixth point is discernible from our vantage point, but was not clearly articulated until almost 1950: most of the children came from poorer neighborhoods. Before World War II, physicians only hinted that these children lived in "unsupervised" circumstances, where toddlers might chew paint and go largely unnoticed. The implication was that parents were off working.

Boston Cases

In 1926 Charles F. McKhann, a pediatrician at Boston's Infants' and Children's Hospitals, published the details of three children with lead poisoning but stated that seventeen cases had been diagnosed and treated over a three-year period. McKhann, closely following Ruddock's formulation, explained:

> The disease is usually secondary to a perverted appetite. In this condition, which is known as pica (Ruddock, 1924), infants and children may ingest sand, coal, cloth, hair and paint, the last chewed from toys, cribs and woodwork. The derangement of appetite may be only a habit, or it may result from gastro-intestinal disturbances, intestinal parasites, mental deficiency or neurosis. In any event, pica, in our experience, is the

most frequent forerunner of lead poisoning, as it is of relatively common occurrence and may result in the repeated ingestion of small amounts of lead. Weeks may elapse before symptoms arise, and the perversion of appetite is passed over lightly or not mentioned by the parents who have become accustomed to the strange habits of the child.[13]

McKhann turned to Joseph Aub's research for treating his patients. Aub had shown that calcium enhanced the body's normal capacity to eliminate lead from the system. With this insight, McKhann placed his patients on a diet rich in calcium.

From reading McKhann's account alone, it is not possible to identify with precision the source of paint in each of these seventeen cases. In the three cases that McKhann detailed, one girl "was eating the paint from the crib"; a boy "had gnawed at the crib and furniture"; another boy "for one year . . . had been biting the window sills and bars of his crib." The following year, the *Monthly Bulletin* of Boston's Health Department reported the fatal cases:

> For this year there has been reported to this department on death certificates four deaths of children from lead poisoning, all such causes of death having been certified by the medical examiner. These deaths were due to a childhood habit of sucking paint from cribs with the consequent ingestion of lead and subsequent lead poisoning and death. It would thus be well for mothers and others entrusted with the care of children in cribs to watch for this common habit in early child life and to take steps to correct it wherever it is found. [two paragraphs later] Here is one cause of death in early childhood that can positively be prevented if we watch the habits of the child with its crib, high chair, or other painted article which comes within its reach.[14]

From the point of view of Boston's Health Department in 1927, the major risks to children were painted cribs, other furniture, and objects. This warning to parents to beware childhood pica was the first published public health alert about lead paint in the United States.

In 1926 L. Emmett Holt (Babies' Hospital of New York City) and John Howland (Johns Hopkins, Baltimore) included a short paragraph on lead poisoning in the ninth edition of their standard pediatric textbook: "An infrequent cause of convulsions in young children is an encephalopathy due to lead poisoning. We have seen thirty or more such cases. The condition is a serious and often fatal one. The poisoning was usually caused by the child's nibbling and swallowing the paint from his crib or furniture."[15]

A third report in 1926 from L. W. Holloway, a physician from Jacksonville, Florida, described eight cases. The source of lead in these cases also was not entirely clear. In the introductory paragraphs, Holloway summarized Ruddock's view of the importance of pica and provided a list of potential sources of household lead. In the section of the paper dealing with his patients, Holloway stated: "The exposure to painted objects ranged from four months to sixteen months."[16] In two of the children there had been an additional acute exposure to lead while their homes were scraped, sanded, and painted.

Bureau of Labor Statistics, 1927

In 1927 the U.S. Bureau of Labor Statistics published a monograph written by Frederick Hoffman, "Deaths from Lead Poisoning." As would be expected, virtually the entire volume dealt with industrial lead exposures. For the years spanning 1914 to 1924, Hoffman included reports of nineteen deaths in children under eighteen years of age that had been collected by the Division of Vital Statistics of the Bureau of the Census. He listed the source of lead in nine children: "ointment," "eating paint," "eating paint off toys," "eating paint and enamel off toys," "playing in a paint shop," "chewing lead foil," "gnawed lead paint from the side of bed," "eating paint from window sill and paint can," "eating enamel off bed," and "face powder."[17]

By 1930 McKhann had seen fifty cases. The public first learned of these thirty-three additional children in the August 1930 number of the *Statistical Bulletin*, published by the Metropolitan Life Insurance Company. The article was based on a survey sent to pediatricians asking about childhood lead poisoning. The statistician, Louis I. Dublin, received thirty-three replies. Of those who replied, McKhann had the most experience. Dublin warned, "Lead poison is a real source of danger to infants and young children, and education of parents concerning this hazard would be a definite, forward step in public health education."[18] From the results of this survey, he concluded: "All believed that wide publicity should be given to this fact through the press or the 'popular' literature of health departments and private health agencies, with special insistence upon the dangers inherent in cribs and toys painted with material which contains lead."[19]

Lead Industries Association's Response

Albert Russell, an assistant surgeon of the U.S. Public Health Service, responded to Dublin's challenge on November 19, 1930, and issued a statement on childhood lead poisoning that served as the background to a front-page story in the *United States Daily* the following day, under the headline "Lead-free Paint on Furniture and Toys to Protect Children":

> Lead poisoning as a result of chewing paint from toys, cradles, and woodwork is now regarded as a more frequent occurrence among

children than formerly. . . . [two paragraphs later] The most common
sources of lead poisoning in children are paint on various objects within
the reach of a child and lead pipes which are used to convey drinking
water. Various manufacturing companies, however, are now beginning to
make paints for indoor purposes which are lead-free and lead is being replaced in pipes by other metals.[20]

The next day Felix Wormser, secretary of the Lead Industries Association, wrote
to R. R. Sayers, chief surgeon of the Bureau of Mines, the federal government's
agency overseeing lead.

The Lead Industries Association (LIA) was a trade association formed in
1928 to promote the lead industry and lead products of all kinds, including lead
pigments. Most of the activities of the LIA dealt with industrial concerns and
marketing. Soon, however, reports of children poisoned from gnawing lead paint
forced themselves upon this organization. The LIA was not a public health
agency and certainly not knowledgeable about issues of children's health. Nevertheless, LIA officials reacted swiftly to the reports from Boston. In his letter
to Sayers, Wormser inquired: "As we are naturally deeply interested in all au-
thentic cases of lead poisoning we should very much like to know of any records
which the Public Health Service Department might have of children who have
been poisoned by chewing upon cribs, cradles, toys, etc. We are inclined to doubt
the accuracy of this statement through previous experience in following down
similar publicity adverse to lead."[21] Sayers telephoned Albert Russell and asked
for published papers supporting the statement that had served as the basis for
the United States Daily article. On November 26, Russell responded to Sayers,
summarizing several papers: Blackfan (1917), McKhann (1926), Ruddock (1924),
and Holt (1923). He mentioned, without specific journal citation, one of the
Queensland papers and Asian cosmetic cases.[22] Three days later, Sayers forwarded
Russell's information on to Wormser.[23]

Wormser, who initially had been skeptical of the validity of the article in
the United States Daily, now took both the article and Russell's message to heart.
The following day—November 30, 1930—Wormser and the Lead Industries Association sent out a survey to children's furniture manufacturers and toy companies inquiring whether they were using lead-free paints as the newspaper article
had suggested. The results of the survey indicated that most toy and children's
furniture manufacturers had stopped or planned to stop using lead-based paints.[24]

The only record of the survey occurs in a publication of the Prudential Insurance Company that Frederick Hoffman compiled in 1933. Hoffman included
the text of the survey and its results in the section of his monograph immediately following his brief enumeration of deaths from lead poisoning in boys and
girls under the age of eighteen years. Many of these children were infants and
toddlers who had chewed paint from cribs and furniture. Hoffman included the

text of the LIA's request: "We are conducting an investigation to ascertain if any lead paint is being used to paint or decorate cribs, children's beds or furniture. Will you, therefore, kindly let us know if it is your practice to use any white lead in painting this type of furniture."[25] Hoffman also included twelve "bottom-line" replies from manufacturers. There is no text of the responses, identification of the companies polled, or the proportion of those polled who responded. Ten manufacturers stated that they did not use lead-based paint on cribs or other children's furniture. One company said that it used "very little of this lead paint," and one manufacturer referred the LIA to the Glidden Company. What Hoffman's account demonstrated was that the LIA identified a potential health risk, investigated the concern, and disseminated the results both to investigators in the field and to its membership.

When the LIA investigated the *United States Daily* story and conducted its survey, there were several dozen published cases on childhood lead poisoning in the American medical literature. Only a very few children were known to have acquired lead from sources other than cribs, toys, furniture, or objects within reach of an infant (Ruddock, 1924, two cases; McKhann, 1926, one case). All three had also chewed paint from cribs. It was possible that some of the fourteen cases for which McKhann failed to specify a source might have gnawed paint from other sources, but the summaries published by the Boston Health Department and the Metropolitan Life Insurance Company indicated that both believed that cribs, furniture, toys, and objects were the primary problems for children. The Metropolitan Life Insurance Company's unpublished survey indicated that McKhann had treated another thirty-three children. When the Metropolitan Life Insurance Company issued its plea for public health education, it called for "insistence upon the dangers inherent in cribs and toys painted with material which contains lead."[26] In 1930 the White House Conference on Child Health alerted participants only about lead paint on toys.[27] The public health authorities in Boston, a prominent insurance company, and officials in the U.S. Public Health Service all shared the view in the fall of 1930 that cribs and toys painted with lead paint were the primary hazards to children.

Research and the Lead Industries Association

Nearly two years before the *United States Daily* story and the survey of manufacturers, the LIA voted to continue funding research on lead physiology at Harvard. At least once each year until 1959, the board of directors heard a report on the research, entertained requests for additional funds, and granted them. In 1932 the LIA discussed the merits of employing its own scientists directly, but, after discussion, Wormser persuaded the board that research carried out by independent university scientists would be cheaper and more "detached."[28] Some members of Wormser's board needed to be coaxed into supporting research. Wormser's argument to them was that the more the public knew about lead, the less the public would fear paint.[29]

Between 1929 and 1944 the LIA supported Joseph Aub's laboratory, including Lawrence Fairhall's research before he left for the U.S. Public Health Service in 1938. Beginning in 1944, the LIA funded Randolph Byers's work at Boston Children's Hospital, and in 1949 the LIA supported research by the Baltimore Health Department, the Johns Hopkins School of Hygiene, and J. Julian Chisholm (also of Johns Hopkins). Aub's findings were pivotal to the understanding of lead in living systems from the 1920s; Byers's work was crucial to the understanding of childhood lead poisoning in the 1940s and 1950s; Chisholm's research would provide the core of understanding from the mid-1950s to the 1990s. All LIA-funded research was published in major scientific and medical journals. There is no evidence that the LIA exerted any restrictive editorial control.[30]

Wormser's network included more than industry leaders and researchers. He also met with pediatricians to learn of their concerns. For example, he traveled to Boston in September 1931 to discuss the babies that McKhann and others were treating,[31] and to Baltimore in 1938 to learn firsthand of the efforts of the Baltimore Health Department.[32] Wormser kept industrial physicians informed of the latest research, and in 1937 he organized a conference that included Aub and Fairhall as speakers.

Aftermath of the LIA Survey

The LIA was not alone in its assessment that manufacturers had removed lead-based paint from cribs, toys, and other children's furniture.[33] In 1935 the U.S. Children's Bureau conducted its own survey. Ella Oppenheimer wrote to Anchor Toy Company (Glidden responded), Newark Varnish Works, Halsam Products, Embossing Company, Sherwin-Williams, A. Schoenhut Company, and Toy Tinkers. The responses detailed how each company was avoiding the use of lead paints.[34] In 1936 the Consumer's Union also sampled the paint on toys sold at Kress, Kresge, and Woolworth's stores. They found none painted with lead-based paints.[35] Three years earlier, H. B. Cushing, a pediatrician at Montreal's Children's Memorial Hospital, told his audience at a meeting of the American College of Physicians about his survey of infants' furniture and toys: "It was easily shown that the enamel used on all the better cots showed practically no lead but some of the cheaper ones, and especially those repainted at home, contained large quantities. Most toys, especially those enamelled, showed no lead, but the cheaper wooden ones, especially if painted yellow or green, had very large amounts of lead."[36]

The medical literature also reflected the elimination of lead paint from toys, cribs, and other children's furniture. In 1933 Boston's Charles McKhann and Edward Vogt stated: "The lead industry and the manufacturers of cribs and toys, informed of the danger to small children from the ingestion of lead paint, have cooperated by substituting other types of pigments for the lead pigments formerly used. New cribs are seldom painted with lead paint, and the better grades of toys are largely free from lead pigment."[37] Similar comments came from the physicians John S. Crutcher, C. M. Jephcott, Randolph Byers, and Elizabeth Lord.[38] Physicians from Baltimore, the city with the most experience with childhood lead poisoning, were emphatic: "We know that the brand new cribs coming from the manufacturers do not contain lead at all. They are perfectly safe to use. We have never had a case of lead poisoning in a crib from the original paint. What happens is that the paint wears off, and it is in the re-painting that danger occurs."[39]

Unpublished correspondence of leaders in the field also reflected the view that cribs and toys were the major risks to children. In 1937 Robert Kehoe wrote to Frederick Hoffman: "My experience, and that of my colleagues at Harvard, leads me to believe that most cases of lead poisoning in infants and children come from chewing objects coated with metallic lead and lead pigments. I am not quite sure, but I believe that every case, except one, in our list of children has had such a causative factor."[40] The following year Kehoe expressed similar sentiments to A. J. Lanza of the Metropolitan Life Insurance Company: "In the course of the past several years I have seen several fatal cases of lead poisoning in children as the result of ingesting lead from toys, play pens, and in one instance from contaminated food."[41]

Paint manufacturers advised consumers of the availability of lead-free paints for children's toys and cribs. For example, in 1937 Henry Gardner wrote to Dr. John M. McDonald of Baltimore's Health Department about the safety of several paints that home owners could use when repainting.[42]

Activities of the Lead Industries Association

The Lead Industries Association was not a disinterested bystander either in the growing appreciation of the lead-paint household hazard or in its hope that research would lessen the role of its products. Press accounts were bad publicity. Minutes of LIA board meetings indicated that Wormser personally investigated cases, writing to physicians or hospitals to verify details. Wormser, who was not a physician, occasionally passed these reports to Aub or Kehoe for opinions whether a particular case represented lead poisoning or some other disease. From these investigations, Wormser believed that some reports were false, and he informed his board of these misdiagnoses.

A reading of two of Aub's letters to Felix Wormser reflects the nature of this relationship. In the case of a child, D.M., Aub thought the child's fever and high white blood cell count indicated infection. Significantly, Aub also concluded: "The bones and paralysis fit in with a possible diagnosis of lead poisoning."[43] In the case of an adult worker, A.G., Aub correctly interpreted the autopsy findings that stated that the man died of a ruptured appendix and peritonitis, tuberculosis, and congenital heart disease. But Aub also told Wormser that the amount of lead in the worker's liver was "too high to ignore."[44] In both cases, lead poisoning coexisted with diseases that killed the patients. Aub was providing Wormser with a sound medical interpretation.

In similar cases, Wormser characterized his activities as "defend[ing] against unjust attacks" or correcting "undeserved publicity."[45] Wormser in addition believed that the lead industry deserved more credit than it received in alerting public health departments to the dangers of burning battery casings.[46] He also thought that the LIA's funding of Harvard's research was the responsible means of objectively evaluating the nature of the risk. Wormser accepted that childhood lead poisoning was an often exasperating but nonetheless legitimate concern that the organization needed to take seriously: "If all other reasons for the establishment of a cooperative organization in the lead industries were to disappear, the health problem alone would be sufficient warrant for its establishment."[47]

Wormser's skepticism played an important role in the history of childhood lead poisoning in the United States. As we shall see, by insisting that every diagnosis be proved by prevailing medical standards, Wormser pushed researchers to become more exacting in their studies. This prodding eventually contributed to the discovery of the hazard from peeling and flaking paint.

In the aftermath of the Boston childhood poisonings, there are indications that the LIA worked with the state of Massachusetts in educating painters about the risk of repainting toys and cribs with lead paint. In the LIA minutes of June 6, 1934, Wormser reported:

> During the year an effort was made by the Massachusetts Department of Labor to establish regulations which would have seriously affected the use of white lead in painting buildings. This subject was discussed by the Secretary [Wormser] with the State Official [Manfred Bowditch] having the matter in hand and a satisfactory adjustment procured. It was particularly important to obtain a hearing and settlement in Massachusetts; otherwise we might have been plagued with an extension of similar restrictive painting legislation in other states, affecting the use of white lead.[48]

There is no record of the proposed legislation, the "satisfactory adjustment," or the "settlement." What is known is that the next issue of the "Revised Rules, Regulations and Recommendations Pertaining to Structural Painting" (1933) for Massachusetts included a boxed statement that had not appeared in previous editions. The box—which was separate from the sections on rules, regulations, or recommendations—contained the sentences: "Many serious and even fatal cases of lead poisoning among infants have been traced to the sucking or chewing of lead-painted surfaces. Toys, cribs, furniture and other objects with which infants may come in contact should not be painted with lead colors."[49] This statement, of course, reflected the views of pediatricians and public health officials.

The minutes of the LIA further indicate that Wormser assisted Bowditch in curtailing manufacturers from using lead-based paints on toys. In 1935 Bowditch asked Wormser to put pressure on a toy manufacturer who continued to decorate with lead-based paints. The minutes indicated that the LIA's board authorized Wormser "to assist Mr. Bowditch in discouraging the use of white lead, or any lead paint in painting children's toys and furniture."[50]

Chapter 6

Baltimore, Boston, and Robert Kehoe, 1930–1940

B ETWEEN 1930 AND 1940, two American cities—Baltimore and Boston—reported significant numbers of cases of childhood lead-paint poisoning. Pediatricians from other cities continued to report sporadic cases of lead poisoning from
sources other than lead paint: burning battery casings[1] and nipple shields.[2] Some
pediatricians reported cases primarily to discuss X-ray findings,[3] autopsy findings,[4] or seasonal incidence.[5]

In the 1930s, lead-based paints emerged more prominently. Holt and Rustin
McIntosh provided pediatricians with the now common lengthy list of potential sources in the eleventh edition of *Holt's Diseases of Infancy and Childhood*
(1940), but they concluded: "The most common source of the metal in children is from gnawing lead paint from toys, furniture, railings, or sills."[6]

The 1930s witnessed three advances in the diagnosis of childhood lead poisoning: bone X-rays, quantitative urine tests, and quantitative blood tests. Of
these, bone X-rays had the greatest influence in the decade. Until then, the diagnosis of lead poisoning had been based almost entirely on clinical signs and
symptoms. Because every symptom of lead poisoning—encephalopathy, anemia,
colic, peripheral neuropathy—could be caused by other diseases, the diagnosis
of lead poisoning had proved difficult for industrial physicians. It was even more
exacting for pediatricians, simply because toddlers could not volunteer information about lead exposure. Often the first sign of lead poisoning was encephalopathy, an event that almost never occurred in factories in the 1930s because
workers would complain of less serious symptoms first. X-rays provided a means
of confirming lead exposure. It is in discussions of X-rays that we find published
cases of lead poisoning in this period.

In 1930 Edward Vogt, a radiologist at Infants' and Children's Hospitals in

74

Boston—where Charles McKhann also practiced—described dense lines on the bone X-rays of eight lead-poisoned children. These lines occurred in the growth plates of bones and could, therefore, be seen only in growing children. Vogt mentioned that the X-ray findings in children with rickets were nearly identical.[7] In 1931 John Caffey (Babies' Hospital in New York City), who would become one of the nation's leading pediatric radiologists, added detailed discussions of three cases and the first studies in animals.[8] Also in 1931, Edwards A. Park, chairman of the department of pediatrics at Johns Hopkins, described the X-rays of three lead-poisoned children.[9] Over the next several years, physicians in Boston and Baltimore made use of this new diagnostic aid.

Boston Cases in the 1930s

McKhann and Vogt collaborated on childhood lead poisoning.[10] When they summarized their findings in the early 1930s, they claimed they had seen thirty-two children with lead poisoning since 1929. These most probably represent the unpublished cases mentioned in the Metropolitan Life Insurance Company's *Statistical Bulletin* (August 1930). In their 1930s papers, McKhann and Vogt provided lists of potential sources for domestic lead poisoning that included nipple shields, water, and face powder, ending with the comment: "The most common cause of the ingestion of lead appears to be the habit of small children of chewing paint from toys, cribs or woodwork of the house [citing Ruddock]."[11] In their published accounts, however, McKhann and Vogt gave only two specific case histories: one child who sucked on a nipple shield[12] and one child who for four and a half months "had been chewing paint from the woodwork and furniture of the house."[13] In 1934 Vogt and McKhann published their final article on childhood lead poisoning. By then they had treated ninety-five children over nine years, nineteen in the previous year. In other words, this last article included forty-six cases that they had not published earlier. Once again they did not detail the sources of lead for each case, only mentioning nipple shields and ointments, water and food, insecticides, and battery cases. As in previous studies, Vogt and McKhann concluded: "Lead poisoning in children is due usually to the ingestion of lead paint, chewed by the child from the toys, crib, or woodwork of the house."[14]

Robert Kehoe and the Kettering Laboratory of Applied Physiology

From 1930 to the mid-1960s, Robert Kehoe was the acknowledged American authority on the medical consequences of industrial lead exposure.[15] Like Joseph Aub before him, Kehoe focused his research on industrial lead poisoning.

Nevertheless Kehoe's ideas, resting solidly on Aub's foundation, informed pediatricians about toddlers poisoned at home.

After the initial funding for the Harvard research from the National Lead Institute ended, the newly organized Lead Industries Association continued to fund the work of Joseph Aub and Lawrence Fairhall. Fairhall eventually moved to the U.S. Public Health Service in 1938, and Aub shifted his research energies to cancer and other health problems, but LIA funding to Harvard persisted until the end of the 1950s. Aub[16] and Fairhall[17] published articles on lead poisoning, and both advised leaders in the lead industry. Despite his continuing interest in lead poisoning, Aub ceded to Kehoe his central position in the history of lead poisoning in the United States. Although they did not collaborate and were in fact somewhat jealous rivals, Kehoe nevertheless built upon Aub's experimental base.[18]

Kehoe's approach to lead research differed from that of Aub. Reflecting a trend toward applied research, Kehoe more directly studied problems that confronted lead workers. As such, most of his research was conducted on humans, usually lead workers themselves. In contrast, Aub's work had been in the tradition of basic research, focused on the metabolism of lead in the living organism from ingestion to excretion. Aub conducted his research on animals. He did not normally address patient issues, except for the development of calcium therapy, which remained only one of two approaches to therapy (Kehoe developed the other) available to physicians until the late 1940s.

The Kettering Laboratory for Applied Physiology in Cincannati, where Kehoe conducted his studies, joined Harvard as the only other laboratory in the country with a sustained research program on lead. Most of Kehoe's research dealt with adults in the industrial setting, but he also investigated lead exposures of everyday citizens. In this effort, he occasionally studied infants. Kehoe also kept abreast of childhood lead poisoning, and from time to time he expressed opinions on the particular lead risks that infants faced in their homes.

The Kettering Laboratory was funded by the Ethyl Corporation.[19] This association with industry raises questions about whether Kehoe's research findings were biased, withheld from publication, or even doctored to support industry positions. To provide academic integrity, the laboratory was insulated within the walls of the University of Cincinnati. Still, some historians have argued that the dominating and authoritative nature of Kehoe's relatively well funded research may have prevented or delayed other researchers from studying lead health risks.[20] Other scholars have viewed Kehoe more favorably. Christopher Sellers has interpreted Kehoe's research as pivotal both to the development of industrial medicine in the United States and to a wider concern in the nation about the dangers of toxic chemicals in the environment.[21] Christian Warren has argued that Kehoe bucked LIA secretary Felix Wormser's dismissal of reports about childhood lead poisoning at a key point in the 1940s.[22]

Kehoe's scholarly output was considerable. He published often and in major medical journals, including *Journal of Medicine, Journal of the American Medical Association, American Journal of Clinical Pathology, Surgery, Gynecology, and Obstetrics, Journal of Industrial Hygiene, Medical Clinics of North America,* and *American Journal of Diseases of Children.* His unpublished papers are also extensive. He was cited constantly for decades by everyone in the field. Even critics in the 1960s still recognized him as an authority.

Despite his industrial focus, in 1930 Kehoe was one of the first to identify lead-painted cribs and toys as a danger to infants: "In the non-industrial population poisoning is frequently occasioned by the ingestion of lead with drinking water and wines and food, and in the case of children especially, by chewing or sucking toys, furniture, or other objects painted with lead paints. That cases of the latter type occur is sufficient reason for abolishing the use of lead paints on toys, beds, playpens, and furniture commonly used by children."[23] Five years later, Kehoe once again expressed his concern in print: "There is every reason for suspecting the existence of significant and dangerous lead exposure in the case of children with a history of pica. The occurrence of lead-containing commodities and the use of lead paints on furniture, toys, and other objects within the reach of small children is much too common to ignore. The existence of symptoms even slightly suggestive of plumbism should result in prompt investigation of the child and his surroundings."[24]

Although Kehoe addressed workers in the workplace, his understanding of lead in the environment and its role in human disease influenced the way in which pediatricians viewed childhood lead poisoning acquired at home. Kehoe believed, as did every industrial physician before him, that lead poisoning was a disease of stark symptoms: seizures, coma, peripheral neuropathy, abdominal pain, and anemia. Kehoe also shared the commonly held view that a diagnosis of lead poisoning required the presence of one or more of these symptoms. His laboratory developed techniques for the detection of small amounts of lead in the urine and stool,[25] but he strongly believed, in keeping with most careful physicians, that a lab test did not define a disease. Only a patient's symptoms could inform a diagnosis. This view was in keeping with practice in other diseases. For example, the presence of the streptococcus in the throat did not make the diagnosis of rheumatic fever; this designation occurred only if a child developed symptoms of heart disease, chorea, arthritis, rash, or nodules.[26]

Symptoms alone were not sufficient for Kehoe to make a diagnosis with confidence. He required identification of lead in the environment, such as working in a lead factory or chewing a lead-painted toy. And a physician needed to confirm that lead had actually entered the patient's body. Here Kehoe used his urine and stool tests. Exposure, symptoms, objective physical findings, and laboratory confirmation were the hallmarks of Kehoe's careful approach.[27]

Kehoe also investigated lead in the environment. He found evidence of lead in the urine, blood, and stool of every living person: in Mexican peasants living far from industry in homes without lead products;[28] in Cincinnati's healthy men, medical students, and infants; in infants and adults who had died from diseases other than lead poisoning;[29] and in workers in the lead industry.[30] The primary source of the lead in everyday life was food; in fact Kehoe found lead in every type of food he tested.[31]

Despite the presence of lead in every living person, virtually none developed symptoms. This striking observation led Kehoe to conclude that exposure to lead was a benign consequence of modern life. Every study pointed to people's leading normal lives without deleterious effects from the lead encountered in daily living. Lead in everyone's urine and stool meant that everyone, even newborn babies, excreted lead, the body's normal way to eliminate the metal.[32] This, then, became Kehoe's preferred treatment: remove the poisoned worker from the source of lead, either by sending him home to recover or by moving him to another job with less exposure. Charles McKhann, who closely adhered to Aub's high-calcium regimen, disagreed with Kehoe's treatment suggestion for children, and McKhann and Kehoe hashed out differences in an exchange of letters.[33]

Kehoe interpreted his evidence to mean that there was a safe amount of lead that everyone could ingest each day without developing the symptoms of lead poisoning. He measured the dietary intake of citizens who were not lead workers and found that, on average, their daily food contained between 160 and 280 micrograms of lead. The daily diet of rural Mexicans contained nearly as much: 100 micrograms.[34]

Lead workers, of course, were exposed to far greater amounts, and Kehoe set out to determine just how much lead a worker could ingest each day without becoming sick. He gave volunteers up to 2000 micrograms/day for months without provoking clinical signs of lead poisoning. When he measured the blood lead levels in these men, they were in what he interpreted as the normal range of 60–70 micrograms/100 cc whole blood.[35] Kehoe also found that workers in tetraethyl lead plants and gasoline stations did not absorb enough lead from fumes to develop symptoms.[36]

Because Kehoe had collected the best data on lead poisoning in humans, pediatricians wrote to him asking for advice. For example, in 1937 Kenneth Blackfan, who had reported America's initial case in 1914, asked Kehoe's opinion about the range of concentrations of lead in normal blood and cerebral spinal fluid.[37] Industry also sought Kehoe's opinion. Pepsodent asked about lead in squeezable toothpaste tubes;[38] Loew Brothers Company inquired about the danger of fumes;[39] Univis Lens Company asked about the dangers of painters who put brushes into their mouths.[40] Health Department officials from Cincinnati and other cities often sent cases to Kehoe, asking his opinion whether a particular child's death had been caused by lead.

To present-day eyes, Kehoe's argument that lead absorption was not a health problem unless it provoked symptoms seems dated. Today many pediatricians embrace the view that any amount of lead in the human body is excessive. The concept of lead poisoning has changed so radically that it is difficult to imagine that any sensible investigator would administer 2000 micrograms of lead daily and confidently assert that no damage was done. Yet this was precisely what Kehoe did and for good reason. In the context in which Kehoe worked, his experiments—meticulously performed and honestly interpreted—had compelling logic. Lead, which everyone ate and breathed, did not produce lead poisoning as physicians then defined it. Even workers who had greatly increased exposures did not develop disease unless the exposure became excessive. An industrial physician knew when that line was crossed, because the worker developed symptoms. Only decades later did physicians learn that lead could produce ill health that did not result in the classical symptoms of lead poisoning.

Kehoe's well-articulated view of lead poisoning built upon Aub's animal studies. Together they served pediatricians well in providing a fairly comprehensive view of lead in the human economy. Of course Kehoe did not give babies 2000 micrograms of lead each day, but he and others believed that infants and toddlers metabolized lead in roughly the same fashion as adults. For example, Kehoe knew that the foods children ate contained lead, even breast milk.[41] He knew that children were able to eliminate lead in their stool and urine, proving that children had the means of ridding their bodies of lead.[42] He knew that most children did not develop lead poisoning. Only those who had an excessive exposure were at risk, just like the few lead workers who encountered an exorbitant amount of lead on the job.

Kehoe published his concern about cribs and toys in his first article of a general nature on lead poisoning (1930). It was in and around cribs, toys, playpens, and other furniture that children spent the most time. These were the areas that Kehoe warned might provide danger. Although some physicians added woodwork to this list, he did not include windowsills or porch railings in his warning. It may be that Kehoe, who was aware of the Queensland epidemic, believed—as the Australians did—that woodwork was only a danger after baking in the tropical sun.

Kehoe's industrial experiments revealed that it required months of continuous exposure to lead before symptoms developed. This observation also informed his view of childhood lead poisoning. The risk to infants and toddlers came from long exposures, not from single high-dose exposures, unless an infant was present when a painter scraped and sanded. The reports of pediatricians from many hospitals provided supporting evidence for these long-term exposures. Virtually every report told of children chewing, gnawing, or nibbling for months or even years.

Baltimore Health Department

Baltimore soon outstripped Boston in identified cases of childhood lead poisoning. Baltimore's Health Department was particularly strong in areas of educational outreach into the community. For example, the department published the monthly *Baltimore Health News*, broadcast a weekly radio show, "Keeping Well," wrote articles for the local press (615 in 1933, spanning 5,483 column inches), persuaded fifty-one movie houses to carry Health Department educational trailers, and delivered over one hundred public lectures every year.[43]

Once the dangers of domestic lead exposure became known, the Health Department quickly got the word out. A Christmas Day radio broadcast in 1934 gives the flavor of the public health message: "Everyone knows that youngsters under three will put nearly everything to or into their mouths. Examine your children's toys for sharp edges or rough corners and warn the child of the danger in licking or chewing the paint off of playthings. Lacquer and paint may contain almost any kind of chemical, especially lead which is poisonous."[44] The department also responded to inquiries about safe paints for children's furniture.[45]

Battery Burning Epidemic

Baltimore's leadership in childhood lead poisoning did not begin with lead paint. In 1932 Huntington Williams, Baltimore's health commissioner, reported a major epidemic of lead poisoning among poor children. In order to cook during the Depression, many families burned wood casings from storage batteries. Soaked in lead-containing fluids, these casings gave off high-dose lead fumes in addition to heat.

This tragic clustering of cases affected the history of lead poisoning in the United States in a number of ways. Among the most important was that it sparked Williams's interest in the subject, a concern that continued until he left office in 1962. Baltimore became the leading city in the nation in efforts to understand childhood lead poisoning and to combat it.[46] Through a careful study of Baltimore, it is possible to see how medical and epidemiological knowledge evolved and the results of various public health measures.

Until the battery case–burning epidemic, the Baltimore Health Department had reported just two lead-paint cases in children who had "chew[ed] paint from window sills, beds, tables, chairs, and other pieces of furniture over a considerable period of time."[47] In comparison, the magnitude of the new outbreak was overwhelming. In just five weeks, the battery epidemic sickened forty children.[48] So many cases of lead poisoning coming on the heels of the new X-ray techniques permitted Edwards Park ample opportunity to employ the method.[49]

The epidemic also prompted the development of a blood test for lead. Huntington Williams arranged for Emanuel Kaplan to learn a new technique for measuring lead in blood from chemists at the DuPont Chemical Company,[50] and in 1935 the Baltimore Health Department became the first in the nation to offer this process as a diagnostic test.[51] Offering free sampling of blood presented a unique opportunity: the department pioneered in tracking serious cases of lead poisoning. By 1942 it had sampled 1,400 specimens, or about one each day. Most came from adults who had lead exposures in the workplace.

Over the next decades chemists and pediatricians developed various ways of reporting the concentration of lead in the blood. I will use the current method, micrograms/100 ml of whole blood, or micrograms/dl, so that it will be possible to compare findings across several decades.

In 1942, when Emanuel Kaplan and John McDonald summarized the first years of blood testing, they were able to conclude that children formed a substantial group of victims. When battery casings cases diminished, lead paint—gnawed at home—emerged as the primary source of lead for ninety-nine children between 1935 and 1940: "Practically all had a history of pica associated with the chewing of objects painted with lead-containing paints."[52]

Blood Lead Sampling in Practice

Blood lead tests eventually became the primary way that pediatricians defined lead poisoning, determined exposure, measured absorption, and monitored therapy. The reason blood testing took several decades to achieve this status is evident in the demands of the test: 10 cc of blood, very difficult to obtain from an infant, and hours of a chemist's time. Blood lead testing did not achieve its preeminence until the 1970s. Even then, "micro" methods, which permitted sampling from a simple finger prick, were not available everywhere.

Evaluating childhood lead poisoning was a very different process in the 1930s and 1940s. Blood testing was generally available only in Baltimore's Health Department. On occasion, some research laboratories—Kehoe's Kettering Laboratory, for example—would aid a health department by measuring lead in a child's blood. For the most part, the blood lead level was a research tool.

More important is the way in which physicians and public health officials in Baltimore used blood lead analysis. Following Kehoe's experience with industrial lead exposures, Baltimore public health officials did not believe that the blood test defined the disease:

Lead absorption is not synonymous with lead poisoning. Experience has demonstrated that individuals in industrial lead exposures may have abnormal lead levels with no accompanying symptomatology. A high blood lead level is not, of itself, diagnostic of lead poisoning but must be correlated with other findings, both clinical and laboratory, as well as with a history of definite exposure to lead. No direct correlation exists between the degree of elevation of the blood lead value and the severity of the symptoms.[53]

In other words, the blood test was an aid to diagnosis, not the diagnosis itself. For Baltimore Health Department officials, lead poisoning remained a disease of dramatic symptoms. Without clinical signs of encephalopathy, colic, palsy, or anemia, a physician would not make a diagnosis.

This understanding had important consequences for the history of child-hood lead poisoning. Kaplan and McDonald sampled blood from 177 children whose lead levels ranged between 10 and 79 micrograms/dl. By our present-day standards, all had unacceptably high blood lead levels. But to Kaplan and McDonald none of these children were lead poisoned, because they did not have symptoms.[54] Those children who were diagnosed with lead poisoning had blood lead levels between 80 and 700 micrograms/dl, with most falling in the range of 100 and 300 micrograms/dl. No child was diagnosed with less than 80 micrograms/dl.

As with any new laboratory test, physicians struggled to determine what constituted "normal," in the sense of both an arithmetic average and a "range of normal." Beginning in the late 1930s, a number of researchers published blood lead values of people considered "unexposed," for example, adults who were not employees within the lead industry or children who did not have pica. Most of the studies were of adults. Kaplan and McDonald measured the average value of unexposed individuals at 30 micrograms/dl, with a range that extended up to 50–60 micrograms/dl.[55] Robert Kehoe determined that rural Mexican indians averaged 23 micrograms/dl; American students, 27 micrograms/dl.[56] The level was twice this, or 54 micrograms/dl, for citizens of Glasgow, Scotland.[57] It was still higher in Manchester (62 micrograms/dl).[58] A Philadelphia study described a wide range of normal, 0–90 micrograms/dl, with an average of 25 micrograms/dl.[59]

Harold Blumberg and T. F. McNair Scott, chemists who developed the blood test for Baltimore's Health Department, also described a wide range of values that they considered "normal," concluding, "non-pathological blood lead values [5–100 micrograms/dl] are considered clinically negative and eliminate lead poisoning as a diagnostic consideration."[60] When Huntington Williams reviewed the experience of the Baltimore Health Department in 1952, he stated that the upper limit of normal blood lead was 50–60 micrograms/dl.[61]

Despite these hurdles in interpreting the meaning of blood lead determinations, the Baltimore Health Department by 1937 had identified fifty-seven cases of childhood lead poisoning with twenty-two fatalities. In the first years, the Health Department investigated the homes of children with blood lead levels above 65–70 micrograms/dl.[62] These investigations revealed "that in each of the above cases of lead poisoning the child had a perverted appetite which manifested itself in chewing paint from cribs, high chairs and woodwork painted with a lead-containing pigment. Laboratory examinations of paint scrapings, taken from the suspected articles, proved the source of lead beyond a doubt. Children's furniture, especially the crib, was most commonly involved." The department outlined the way in which it believed the poisonings came about: "In every instance the furniture had been reconditioned in the home with lead-containing paint. Thus it is clear that parents are frequently unaware of the paint-eating habit in their children. New cribs and other children's furniture are seldom painted with a lead-containing material, but the repainting of these articles at home with a paint of unknown composition may result in a fatality. Only too often are parents fearful of wet paint but oblivious to the danger of dry paint which contains lead."[63] A summary of the Baltimore Health Department's views can be found in the transcript of a 1935 radio address, "Children Who Eat Paint":

> In most cases this serious poisoning has occurred in the child's own home and is the end result of a habit of chewing paint from toys and cribs or other furniture. Any infant, when given a toy, will put it into his mouth. Instinct tells him that it may be something to eat. During the teething stage when the erupting dentition is causing the gums to be swollen, children will seek relief by biting or gnawing on anything they can reach. This practice is abandoned by most children as soon as the teeth have erupted, but occasionally a child develops a habit of chewing on his toys or on the furniture or woodwork. . . .
>
> Much can be accomplished in preventing your children and mine from ever reaching this condition. That, in fact, is the real purpose of this radio talk. Only a few simple rules need be followed:
>
> 1. Discourage your child, as far as you can, from putting toys and other objects into his mouth. Keep instinct from becoming habit.
> 2. If you find that he considers his bed to be some palatable delicacy, wrap the bars of his crib with cloth bandages.
> 3. If you find that even after the child's teeth have erupted he still continues to gnaw on his crib or the furniture or to chew the paint from his toys, then consult your physician. He may find that dietary or other conditions need correction and will be able to give helpful advice in habit training.
> 4. Make sure that the child's furniture, his crib, and toys have been finished with a paint which does not contain lead. . . .
>   Of course, a child is much more apt to chew on his toys than on his

crib, but toy manufacturers have recognized this hazard and most playthings are colored with harmless vegetable dyes and the others are finished with paints containing a non-poisonous zinc base. . . .

In summary, then, let me say that children who eat paint from their cribs or playthings may develop a serious illness due to lead poisoning. Two simple instructions, if followed, will safeguard your child from this catastrophe: First, be persistent in your efforts to keep your child from chewing on painted objects and second, make sure that those objects, such as his cribs and toys with which he has daily close contact, are finished with paints containing no lead pigment.

If it were possible for this simple message to reach the parents of every child in Baltimore, no additional cases of lead poisoning in paint-eating children need ever occur and a dozen lives would be saved each year. [64]

In 1939 the *Baltimore Health News* carried a similar message:

There are two things that we can do to help. One is to be sure that we use lead-free paint in refinishing children's furniture, toys and other things with which they are apt to come into intimate contact. Although there are in this country few laws which prohibit the use of lead in painting children's furniture, most manufacturers knowing of the danger have given up this material for decoration. Hence, it is repainted furniture that is apt to be the most dangerous. The other thing we can do to prevent the occurrence of lead poisoning is to discourage children putting things in their mouths. This is a natural course of action for babies, most of them giving it up by the time they are one or two years old. Up to that time we can choose for them the toys and articles in their immediate environment, but after they begin running around the house and yard it is impossible to see every thing that they do and choose everything that they pick up. Hence, if we can break the habit of putting things in the mouth by the time they reach the run-about age, it will be of great value in reducing occurrence of lead poisoning. [65]

Despite the clear understanding of the Health Department and city officials about the dangers of lead paint, Baltimore chose to apply white lead paint to the walls and ceilings of municipal office buildings and the Baltimore City Hospital.[66] This decision exemplifies their understanding of the nature of the risk posed by lead paint. Cribs, toys, and children's furniture constituted the danger. Lead paint could be applied to walls without endangering occupants.

Public Health Measures

In the 1930s and 1940s public health officials developed strategies to combat household lead poisoning. The clear message in every publication on childhood lead poisoning was that chewing on lead-painted cribs, toys, and other objects should be avoided. This advice was directed particularly at the parents of children with aggressive eating behaviors. Writers in many medical publications believed that the lead-paint companies and manufacturers of children's toys and furniture had responded to this threat by eliminating lead pigments from their products. The danger lay in repainting these items with inappropriate paints. For example, in 1931 the surgeon general observed that "generally manufacturers of [babies' toys and cribs] are seeing to it that lead paint is not used for this purpose, but warning is necessary that parents, especially in repainting cribs, should use paints which are free from lead."[67]

In keeping with public health initiatives of the period, health department officials relied largely on patient (and in this instance) parental education. The American Public Health Association's warning was typical:

> Doctors are now reporting cases of lead poisoning in infants and children apparently due to biting paint from cribs and playthings. It is likely that many more cases are caused in this way than become known. Although lead paint has many wide fields of usefulness, babies' toys, beds, and carriages are not the places to put it. We assume that the manufacturers of such articles will not use anything that might be dangerous, but a warning to parents may be needed. *Train the children as early as possible that food is the only thing meant to be eaten. In re-painting articles that children can get into their mouths the use of lead paints should be carefully avoided.*[68]

One pediatrician from San Mateo, California, explained his advice to parents: "The pediatrician has the greatest responsibility, also the greatest opportunity, in this disease to practice good preventive medicine. Advice to mothers to get beds that are stained instead of painted; the avoidance of lead-painted toys, and the discouragement of buying lead-containing colored crayons."[69] Holt and McIntosh's textbook in 1940 urged: "Parents should be educated to recognize the possible harm of pica, paint chewing and other common methods of acquiring lead."[70]

Many home safety advocates wanted to keep attention tightly focused on the toddler's intimate environment—toys and cribs—because cribs were the places where infants spent the most time and where parents might leave them unsupervised. For example, F. H. Lewy, a physician at the University of Pennsylvania, explained:

> It has been stated that woodwork, furniture and many other painted objects, because of their larger surfaces, offer a much larger hazard than toys; and yet they do not seem to play such an important part in infantile plumbism as toys do. The majority of children observed with lead

poisoning was younger than eighteen months—in other words more or less confined to their given surroundings. The main stress should therefore be laid on preventing the avoidable risk inherent in toys, cribs, cradles and beds painted with enamels containing white lead, lead-chromate, or other lead compounds.[71]

Some safety advocates focused directly on the dangers of painted toys simply because infants had greater opportunities to chew on familiar objects:

> While it may seem that furniture and woodwork about the house, coated with lead-content lacquers, enamels or paints, may constitute a greater hazard than toys, actually it has been found that this is not true. The greatest hazard lies in toys small enough to be placed in the mouth or at least light enough to be picked up and licked. Painted surfaces such as those of cribs, cradles, play pens and beds also may constitute a hazard in this respect. Respectable manufacturers of toys and children's equipment use only non-poisonous coloring and label their products accordingly.[72]

Canada before 1940

Before 1940, Canadian physicians reported forty cases of domestic childhood lead-paint poisoning. All reports came from either the Children's Memorial Hospital in Montreal or the Hospital for Sick Children in Toronto. In 1932 H. S. Mitchell reported two cases, giving furniture as the source of one.[73] The following year a symposium on lead poisoning was held at the hospital in Montreal as part of the annual meeting of the American College of Physicians. Six physicians contributed papers. H. B. Cushing discussed seventeen children (almost certainly including Mitchell's cases) who had been admitted to the hospital in the past year.[74] He told his audience that he had investigated the nature of paint used on furniture and toys:

> I went to several leading paint companies of the city and all assured me that none of their paints contained poison, in fact might even be used as infant food. However, by calling on different experts I gathered the following information. Formerly white lead was used as a basis in most paints. In recent years this has been displaced by other substances. The outdoor paints always contain large quantities of white lead to give them greater durability, but the better paints used indoors do not contain any lead and are made of zinc or titanium. . . . The next step was to analyse the paint from various infants' cots and toys and ascertain if it contained lead. It was easily shown that the enamel used on all the better cots showed practically no lead but some of the cheaper ones, and especially those repainted at home, contained large quantities. Most toys, especially those enameled, showed no lead, but the cheaper ones, especially if painted yellow or green, had very large amounts of lead.[75]

Cushing closed with a comment about preventing childhood lead poisoning by persuading painters and manufacturers not to use lead paints on toys: "Many countries in different parts of the world prohibit the use of lead in indoor paints and paints for toys, etc., but I am not aware of any such laws in any country or state in North America. We would be horrified if we saw a mother give a child a piece of broken glass or a sharp razor to play with, yet obviously these would be far less dangerous than to give them cheaply painted toys, or a cheap yellow pencil. With this in mind, we are wondering if some steps should not be taken to try to prevent this form of lead poisoning."[76]

In 1935 John Ross and Alan Brown, physicians at the Hospital for Sick Children in Toronto, published their experience with childhood poisonings. One section of their paper dealt with lead. In two years, the hospital had treated twenty-three children. The authors identified repainted cots and cribs as "probably the most common source," but also mentioned playpens, kitchen chairs and tables, windowsills and veranda railings, crayons, and painted toys.[77]

Ross and Brown ended with a suggestion about prevention: "Lead poisoning is a preventable disease in children and lead-containing paints are the chief source of the poison. In order to adequately prevent this condition, the elimination of these paints from the immediate environment of the child during the second and third years of life is essential. . . . The principal hazard occurs from repainted furniture in the poorer class homes."[78] The two authors identified repainted furniture as the problem and specifically mentioned that all exterior paints and many interior paints contained considerable lead. Because lead-free paint was available in Canada, this was the product they recommended to home repainters. They ended the section on lead with the following sentences: "It would seem advisable to prohibit the use of lead containing paints for toys, children's furniture, and for interior work. Such regulations have been in force in France since about 1915."[79]

How significant were the Canadian studies for the development of ideas about lead poisoning in the United States? The Montreal symposium was part of the annual meeting of the American College of Physicians. We have no way of knowing who attended this session of the larger meeting, but it is fair to say that at least some physicians from the United States had access to the ideas presented. For the most part, the pattern of cases in Canada approximated those in the United States: the source of the poisoning was found in the interior of homes, on painted cribs and toys, gnawed for considerable periods of time. Cushing's analysis of the lead content of paint sold in retail stores and the amount of lead in paint on children's furniture and toys reflected the general view in the United States that manufacturers were eliminating lead paint on new products and that the risk was shifting to home owners who repainted furniture.

The experience of Toronto's Hospital for Sick Children was not presented to an audience of physicians from the United States, and its relevance to the history of lead poisoning in this country is harder to assess. Ross and Brown's concern for lead paint on toys and children's furniture mirrored similar sentiments in the United States, including those of the Lead Industries Association. Their recommendation of a prohibition on lead paint on "interior work" was unique in the medical literature in North America. No physician or public health official in the United States published such a recommendation in the 1930s. Did physicians in Canada or the United States take note of this exceptional and isolated suggestion? It appears not. I have found only one citation of this article in the literature on childhood lead-paint poisoning before the seminal paper that Huntington Williams and colleagues in Baltimore wrote in 1952.[80] The single citation came in another Canadian paper.[81]

Part III

Peeling and Flaking Paint

Chapter 7

A 1950s
Transformation

IN 1952 HUNTINGTON WILLIAMS, Baltimore's commissioner of health, described a revolution in thinking about childhood lead poisoning.[1] In the mid-1930s the city's Health Department had begun an educational campaign to warn families about toddlers gnawing on painted furniture and about the dangers of placing children within reach of lead-painted objects. The *Baltimore Health News*—which had a circulation of over 10,000, including 1,800 local physicians and 6,000 teachers—devoted issues to lead poisoning in 1937, 1949, and 1951. The Health Department widely circulated a leaflet, "Lead Poisoning in Children, a Disease You Can Prevent," to parents. In addition, the department discussed childhood lead poisoning in radio and television programs and in the local press.[2]

The Health Department understood that manufacturers of cribs, children's furniture, and toys had responded to this danger by using lead-free paints on new products. Officials' concern was that parents would repaint cribs or toys with lead-based paints. Indeed, the repainting issue was part of the public health campaign. With these efforts, the number of lead-poisoned children in Baltimore in the early 1940s held steady, between eight and fifteen each year.[3]

Huntington Williams's 1952 paper upset the view that childhood lead poisoning was successfully limited to repainted cribs and toys. In 1948 Baltimore's cases had jumped to thirty; in subsequent years they remained at this far higher level.[4] This prompted the Health Department to rethink the disease. What emerged was a sea change in how pediatricians, public health officials, industry, and politicians thought about childhood lead poisoning.

The Baltimore Plan

In 1939 Baltimore initiated a program of slum reform that became known as the "Baltimore Plan." A key element of this urban renewal agenda was the transferral to the Health Department in 1941 of the powers to inspect housing, to enforce existing health provisions, and to initiate new health standards.[5] What followed was a shift in emphasis in the department to health issues associated with decaying housing. As Williams explained to a national meeting of the American Public Health Association later that year: "Until a few years ago the problem of improving the housing for the poorer segments of our urban population was not widely accepted as a health officer's responsibility in this country."[6] Getting Health Department inspectors and nurses into the homes of Baltimore's poor provided Williams with a firsthand appreciation of the massive health problems facing those least able to help themselves. From 1941 through 1950, the Baltimore Plan focused on the pressing hazards facing "rock bottom slum dwellings": sanitation; repair of holes in floors, walls, ceilings, and roofs; overcrowding; fire and electricity safety; rat control; inadequate lighting; toilets; water; kitchens; drainage; garbage; and trash.[7]

Despite the Health Department's keen interest in childhood lead-paint poisoning, Williams did not include paint or other wall coverings as part of the Baltimore Plan during the 1940s. As late as 1947, a detailed presentation by the Citizen's Planning and Housing Association of Baltimore did not mention paint as a health issue.[8] Certainly this omission did not indicate a waning of interest. Rather, it represented the way in which Williams and the Baltimore Health Department viewed the relative risk posed by lead paint.

Beginning in 1936, members of the department had investigated the homes of lead-poisoned children to locate the source of lead paint.[9] In late 1948 home investigators found evidence that upset the older consensus that cribs and toys were the main danger. As Williams described: "The most common cause of lead poisoning is apparently the habit of chewing paint from cribs, toys, furniture, woodwork such as windowsills, and the eating of painted plaster and fallen paint flakes."[10] The first items on Williams's list, of course, were familiar; what set the Baltimore experience apart was the identification of plaster and fallen paint flakes. Williams went further. He identified the setting: "The problem in Baltimore at present involves chiefly slum or blighted-area properties. The cases are concentrated in two areas which are of known slum status and where the houses are old and have had many coats of paint, usually lead paint, applied throughout several decades."[11] Williams also identified the population of children at particularly high risk: "The annual attack rate for the age segment under 5 years during the period 1931–51 was 7.5 times as high among the Negro population

(71 per 100,000) as it was among the white population (9.5 per 100,000). . . . The racial difference in incidence is believed to be due to environmental factors probably resulting chiefly from economic disadvantage."[12]

A New Hazard, a New Response

Flakes of peeling paint in decaying, poorly maintained urban housing created a major health hazard that had not been previously recognized. It demanded an entirely different response from industry and public health officials. Baltimore led the nation, but Baltimore's experience was not an isolated one. How Baltimore and several other cities, universities, medical and public health organizations, and the lead industry moved from thinking about childhood lead poisoning as a contained problem to a major new public health menace in the space of a few short years, and how industry, public health officials, and university researchers fashioned a new, more appropriate public health response is a fascinating story. The transformation occurred in several urban and university settings, and important to it were the Lead Industries Association and especially its director of health and safety, Manfred Bowditch.

Randolph Byers and Elizabeth Lord

To set the stage for the transformation, we begin in 1943, when Randolph K. Byers, a child neurologist at Boston Children's Hospital, and Elizabeth Lord, a psychologist, published a paper that aroused controversy both at the time and in later decades, but for largely different reasons. Byers and Lord wrote their article to refute the commonly held notion that successfully treated lead-poisoned children suffered no long-term neurological problems. They started with the views of Charles McKhann, who had diagnosed and treated some of the patients whom Byers and Lord had under study: "The neurological manifestations of lead poisoning usually subside without serious consequences if the ingestion of lead is stopped and the removal of lead from the circulation and its deposition in inert form in the bones can be hastened."[13] Byers and Lord identified 128 children who had been diagnosed with lead poisoning at Boston Children's Hospital over the previous ten years. They weeded out those who now lived too far away and those who were known to have had major neurological consequences at the time of poisoning. This left 59 children who had been discharged from the hospital as "cured." They selected 20 for their study.

What caught the attention of industry leaders in Byers and Lord's study was the children's source of lead. Eighteen were known to have chewed lead paint exclusively. Of those, Byers and Lord identified the source—by chart review— of fifteen: eleven of the fifteen had gnawed cribs, toys, or other furniture; eight had chewed windowsills or railings. This finding implied that children were still getting lead from repainted cribs and toys but that windowsills figured far more prominently than in earlier studies.

What also caught industry and medical attention was Byers and Lord's conclusion that all the children but one had learning difficulties when they enrolled in school some years later. In decades to come, some researchers referred back to this study as an early statement that *asymptomatic* children with lead exposure had long-term neurological deficits. A close reading of the paper reveals that all of the patients Byers and Lord reported had evidence of encephalopathy. Indeed, that is how they came to be admitted to the hospital. Like most researchers in the 1940s, Byers and Lord did not measure blood lead levels. Nevertheless, it is reasonable to assume—on the basis of reports from Baltimore— that these overtly symptomatic children all had blood lead levels in excess of 100 micrograms/100 cc whole blood. What this study showed, then, was that many children who had lead exposure sufficient to provoke easily perceived cerebral symptoms had neurological impairments that made success in school difficult. Byers and Lord did not address the possibility of impairment in asymptomatic children, nor did they attempt to sort out the role of lead exposure among other significant variables for school performance, such as poverty, broken homes, or family violence—issues with which researchers in the 1970s and 1980s would begin to grapple.

This study, and the *Time* article it sparked,[14] provoked a response from Felix Wormser, secretary of the Lead Industries Association, who did not believe either major conclusion of the study. Wormser immediately wrote to Robert Kehoe and asked his opinion: "[The study] drew some amazing conclusions alleging that lead poisoning in early childhood had left effects showing up years later. . . . As you know, it is our belief here, based on careful investigation, that no crib manufacturer in the United States today is using any lead paint on cribs, nor has he used any for years."[15] Wormser also raised methodological issues with the paper. He did not believe that Byers had correctly diagnosed lead poisoning, because he had not identified lead in the children's bodies. And Wormser criticized Byers for not checking the children's homes for lead paint. Of course, since Byers had not cared for these patients when they first entered the hospital years earlier, it was not possible for him to address these shortcomings.

Wormser also criticized Byers's reliance on X-rays to make the diagnosis of lead poisoning in children. This was a complicated story that entailed a thorough understanding of lead metabolism in bones and the physics of X-rays.[16] Wormser thought he had identified a major flaw in Byers's method, and he spent considerable energy in attempts to substantiate this claim. The issue was whether the "lead lines" on the X-rays of bones were the result of lead at the site of the line or simply reflected a shadow indicating bone injury that could have other causes in addition to lead. There was no doubt that Byers and Lord's study prodded Wormser into action.

Kehoe's reply to Wormser was also unsettling. Kehoe accepted the observation that lead poisoning could result in permanent injury, and he believed that lead-based paint might well be the source.[17] In an effort to persuade Wormser, Kehoe sent him papers and a bibliography about the Queensland epidemic.[18] Wormser read these papers and objected to many of their conclusions as well, but this exposure to Queensland's experience may have added momentum to the changes beginning to take shape in his thinking.[19]

Wormser's zeal to discredit Byers's paper irritated Kehoe, and he discussed his concerns with Wormser's superiors at the Lead Industries Association. J. H. Schaefer reined Wormser in, and this mild rebuke may also have added energy to Wormser's transformation.[20] In any event, Wormser kept his board well informed on his activities.[21]

Wormser then met with Byers to discuss his concerns. What emerged from the meeting was an agreement that the LIA would fund a new study. Byers agreed to be meticulous in establishing the diagnosis of children he suspected of being lead-poisoned, and he agreed to visit the homes to verify the source of lead paint.[22] This LIA-funded study set into motion fundamental changes in thinking, similar to ones occurring in Baltimore. Byers's new study did not get under way for two years because of the terminal illness of one of the researchers and Byers's stint in the army.[23]

This close attention to details sharpened Byers's analysis. For example, fifteen years later, Byers judged that around one-third of cases diagnosed as lead poisoning at Boston Children's Hospital had almost certainly been incorrect.[24]

In his unpublished memoirs written in 1986, Byers gave a colorful account of his dealings with the LIA in the 1940s:

> The second result was that I was waited on by several members of the Lead Industries Association and threatened with a suit for a million dollars. At the invitation of the lead people I went to meet them at the Ritz for lunch to discuss the matter. Dr. Crothers who had urged my publication went with me. When we were through, the lead people gave me a grant which they continued for eight or ten years to continue and expand my studies. This fortunate result may have been abetted by the four or five martinis the lead executives each drank, but more likely it resulted from the quiet skillful backup given my work by Dr. Crothers. After that I met with executives from the the lead industry each year and in spite of three to five martinis for each of them and one for me, they gave me a grant of several thousand dollars annually to continue my investigation, resulting in a second paper about 1955. Mr. Manfred Bowditch administered the fund and visited me two or three times a year, helpful he was.[25]

Although his account contained a threat of a lawsuit, Byers's tone was anything but intimidated.

As the result of lunch at the Ritz, letters from Robert Kehoe, pressure from his superiors at the LIA, and a reading of papers from the Queensland epidemic, Wormser came to believe that there was enough substance in Byers and Lord's paper to warrant additional research. But he did more. He persuaded the LIA to create a Safety and Hygiene Program that would in part address the child-hood lead-poisoning issue.[26] In addition Wormser proposed a joint symposium with the American Medical Association on lead poisoning that was held in September 1947.[27]

The LIA also funded the work of Alsoph Corwin of Johns Hopkins to study the therapeutic effects of British Anti-Lewisite, or BAL, in the treatment of lead poisoning.[28] A few years later, the LIA would serve as a clearinghouse of information on EDTA, the new and more effective therapy.[29] The availability of therapy should not be underestimated in the transformation of thinking about childhood lead poisoning: therapy gave additional energy to seeking out cases.

Wormser resigned as secretary of the LIA in May 1947. In early 1948 the LIA appointed Manfred Bowditch as its first director of health and safety. Bowditch would be instrumental in the changes in attitude and approach to come.

Upsurge of Cases in Baltimore in 1948

Baltimore's increase of cases of childhood lead poisoning in 1948 prompted an analysis in January 1949. Charles Couchman, a coauthor with Huntington Williams on the 1952 paper, scrutinized the cases and concluded: "Investigations were made of 30 of the confirmed cases and these disclosed that all took place in rented property. In two-thirds of these properties the children had easy access to dried paint which was flaking or easily chipped from surfaces."[30]

On February 4, 1949, Manfred Bowditch, hearing of Baltimore's analysis of cases, wrote to the Health Department requesting information.[31] He visited Baltimore in March.[32] In May the Baltimore Health News reported the increased number of lead-poisoned children and the new source of lead: "There were 31 such cases in 1948, considerably more than the number recorded in any prior year. These cases were carefully investigated and were found to have resulted chiefly from chewing painted surfaces such as window sills, or from the eating of dried paint flakes which had cracked or chipped from repainted indoor wood-work areas."[33] This was the first published account of the hazard of paint flakes. The Baltimore Health News article also included "Suggestions for Parents," which contained a warning not to allow children to eat paint flakes and urged parents to repaint only with lead-free paints. The paint-flake recommendation had not previously been included in the many educational efforts.[34]

In July, the Baltimore Health Department conducted a second analysis—this time of cases from early 1949—and concluded that more than 80 percent of lead-poisoned children were African American and that most were receiving well-baby care in department clinics. This suggested a means of educational intervention, and the department promptly issued a pamphlet, "Lead Poisoning in Children."[35] Later that month, Huntington Williams enthusiastically welcomed Bowditch's offer to fund a third study.[36]

The Watt Report

In the summer of 1949 Dr. Anna Baetjer and Mary Watt, a medical student, investigated sixty cases from the records of the Baltimore Health Department. This LIA-sponsored study included department records, blood lead determinations, hospital records, and home visits. The project was the most comprehensive epidemiological study to date on childhood lead poisoning.[37] The Watt Report documented that lead-poisoned children got into lead-paint flakes and peelings from walls, ceilings, and woodwork in poor repair. Huntington Williams received the report on October 3.[38] Manfred Bowditch received the report after Williams.

By December 1949, there was evidence that Bowditch had circulated the findings of the Watt Report to Randolph Byers and Joseph Aub in Boston, Drs. Weech, Dodds, and Kehoe in Cincinnati, Drs. Alfred G. Langmann and May R. Mayers in New York City, and Drs. Donald B. Armstrong and George Wheatley of the Metropolitan Life Insurance Company.[39] Wheatley was also chairman of the Committee on Home Accidents of the American Academy of Pediatrics. The American Academy of Pediatrics and health officials in Baltimore, Boston, Cincinnati, and New York would form a partnership with the LIA to forge a new public health approach to childhood lead poisoning.

In 1949 Maryland's state legislature—prompted by Baltimore's cases—passed a "Toxic Finishes Law," which contained the following provision: "It shall be unlawful for any person to manufacture, sell or offer to sell, any toy or plaything, including children's furniture, decorated or covered with paint or any other material containing lead or other substance of a poisonous nature, from contact with which children may be injuriously affected."[40] Though well-intentioned, the law was repealed a year later, with the approval of the Maryland State Board of Health and the Baltimore City Board of Health, because of the ambiguities of its definitions ("injuriously"), its lack of enforceability, and its failure to define acceptable levels of lead for paint.[41] An editorial in the *Baltimore Sun* explained:

> The law, according to the State Health Department, only caused confusion among manufacturers, retailers, and parents and was not likely to

prevent a single case of sickness or death. It turns out that the children who have had lead poisoning have never got it through chewing on new furniture or toys. They have got it through chewing on objects which have been repainted, frequently by parents, with lead-based paints intended for outdoor use. Repainted cribs and inside window sills are two of the most common hazards along this line.[42]

In its repeal of the statute, the Maryland state legislature acknowledged that the LIA had agreed to fund a much larger study of Baltimore through Johns Hopkins's School of Public Health.[43] Unfortunately, this project was delayed at Hopkins because of staffing shortages.[44]

Between 1949 and 1951 Bowditch devoted much energy to childhood lead poisoning. Occasionally in his correspondence, Bowditch referred to the Baltimore cases as a "headache." Although this was certainly a pejorative phrasing, Bowditch's activities did not indicate that he was insensitive to childhood lead poisoning or that he dismissed the problem; rather, he was at the heart of the 1950s transformation.[45]

The Watt Report had a profound effect. The reaction of May Mayers of New York is particularly telling. Mayers was a prominent industrial hygienist who had published extensively on lead poisoning in the workplace. She had served on the Lead Poisoning Committee of the American Public Health Association and in 1950 was chief of the Medical Unit of the New York State Department of Labor. It was no surprise that Bowditch chose to send her the report. Mayers wrote to Bowditch about the way in which the Watt Report altered her thinking: "For the first time, I am beginning to be really concerned that there may be many more children who develop lead poisoning and die of it throughout the country than we had hitherto suspected."[46]

The Baltimore Health Department alerted other health departments about peeling paint and inquired about cases: St. Louis,[47] Detroit,[48] Richmond,[49] Washington, D.C.,[50] Philadelphia,[51] and Oak Ridge, Tennessee.[52] In June 1950, the New York City Health Department concluded that at least one child had died from "the habit of eating paint peelings."[53]

As Bowditch learned of cases in one city, he passed the information along to other health departments.[54] In November 1950 Bowditch traveled to Cincinnati, where he learned that cases had doubled that year.

Manfred Bowditch's flurry of activity continued while the 1950s transformation progressed. But the problem of childhood lead poisoning could not be fully addressed without an understanding of another, larger issue—the state of urban housing.

Chapter 8

The Urban Ecology

How did the new ecology of childhood lead-paint poisoning alter the lead landscape? Key questions are: Why did the issue of peeling and flaking paint from walls and ceilings emerge in the late 1940s? Did decaying paint from walls represent a new hazard or did physicians and public health workers simply see the problem differently? In the latter view, what happened was merely a change in perception. Certainly, after 1950, physicians and public health departments virtually dropped concerns about cribs, toys, and children's furniture. Lead paint had not been used on such items since the 1930s, of course; only in repainting did cribs and toys persist in creating a hazard. Once Huntington Williams, Manfred Bowditch, Randolph Byers, and Robert Kehoe reformulated childhood lead poisoning as a manifestation of "inner-city blight," all urban public health officials followed suit.[1]

But more is at issue here than a change in perception of observers. It is likely that there were more decaying urban walls and ceilings after World War II. The timing of the "sea change" was fairly precise. There was no published description of household lead poisoning from peeling or flaking paint in the United States until the May 1949 issue of the *Baltimore Health News*.

Beginning in 1936, Baltimore had investigated the homes of children diagnosed with lead poisoning. One assignment of the home visitor was to determine the source of lead and to educate the family on how to avoid future poisoning. In every published case, these visitors determined that the source of paint had been cribs, toys, other children's furniture, or woodwork.[2]

When home visitors investigated the dwellings of children poisoned in the late 1940s and early 1950s, they described lead paint peeling off in sheets—in one well-publicized dwelling, hanging like stalactites. Williams applauded the work of these home visitors: "One of the most promising advances in the prevention of child plumbism was the assignment several years ago of a public health nurse supervisor to investigate lead poisoning cases. With the knowledge gained by intimate association with the problem, the supervisor was able to interest other public health nurses. They not only make home visits and disseminate information in the most-affected areas of the city, but may take part in well-baby clinics, where mothers are told of the dangers connected with pica."[3]

Flaked paint was everywhere in many apartments. In Baltimore, visitors noted, "usually the children lived in old rented properties where lead paint had been used for many years on window sills and frames and where it had often flaked and scaled."[4] Similar inspections in Chicago revealed that "the home visits provided an excellent opportunity to study the environments of these children. Most of the homes were dilapidated. In 19 instances there were large amounts of peeling or chipped paint, plaster, and putty."[5] The pattern was the same in New York City: "Most apartments are in bad repair with paint peeling from walls and loosened plaster falling on floors."[6] A colleague of Robert Kehoe, Hugo Smith, noted that slums in Cincinnati fared no better: "No new paint has been added to these homes; instead, the explanation for the appearance of saturnism is the fact that the paint has been allowed to crumble and peel."[7] It is hard to believe that home visitors would have missed such vivid hazards had they been present in the 1930s or early 1940s.

Decorating Walls with Lead Paint

To make sense of this dramatic change, we need to learn when American urban dwellings were first painted. This is not as simple a question as it might seem to answer. Urban reformers exerted considerable energy defining the unhealthy aspects of tenement living. Most often they focused on the pressing issues of sanitation, fire safety, garbage, and clean water. In the last decades of the nineteenth century and the early years of the twentieth century, interior decoration emerged as an element of tenement-reform ferment, but these concerns figured far down the list of most reformers.

In the early 1950s, when lead poisoning emerged as a hazard to children living in the urban slums, home visitors discovered that the homes of afflicted toddlers had not always housed the poor. In fact, the paradox of childhood lead poisoning was that the most dangerous places for poor children in the 1950s were the former homes of well-to-do dwellers who had lavished walls with many coats of expensive lead paint decades earlier.

Lead paint had been used for some interior decoration in the nineteenth century, sharing walls and ceilings with wallpaper.[8] When paint was selected, painters and homeowners preferred lead paints for their vivid colors, ease of spreading, and durability. Changes in fashion in home decoration are complex enterprises to follow precisely, but walls were increasingly painted in many homes in the 1890s. In part this had to do with the availability of ready-mixed paints for home use.[9] At the U.S. Bureau of Mines, Paul Tyler, noting the great increase in the use of paint for decoration inside homes, in 1936 concluded: "A definite vogue in favor of painted walls was observed over a decade ago. Other wall coverings, including wall paper and cold water paints, have been replaced by oil paints in private dwellings and even more extensively perhaps in apartments and offices where repeated changes in tenants call for frequent redecorating. The rapid growth in sales of interior paints coincided roughly with the boom in apartment building."[10]

In considerable measure, the middle class perceived paint to be more sanitary than wallpaper. The importance of germs and infectious diseases cannot be overly stressed here. Germs could more easily be washed from a smooth painted surface than from an absorbent wallpaper. One might ask, of course, for proof that any inhabitant of a wallpapered room ever contracted a disease simply because of germs on the wall. But in the eye of public health officials, germs needed to be combated wherever they lurked. Reformers' recommendation was to paint walls, ceilings, and even floors with washable paint.[11] Paint manufacturers quickly seized on this change, and the interiors of homes, schools, and hospitals were all painted. Wallpaper was stripped from many homes.

For example, Maria Elliott, an instructor of household economics at Simmons College, in 1907 recommended: "Wall paper is made of organic material, is put on with paste which is subject to decay. It is absorbent and liable to be destroyed by thorough cleaning. Hard finish in plain color or in fresco is non-absorbent, repels dust and may be frequently cleaned."[12] Henry Gardner, director of the Scientific Section of the Paint and Varnish Manufacturers Association, also trumpeted the sanitary advantages of the painted surface: "From the standpoint of sanitation and hygiene, properly painted walls are superior to papered walls upon which bacteria may in some instances be harbored, where, for example, it has been the practice to repaper without taking off the old paper which, having been glued with organic pastes, acts as a culture medium. . . . In hospitals where it is necessary to maintain sanitary conditions, the walls are invariably painted with paints that can be frequently washed. It is just as important that similar precautions should be taken in the home."[13]

Switching from wallpaper to paint was primarily a middle-class phenomenon. In tenements, the walls often had never been decorated. In the late nineteenth century, reformers in New York City recommended that the floors and ceilings of tenements be whitewashed at least once a year. Cheap whitewash, which was easily applied and did not contain lead or other pigment, served the dual purposes of cleanliness and the psychological and safety value of brightening the otherwise dark buildings. Reformers such as Jacob Riis often spoke on the evils to health—physical, psychological, and spiritual—of darkness.

This is not to imply that homes of the poor were free from lead paint. After the turn of the century, reformers advocated either paint or whitewash on tenement walls and actively discouraged wallpaper for both sanitary and aesthetic reasons. Lead paint was viewed as superior.[14] The United States government recommended lead paint in federally funded buildings until after World War II.[15]

There was a lot of lead in paint at the turn of the century. When Alice Hamilton surveyed the paint industry in 1913, she observed that lead paints could be up to 60 percent lead carbonate.[16] Interior lead paint flatted with turpentine bubbled and cracked, but changes in paint chemistry in the twentieth century substituted linseed oil, which allowed for longer wear.[17] Nevertheless, depending on sunlight and wear and tear, all walls and ceilings would eventually crack and require repainting. This required scraping and sanding, which was the hazard that Hamilton and other industrial hygienists had described. Not all the paint would be removed in this repainting process, so that over the decades lead paint built up in layers.

There is evidence that painters used less lead pigment by the late 1920s. The Bureau of Mines reported that "sales of white lead declined almost 60 percent from 1927 to their low point in 1932." The Depression played a part in this decline, but zinc pigments fell much less and titanium pigments actually doubled.[18] Health concerns for painters also contributed to the decline in lead paints, especially after painters began using spray equipment. Zinc pigments were not as vivid and hence lacked aesthetic appeal, but they were cheaper and could be sprayed. In 1936 Hamilton noted that lead pigments were used far less commonly.[19] In some cases, zinc-based paints covered older lead-based paints. In others, a combination lead-zinc pigment paint was used. Lead did not disappear from paints in the 1940s. Exterior walls required lead paints for resilience.[20]

In Britain, tenements were older, but the same trend can be seen in using interior paints containing less lead pigment. For example, when analyzing the paint from walls in flats where children had been lead-poisoned, British observers concluded: "Children inhabiting homes built between 1930 and 1965 were mostly exposed to paints with less than 1% of lead, and conversely children inhabiting pre-1855 homes were exposed to paints containing 5% lead."[21] Lead paints for interiors could still be purchased, but the trend was toward reduced lead paint on the inside of the home.

The high-dose lead paint, then, was spread on walls and ceilings early in the century, and much of it remained there in 1950. In every city that investigated this newly perceived hazard, public health officials concluded that the paint had been applied before 1940. As Julian Chisholm described: "The interior wood-work, painted plaster and wallpaper of houses built prior to 1940 and still in use may contain layers of lead pigment paints which have never been removed."[22]

The "Blighted" Inner City

What happened after World War II to alter the calculus of the hazard? Lead paint did not present a danger to children if walls and ceilings were maintained properly and repainted regularly. That is, painted surfaces were not a worry un-less a child gnawed them. Unlike cribs and toys, walls and ceilings were hard to chew. Woodwork was different: a toddler might pull up to look out a window and find the sill just at mouth level. Active chewing was easy to spot, and health officials urged parents to be on guard for it.

What Huntington Williams described was not children gnawing on walls. Rather, he observed toddlers passively ingesting paint flakes strewn over their homes. What had happened to the maintenance of these buildings? This is a difficult question to answer generally, but in many cities the owners who had maintained painted walls before World War II moved out after the war as part of the flight to the suburbs. Middle-class apartments were subdivided into smaller rental units. A common complaint was that buildings received little or no main-tenance.[23] When paint on walls and ceilings deteriorated, it was not scraped, sanded, and repainted. It was simply left to peel and flake. Often housing codes did not address paint, so landlords had no obligation to repaint. Former middle-class neighborhoods evolved into slums.

In an effort to improve urban housing, the American Public Health Asso-ciation issued guidelines on housing and health throughout the 1940s. These focused on sanitation, heating, electrical safety, fire safety, structural integrity, and gas poisonings. So pressing were these concerns that at no point did its Com-mittee on the Hygiene of Housing address painted walls. Huntington Williams, who was quite familiar with the health hazards associated with lead paint, was a member of this committee.[24] Only in 1951 did lead paint join other housing concerns as a component of the Baltimore Plan.

Margaret Galbreath, a visiting nurse in Baltimore, reflected on the deterio-rating homes that she was investigating:

> Most of the cases occurred in rented housing units where predominantly the landlord lived elsewhere. Most frequently we found flaking, scaling paint; broken wall surfaces; torn wallpaper. There was a lack of supervi-sion by the owner or agent. In many instances the tenant made his own repairs and did his own decorating, sometimes without notifying the landlord. Tenant responsibility was not encouraged. . . . Frequent re-painting without scraping or burning away the old paint makes the new

paint buckle and scale. Soon comes a time when paint and wall part company.[25]

Julian Chisholm, in his detailed study jointly funded by the Lead Industries Association and the National Institutes of Health, agreed with Galbreath's assessment: "All [cases] dwelled in the urban slum areas of Baltimore."[26] A physician from Chicago, Arnold Tanis, commented, "Almost without exception these children come from families in the poorest economic groups, whose homes or apartments are in poor repair, often with paint peeling off the walls."[27] David Jenkins and Robert Mellins, also of Chicago, stated that "the homes were for the most part dilapidated, submarginal apartments."[28] Cook County Hospital's Joseph Greengard and colleagues noted the declining status of the neighborhoods where lead-poisoned children resided: "They live in old houses, badly deteriorated and divided into multiple units, with consequent severe overcrowding."[29] Harold Jacobziner, assistant commissioner of the New York City Department of Health, reported: "All patients lived in substandard housing, where paint peelings and painted plaster are freely available."[30] Hugo Smith detailed a similar process in Cincinnati:

> A preponderance of nonwhites merely reflects the population residing in the older, more disheveled dwellings in the impoverished areas of our cities from which virtually all cases of pediatric plumbism come. Interior surfaces within buildings in these areas have, over the years, received numerous coats of paint, many of which contained lead, and with the influx of an economically poor population the walls and ceilings have fallen into disrepair, providing a readily available exposure for any inadequately supervised toddler who, due to a variety of poorly understood factors, continues to explore with his mouth.[31]

In 1959 Jerome Trichter explained to New York City's Board of Health how lead poisoning had emerged as one problem of the city's slums:

> I want to point out that the greatest proportion of these slum buildings are in Manhattan. These people, therefore, come to Manhattan. The in-migrating Negroes and Puerto Ricans are generally forced to come to the Manhattan slums for a living place and unless halted this will continue. The middle-income group is a problem also. One wouldn't expect this to be so but a similar situation exists here. . . . One hundred thousand of these families live in substandard dwellings or under seriously over-crowded conditions. . . . The high cost of construction absolutely precludes any substantial increase in the number of such buildings which are likely to be put up by private realty operations. Middle-income families have no place to go in New York City and the result is they go to other communities outside the city. I think Manhattan already is as close to being a two-class town as it can be. . . . We have had a cessation

of housing construction in New York City because of the war. Our costs go up and people do not build. Then there is deterioration of buildings and many are vacated or condemned. Finally, there is condemnation for public use or occupancy. With this come the demands of war prosperity. New people come to New York for opportunity that exists here and because we have prosperity. If there weren't jobs for the people, they wouldn't come, and they are needed here to fill important gaps in the labor supply. This, coupled with the natural increase in population, results in great overcrowding. Because of prejudice, real and promoted, people move out. This results in more overcrowding elsewhere. Long-time residents move out of the changing neighborhood. Buildings are converted from one and two-family occupancies to extremely profitable rooming houses. These fine buildings now fall into deterioration. There is even a greater exodus of good families and long-time residents. The number of resident landlords decreases. These converted houses are bought up by absentee landlords. City services become strained beyond capacity, including health, fire, police, street cleaning and garbage collection. School classes become overcrowded. Then we have juvenile delinquency, crime, and disease concentrated in the slum. Unscrupulous realtors keep the profit-pot boiling with rumors, scare prices, gossip that the community is going "black" and "sell before it is too late." Finally . . . the situation becomes uncontrollable and the city and that neighborhood begin to rot. This rot is contagious and soon other neighborhoods rot in the same way.[32]

Compounding the problem in New York City was a continuation of rent-control policies, which, many believed, were preventing landlords from making needed repairs. In addition, housing allowances for people on public assistance were insufficient to command better living conditions. To make matters worse, New York City had no bureaucratic means to arbitrate disputes among residents, landlords, and the Board of Health.[33]

Trichter noted that the problem spanned most American cities: "Today some 17,000,000 Americans live in buildings that are beyond rehabilitation, decayed, dirty, rat-infested, without decent heat, light or plumbing." He criticized the failure of governments at all levels to formulate adequate plans, and he predicted that grassroots community groups would spring up to force solutions.[34] As we shall see, local programs in many cities formed one of the public health responses to childhood lead poisoning in the 1950s and 1960s.

Mapping Childhood Lead Poisoning

Home investigations in many cities quickly revealed that most cases of childhood lead poisoning clustered in the same slum neighborhoods. Baltimore was

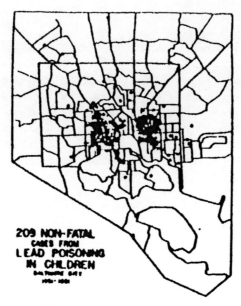

209 Children Survived

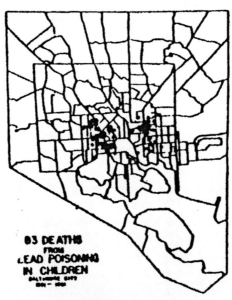

83 Children Died

Figure 6. Baltimore: Occurrence by Months of 292 Cases of Lead Poisoning in Children, 1931–1951. (*Baltimore Health News* [1951], 114.)

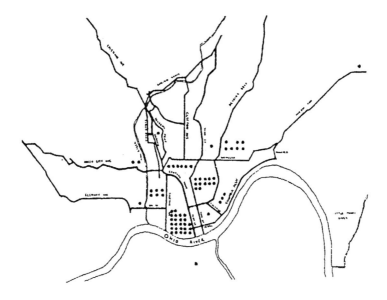

A map of Cincinnati, Ohio, indicating the location of homes of pediatric patients with lead poisoning seen between 1940 and 1957. Of note is the intense concentration in the downtown basin area. Urban redevelopment in this district has resulted in the more recent cases coming from the region in the right center of the city.

Figure 7. Cincinnati: Lead Poisoning, 1940–1957. ("Lead Hygiene Conference," *Industrial Medicine and Surgery* 28 [1959]: 150.)

the first of several cities to represent cases on a map, joined by Cincinnati, Philadelphia, Chicago, and New York City (see figures 6, 7, 8, 9, and 10). [35] These areas coincided geographically with areas where homes had received many coats of lead paint in past decades, areas that public health officials dubbed the "lead belt." Harold Jacobziner explained: "There is a marked concentration of lead poisoning in slum areas in the 'lead belt' and it results chiefly from chewing on flakes of painted plaster from walls, paint peelings from ceilings and window sills."[36]

Race and the "Blighted" Inner City

The residents in these poorly maintained, rented apartments were often newcomers, southern blacks moving north in search of jobs.[37] In New York City,

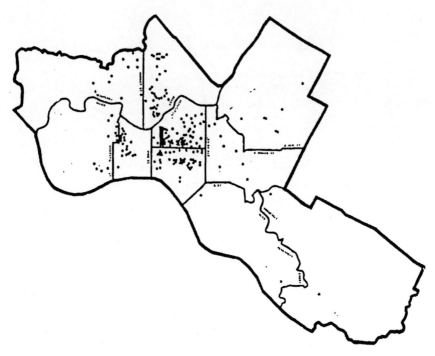

Figure 8. Philadelphia: Spot Map of 219 Cases of Lead Poisoning by Residence of Patients. (*Archives of Environmental Health* 3 [1961]: 577. Reprinted with permission of the Helen Dwight Reid Educational Foundation, published by Heldref Publications. Copyright 1961.)

many of the newcomers were Puerto Ricans. Every city reported that childhood lead poisoning fell disproportionately on minorities. Most public health officials believed that there was no racial susceptibility for lead poisoning among African Americans and accounted for differences in incidence solely in social and economic terms. For example, Huntington Williams called attention to the great disparity of lead poisoning among Baltimore's children: black children suffered at a rate that was 7.5 times the rate of white children. He explained, "The racial difference in incidence is believed to be due to environmental factors probably resulting chiefly from economic disadvantage."[38] In New York City, African American and Puerto Rican children accounted for over 80 percent of the cases.[39] In 1960 Jacobziner claimed that, of the ten cases he surveyed, "all but one are from Brooklyn and are nonwhite."[40] Similarly striking claims were made for Cincinnati, Philadelphia, and Chicago.[41]

These residents had no prior experience with lead paint. In fact, housing for poor blacks in the South was rarely painted. The concern for chewing on lead-painted objects—so much the topic of educational programs in northern cities in the 1930s and 1940s—had not reached the rural South.

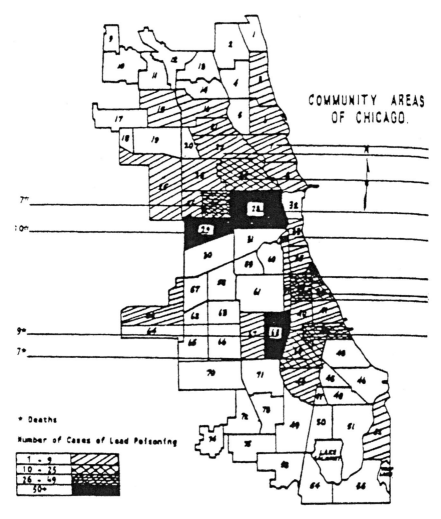

COMMUNITY AREAS OF CHICAGO.

* Deaths

Number of Cases of Lead Poisoning

| 1 - 9 |
| 10 - 25 |
| 26 - 49 |
| 50+ |

Figure 9. Chicago: Lead Poisoning, 1959–1961. (*American Journal of Public Health* 54 [1964]: 1244. Copyright 1964 by the American Public Health Association.)

Pica

Pica remained a hallmark of childhood lead poisoning. In virtually every city, public health officers identified the children at risk as those with aggressive eating behaviors. Home visitors were often astonished to learn that parents did not understand the danger in chewing paint. In Chicago, public health officials observed: "It was somewhat surprising to learn that the chewing of paint was not regarded as a dangerous activity by the parents."[42] Baltimore's physicians were clearly frustrated that public health education was not reaching the population

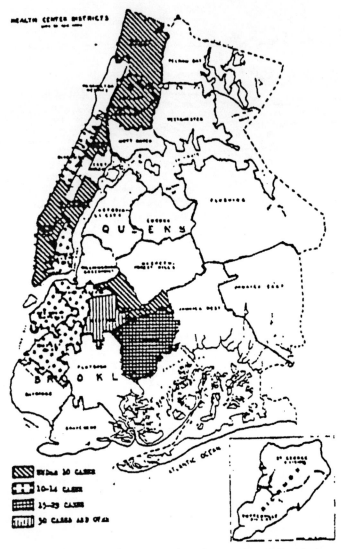

Figure 10. New York City: Lead-Poisoning Cases Reported in 1961. (*Archives of Pediatrics* 79 [1962]: 73.)

most at risk: "These children live in houses where lead-containing paint, used many years ago, is now flaking and peeling from the surface. There seems to be widespread ignorance or disregard of the hazards to the child through the inges- tion of these particles. Despite vigorous education campaigns which have been conducted by the public health department in Baltimore, many parents con- tinue to accept pica as a harmless manifestation of normal infantile development."[43] This failure to monitor what children placed in their mouths also struck Harold Jacobziner and Harry Raybin: "In all cases there was a history of pica and . . . nearly all of the parents were unaware of the harmful effects which may result from the chewing of painted surfaces and objects."[44]

Some public health officials noted the high incidence of pica among African American children who moved with their parents into northern cities. Many southern African Americans viewed eating nonfood items with less concern. For example, in 1942 about one-quarter of Mississippi school children reported that they regularly ate dirt, a practice also reported by a similar percentage of pregnant women. In one study from Baltimore, many mothers of children who had become lead-poisoned had pica behaviors themselves. In these families, pica was considered a habit but not a life-threatening activity.

What is entirely plausible was that African American children from the South continued a custom of eating nonfood items when they moved to northern cities. Instead of dirt, paint flakes became their target. Parents, not previously informed of the dangers of eating paint, failed to appreciate the danger.[45] What this meant was that migrating parents did not respond to eating paint flakes with the same earnestness that families raised in Baltimore did. In other words, paint flakes on floors or furniture did not convey an ingrained sense of urgency. In Washington, D.C., pediatricians and child psychiatrists noted: "In the *cultural* background of many of the Negro mothers pica is acceptable, and from them we learned of their own pica, either past or current, and heard the idea frequently expressed that 'all children eat dirt.' Some expressed surprise when they learned that ingestions might be dangerous, particularly ingestion of paint or plaster. There was generally more acceptance of pica among the mothers of the Negro clinic group than the white mothers."[46] Julian Chisholm described the eating behaviors of Baltimore's children: "the habitual, purposeful, and compulsive search for and ingestion of such unnatural food substances."[47] He observed that "pica in large cities of the United States is most prevalent among families—particularly Negroes—recently arrived from the rural South," and that "as many as 50 percent of mothers of children with pica may also have pica themselves."[48] To make matters even more difficult for public health officers, educational programs aimed at these newcomers—even door-to-door efforts—failed because many occupants moved each year.[49]

Many home health visitors reported that poisoned children were poorly supervised, left to roam without parental vigilance. In Cincinnati, home visitors noted: "Socioeconomic conditions frequently prevent sound child rearing."[50] In Baltimore, public health officials observed: "In many instances the absence of supervision by adults who may be obliged to leave the children to earn a living allow the infant and preschool child opportunity to eat toxic material without restraint."[51] In Washington, D.C., home visitors remarked that "personal

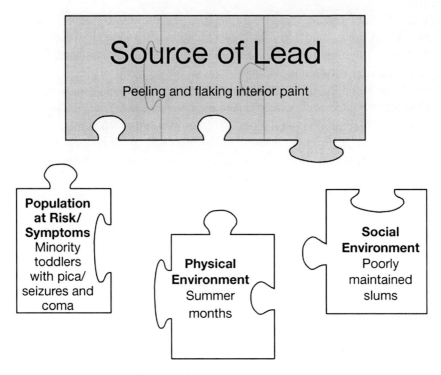

Figure 11. American Childhood Lead Poisoning, 1950-1975

supervision was limited because of the necessity for working parents to be away from home."[52]

The New Ecology of Childhood Lead Poisoning

By the 1960s pediatricians and public health officials embraced the new ecology of childhood lead poisoning. (See figure 11.) Emil Tiboni and Raymond Tyler, who had described the disease in Philadelphia's crumbling slums, stated it well: "[Childhood lead poisoning occurs] in older residential areas where a complex of adverse health, social, educational, and economic factors is present."[53] In a detailed analysis, drawing on nearly two decades of experience with the new ecology in Baltimore, Julian Chisholm described the complicated web that resulted in childhood lead poisoning: "Lead poisoning in the young child is a chronic disease. It results from the impact upon the urban slum child, in particular, of a variety of causative factors—pica and environmental exposure to lead, cultural and behavioral patterns of parents and certain aspects of lead metabolism."[54]

What did not change with this new ecology was the physical expression of the disease. Lead poisoning was a disease of visible symptoms. It took substantial lead to produce seizures and coma. When Baltimore health officials measured the blood lead levels in the children who prompted the reassessment in 1948, they discovered that the values were high, ranging from 100 to 700 micrograms/dl.[55]

Blaming the Victims?

By calling attention to aggressive eating practices and the need for parental vigilance, public health officials focused attention on the role of children and parents in the development of household lead poisoning. Exhorting parents regarding the dangers of repainting household objects also placed a heavy burden on those who were often the least able to change their environments. But identifying peeling and flaking paint as the hazard changed the focus of the public health response. No parent could protect an infant against flakes strewn throughout a decaying tenement. The public health effort needed to shift to cleaning up the blighted inner city and to address the lead content of paint. At the same time, efforts were under way to find a more efficacious therapy with which to treat affected children.

Chapter 9   New Therapies

In the 1950s LEAD poisoning became a treatable disease. Until then, there were two schools of thought on how to manage the symptoms of lead poisoning. The emphasis on symptoms was a key point. No pediatrician or industrial physician advocated any treatment unless easily identifiable symptoms existed. Unfortunately in children, the first symptoms were often seizures and coma. Joseph Aub and Robert Kehoe had provided industrial physicians with differing approaches to lead-sickened workers. In the 1920s, on the basis of animal experiments with lead and calcium metabolism, Aub discovered that most lead was located in the skeleton. Calcium and lead share properties, and Aub found that a diet high in calcium permitted the body to enhance its excretion of lead. Kehoe, in his studies of lead metabolism in workers, discovered that simply removing a worker from the source of lead permitted the body's normal excretion to lower lead to levels that did not provoke symptoms. Neither Aub nor Kehoe addressed therapy in children, but pediatricians usually combined approaches, providing a diet high in calcium (milk) and protective hospitalization. Depending on how much lead a child had ingested, it might take weeks or even months for a child's body to excrete lead to safer levels.

Lessons from chemical warfare in World War II added another approach. A drug developed to neutralize and promote excretion of arsenical war gases, 2,3-Dimercaptopropanal (also known as BAL or "British Anti-Lewisite," lewisite being an arsenical poison), was found after the war to be effective in treating another metallic poison: lead.[1] As might be expected, Kehoe was one of the first to test BAL in adults.[2] He found that the blood level of lead dropped within minutes, with the lead promptly finding its way into the urine. Within hours, however, additional lead left the skeleton, entering the blood, and the blood lead level rose.[3]

Pediatricians in Baltimore were quick to seize on the potential of BAL for the treatment of children. In 1949, within months after the Health Department noted the upsurge in lead-poisoned children, nine toddlers, from eighteen months to four years of age, were admitted to the Harriet Lane Home with severe lead encephalopathy. All suffered seizures; most had lapsed into coma. All had markedly high blood lead levels, ranging from 150 to 510 micrograms/dl. All received BAL for at least four days, some for as long as two weeks. Most children awoke from coma after several days. Two children died. The mortality in the BAL-treated group was considerably less than similarly sickened children in Baltimore who did not receive BAL.[4]

Across town, physicians at the University of Maryland, which also had the benefit of blood lead measurements from the Baltimore Health Department, likewise tested BAL. They compared the mortality rate of children treated for lead encephalopathy prior to BAL (1931–1948) with that of sixteen similar patients who received BAL. These children had blood lead levels from 80 to 730 micrograms/dl. BAL lowered the mortality rate to 6 percent from 26 percent.[5]

What particularly excited these physicians was that most of the survivors seemed neurologically less damaged when compared with survivors who had not received BAL. Psychological assessments of lead-poisoned children were scanty indeed in 1950. The 1943 study of Randolph Byers, who was still investigating the upturn in cases in Boston, and Elizabeth Lord, remained the only study of survivors that included an evaluation of school performance. Although the Baltimore physicians conceded that it was too soon to measure long-range neurological outcomes, their initial assessment of the children treated with BAL indicated that about one-half appeared normal. Significantly, improvement in neurological outcome became the goal of treatment and, over the next decade, the impetus for early identification of cases.

Other pediatricians quickly followed suit. Among the most determined were physicians at Kings' County Hospital, Brooklyn. Their initial studies differed significantly from ones in Baltimore in that the children selected for treatment had milder symptoms of encephalopathy, such as loss of balance. None suffered seizures or coma. In addition, the New York City doctors did not assess their patients for residual neurological damage.[6] Despite these limitations, they were impressed that their patients improved much more rapidly than if they had not received BAL. A follow-up study a year later permitted these physicians to conclude that their patients fared better neurologically than patients who had received the standard calcium treatment.[7]

EDTA

BAL ushered in the new therapeutic era; EDTA revolutionized it. EDTA, or ethylenediaminetetraacetic acid (trade name Versene), is a drug that attracts lead from tissues, renders it harmless and soluble, and permits excretion through the kidneys. The chemical process is called "chelation." EDTA is able to remove more lead from the human body more quickly than BAL.

On June 1, 1950, a three-year-old boy in Washington, D.C., convulsed while pulling on his shoes. His parents had been unaware of any illness until the seizure. They quickly brought him to Children's Hospital, where doctors recorded that he was "semi-comatose." For three days, doctors pondered the diagnosis, suspecting infection. Frustrated, they searched for rarer causes of seizure and coma, and on questioning the parents, they discovered that "the child had eaten the paint from 3 window-sills in the past 8 months." His blood lead level was 417 micrograms/dl. On the ninth hospital day, he received EDTA, apparently the first child recipient. EDTA was not commercially available for use in humans and had to be obtained from Riker Laboratories in Los Angeles. Physicians in Washington had to modify the chemical so that it could be given intravenously. During treatment, the boy suffered problems with blood pressure and kidney function, which caused his doctors to modify their therapeutic plans. Despite these concerns, the boy's clinical improvement was remarkable. In all he received twelve days of treatment.[8] By the end of 1952, these physicians— with a collaborator in Milwaukee—had treated eleven patients, three of them children.[9]

In short order, physicians from around the country used EDTA to treat lead-poisoned patients. Manfred Bowditch and the Lead Industries Association agreed to serve as an information clearinghouse, and by early 1953 physicians had sent Bowditch records of over 125 patients. Deciding how to use the drug was a complicated process, but accomplished with relative swiftness. When EDTA was initially employed, there was no notion of the correct dose, route of administration (oral, intramuscular, or intravenous), spacing of treatment, or duration. There was also no agreement on which lead-poisoned persons stood to benefit. What the LIA registry did was to aid physicians in sorting out these issues before the subsequent reports were published.[10]

There were many technical issues.[11] A crucial one was that there was no measure of the total amount of lead in the body or the amount that needed to be removed so that the danger was diminished. On the basis of research by Aub and Kehoe, physicians understood that most of the lead was stored in bones, where it caused no harm. Physicians differed on what clinical test best reflected the total lead content in the body. Some believed that blood lead was most sensitive, but most hospitals in the early 1950s did not have the ability to measure blood lead. Others argued that urinary excretion of lead was a better clinical measure. This was a more readily available test. When it came time to administer EDTA, pediatricians faced problems that industrial physicians did not. For example, most doctors came to believe that the intramuscular or intravenous route of administering EDTA was better than oral dosing. Yet babies had less muscle mass for repeated injections, and maintaining intravenous catheters was a challenge. Children also developed complications of therapy because of their small size.[12] One of the early investigators of EDTA in children was Randolph Byers, whose research was funded by the Lead Industries Association.[13]

Technical issues aside, all pediatricians believed that the reason to treat children was to end encephalopathy as soon as possible, thus preventing brain damage. The availability of effective treatment motivated pediatricians to seek out and diagnose cases promptly. As Julian Chisholm, the pediatrician at Johns Hopkins who contributed greatly to the understanding of childhood lead poisoning from the mid-1950s through the mid-1980s, explained: "The availability of a new and effective therapeutic agent has resulted in renewed interest in lead intoxication in childhood."[14]

Physicians in the 1950s thus had the choice of two drugs that greatly improved the outcome of lead-poisoned children. Although doctors in Brooklyn advocated BAL until late in the decade,[15] most pediatricians selected EDTA because of a perceived advantage in neurological functioning.[16] In the late 1950s, physicians had yet a third drug, penicillamine, which had been used previously to aid in the removal of excess copper in Wilson's disease. Penicillamine had the advantage of being orally administered.[17] It was not tested in children until the 1960s.

Effective Therapy Makes Accurate Diagnosis Imperative

In the early 1950s, physicians still made a diagnosis of lead poisoning on the basis of symptoms (encephalopathy, colic, peripheral neuropathy, anemia).[18] Laboratory tests, such as skeletal X-rays[19] or the stippling of red blood cells,[20] served only as an aid. Blood lead levels were available for clinicians in very few places, most prominently in Baltimore and to a lesser extent in Cincinnati. Lab tests thus supported the diagnosis but did not make it. In part, this reluctance to rely on laboratory tests was based on the recognition that it remained technically quite difficult to measure lead quantitatively in bodily fluids.

In this period, with lead in the atmosphere and coating most foods, all people, from infancy to old age, had lead in their bodies at levels that we would find wholly unacceptable today. Therefore sampling blood or urine for the presence of lead would almost always yield a positive result. At issue was how much lead, not whether it was detectable. There were several techniques for quantifying lead, but most observers believed that errors readily occurred. In toddlers, measurement was even harder because of the volumes of blood involved and the difficulty of collecting all urine produced over an interval of time (some inevitably lost in the diaper or spilling in a poorly cooperative child).[21]

Effective therapy inserted urgency into diagnosis. Physicians needed a rapid and accurate means of determining the amount of lead in a worker or child suspected of lead poisoning. The urine provided one avenue. Here we must turn to the biochemistry of lead metabolism. One effect of lead is to interfere with the synthesis of heme, a constituent of hemoglobin, which is one way lead causes anemia. With the formation of heme inhibited, a building block, porphyrin, is produced in excess and ultimately excreted in the urine in various chemical forms. Urinary porphyrin became the basis of a clinical test. As would be expected, the initial focus was on the workplace.[22] Later in the decade, physicians investigated another precursor of heme: delta-aminolevulinic acid. This metabolite would serve as the basis for both urinary and blood screening tests in the 1960s.[23]

By the mid-1950s Baltimore physicians employed urinary porphyrin tests to screen children for lead poisoning. With the unique ability to compare the urine test with blood lead levels, they discovered that the urine test was most accurate only at fairly high blood lead levels (over 100 micrograms/dl). This meant that a urine test would not serve as a reliable screening tool for children with moderate exposures, which did not produce symptoms. As we shall see, these lower levels had not concerned pediatricians previously. Effective therapy created a new category of concern.[24]

Even though blood lead levels were not generally available, most researchers believed that this test provided the most sensitive measurement of lead absorption.[25] The increasing reliance on blood lead levels shifted the emphasis in the way a pediatrician determined a diagnosis. Over the next decade, the lead level itself, not symptoms, became sufficient. This test became crucial as pediatricians became aware that lead could be harmful at levels lower than those required to produce symptoms. What blood lead level was "normal," what blood level was needed to produce symptoms, and at what point a child should be treated were questions that pediatricians debated—beginning in the 1950s and extending until today.[26]

In 1959 Lillis Altshuller, working with Robert Kehoe in Cincinnati, suggested another means of assessing the amount of lead in a child's body. Altshuller was concerned that a single measurement of blood or urine would indicate only a "snapshot" of lead. She suggested that measuring lead in "baby teeth" would provide a more accurate measure of lead exposure over longer periods.[27] This method would serve some researchers well in the 1970s.

Treatment Outcomes

Although lead poisoning produced a variety of symptoms, only neurological damage greatly worried pediatricians. Identifying children at risk for brain injury, treating them quickly before lead produced permanent damage, and assessing the extent of injury became hallmarks of patient care.

In the early 1950s Robert Mellins, a U.S. Public Health Service epidemiologist "on loan" to the Chicago Board of Health, and David Jenkins, a psychologist, attempted to assess the neurological outcome of children treated for lead poisoning in Chicago. Neither Mellins nor Jenkins was involved with the children's care during the treatment phase. Approximately four to six months after hospitalization, they carefully reviewed the patient charts, interviewed the parents, and administered psychological tests to the survivors. Chart review revealed that all the children had signs of encephalopathy (as had the children that Byers and Lord had studied a decade earlier). Some children received EDTA, but Mellins and Jenkins were not able to evaluate the effect of the treatment, why only some received the drug, and whether the differing dose schedules had any long-range effect. This failure to detail specific treatments most likely reflected the general hurly-burly that often accompanies the introduction of a "wonder" drug. Mellins and Jenkins found that the survivors lagged behind normal children in language and speech and in visual motor coordination. At issue was whether these children had been "normal" prior to their admission for lead poisoning. Mellins and Jenkins attempted to answer this question by interviewing the children's parents. In interviews—carried out several months after the child had been sickened, diagnosed, hospitalized, treated, and discharged—parents remembered their children as being normal except for aggressive eating behaviors. Mellins and Jenkins accepted the parents' recollections, but later pediatricians and psychologists pointed out that parental memory—always flattering when recalling children—might have been skewed after the trying experience of the illness. This, coupled with the usual tendency of children to regress in behavior when hospitalized, made assessment difficult.[28] Julius Richmond, a pediatrician who later became surgeon general, expressed his concern about assessing the level of development before lead poisoning:

> I think this raises another question in evaluating sequelae of this disorder. If we use such criteria as intellectual quotients as one very important one, it becomes very significant to know what these children were like before they ingested lead, again because of the factor of lack of stimulation. Historical data in this connection are not very valuable, because many of these parents would have regarded their children as being of perfectly normal development when, under usual test measurements, this might not have been the case, even prior to their developing symptoms.[29]

Mellins and Jenkins studied the children again two years after the illness. They found that most had improved in neurological functioning but that many had not recovered to normal levels. Deficits in speech, language, and emotional control were the major lingering effects.[30]

Mellins and Jenkins raised the issue of whether these lead-poisoned children had been entirely normal before their illnesses. In particular, they pointed to the aggressive eating behaviors that they viewed as strikingly abnormal.[31] Other pediatricians and psychiatrists also noted markedly abnormal feeding behaviors in lead-poisoned children.[32] This group of professionals believed that a disturbance in the child's relationship with parents resulted in pica.

These studies had all evaluated children with encephalopathy. What became clearer once blood lead levels became more commonly available was that not all children developed symptoms at the same blood level. At issue was whether neurological damage resulted from the lead alone or from a combination of lead with symptoms of encephalopathy, such as seizures or coma. Physicians in Cincinnati addressed this issue and concluded that symptoms were required for long-range injury.[33]

Baltimore physicians were optimistic about the neurological outcome of lead-poisoned children. They compared the intellectual and visual-motor functioning of sixteen children who suffered encephalopathy, eight treated with BAL and eight treated with EDTA. In both groups, the children functioned in the normal range, but the EDTA-treated group fared a bit better.[34]

There was little question that treatment enhanced survival. Most observers also believed that treatment greatly improved neurological outcomes. At issue were methodological problems that would plague researchers for decades: how to determine the prepoisoning level of functioning; which psychological tests best measure the effects of lead; and how other adverse environmental stresses—poverty, growing up in a slum, broken families—contribute to the failure to reach developmental potential.

Part IV

Industry and Public Health Responses

Chapter 10

One Percent Lead Content for Paint

By the end of 1950 Manfred Bowditch was beginning to understand that a new public health response to childhood lead poisoning was needed and that the LIA should take the initiative in bringing it about: "I continue to work as closely as possible with the pediatricians and others in Boston, Baltimore and elsewhere who are concerned with this problem and all the information I can secure is of potential value in its ultimate solution."[1] The "ultimate solution" that Manfred Bowditch had in mind was a national standard for the lead content of paint for interior use. To accomplish this goal, he used his LIA position to coordinate his contacts across industry, universities, health departments, insurance companies, the American Academy of Pediatrics, and governments on various levels.[2]

In December 1950 Bowditch discussed childhood lead poisoning at a joint meeting of the National Safety Council and the American Academy of Pediatrics.[3] On March 28, 1951, Bowditch met with George Wheatley of the American Academy of Pediatrics, Robert Kehoe, and Dr. Kotte to discuss lead poisoning in Cincinnati.[4] At that meeting, George Wheatley became an "enthusiastic rooter." (Bowditch made the return trip to New York with Wheatley.)[5] Bowditch also helped to engineer a citywide program for Cincinnati.[6]

George Wheatley's enthusiasm was in full evidence on May 23, when he delivered a speech, "Can Accidental Trauma Be Prevented?" at a meeting of the Massachusetts Medical Society. Wheatley included a section on lead poisoning, mentioning the upsurge of cases in Baltimore and Boston. He included his thoughts on prevention: "The cause in young children is usually due to pica and the source of lead is usually lead-containing paint on window sills, play yards, toys, etc., which have been repainted by amateurs. Inside woodwork is rarely painted with a lead-containing paint by professional painters and reputable toy and juvenile furniture manufacturers do not use toxic paints on their products. Prevention must be centered chiefly on educating parents about the danger of permitting children to chew or suck on painted objects or surfaces."[7] Bowditch also kept Wheatley informed of Baltimore's new cases and the activities of the Baltimore Health Department.[8]

Despite Wheatley's awareness of household lead poisoning, he understood that lead represented only a small fraction of home poisonings. In 1953, for example, lead accounted for 1.2 percent of childhood poisonings reported to the Committee on Accident Prevention of the American Academy of Pediatrics. Medicines, kerosene, cleaning materials, and insecticides headed the list.[9]

The Baltimore Plan and Peeling and Flaking Paint

On June 29, 1951, Huntington Williams, using his authority to issue and enforce health-related housing regulations, banned the use of paints containing lead pigments in Baltimore, becoming the first city to pass such an ordinance: "No paint shall be used for interior painting of any dwelling or dwelling unit or any part thereof unless the paint is free from any lead pigment."[10] Two months later, Williams added peeling and flaking paint to the list of health hazards covered by the Baltimore Plan.

In December, Baltimore's ordinance and the peeling and flaking paint that provoked it received comment in the *American Journal of Public Health*. The commentator, seemingly unaware of Bowditch's efforts with leading health departments, was not certain whether Baltimore's experience was applicable to other cities: "The question naturally arises whether babies brought up in the shadow of 'the Hopkins' develop peculiar alimentary tastes not common elsewhere. If such is not the case, perhaps other health officers have been missing something."[11]

Baltimore's ordinance also caught the attention of the U.S. Public Health Service. In a memo to Katherine Bain, a physician in the Children's Bureau, J. O. Dean, assistant surgeon general, proposed that Huntington Williams submit a paper on Baltimore's experience to *Public Health Reports*. Dean, who also appears unaware of LIA efforts, cautioned against endorsing Williams's observations on the peeling and flaking hazard and Baltimore's new ordinance:

> It is the opinion of our industrial hygiene staff that it would be unwise
> for the Service or the Agency to circulate a specific notice on the sub-
> ject because of the public relations problem that a notice from the Ser-
> vice or the Agency would be sure to develop with the lead industry.
> Furthermore, such endorsement of the action taken by the Baltimore
> City Health Department, and in the absence of any more widespread
> evidence that is here available our experts caution against early endorse-

ment of the proposal. They believe, however, that the Baltimore action deserves wide publicity and therefore suggested the *Public Health Reports* article.[12]

Also in 1951, New York City—experiencing an upturn in cases—investigated twenty cases of childhood lead poisoning.[13] A problem, quickly identified by George Wheatley, was that unlike Baltimore, New York City had no centralized laboratory to measure blood lead.[14] Beginning in 1952, members of the health departments of New York City and Baltimore exchanged information.[15]

Manfred Bowditch

On December 19, 1951, Bowditch wrote to Reginald Atwater, executive secretary of the American Public Health Association, informing him of the increase in lead poisoning cases around the country and of the need for an "all-out preventive attack on this very difficult problem." Bowditch volunteered his office as a clearinghouse.[16]

Also in December, Wheatley, representing the American Academy of Pediatrics, met with the American Standards Association—at the suggestion of Bowditch—to work toward a national safe standard for the lead content of paint to be used on "articles such as furniture, toys, etc., or for interior use in dwelling units where it might be chewed by children."[17] A Committee on Hazards to Children (AAP/ASA committee) was organized to deal with standards for lead-based paints, as well as other hazards to children. The LIA participated in this group from the start; Manfred Bowditch served as the secretary of its subcommittee on a paint standard. Even before the AAP/ASA committee had completed its work, Bowditch announced its intent in a speech he delivered at the First Conference on Home Accident Prevention (January 20–23, 1953), sponsored by the National Safety Council, the U.S. Public Health Service, the American Public Health Association, and the W. K. Kellogg Foundation.[18] In addition to Bowditch, the membership of the American Standards Association Committee on Hazards to Children included the American Medical Association, the American Hospital Association, the American Public Health Association, the Child Study Association of America, the Department of Health, Education, and Welfare's Children's Bureau, the Food and Drug Administration, the U.S. Public Health Service, the National League of Nursing, the National Safety Council, the National Society for Crippled Children and Adults, the New York City Department of Health, and the New York State Department of Health. Industry also had broad representation on this committee.[19]

Wheatley and Bowditch's initial agenda was to negotiate a voluntary standard establishing a safe amount of lead to be used in paints covering toys, cribs, and other furniture. This agenda quickly evolved to include interior surfaces of places where children lived.[20] The resulting standard was a consensus achieved among public health officials, industry, and governments. The AAP/ASA committee wanted industry to embrace this standard; enforcement would be voluntary.

From the start of the committee's deliberations, industry members wanted the ASA standard to be a single, national gauge. With several cities and states considering restrictions on the amount of permissible lead in paint in the wake of the peeling and flaking paint hazard, the industry worried that a multitude of differing regulations would make marketing and distributing paint in multiple markets difficult.[21]

The ASA decided that paints with less than 1 percent lead were safe for use on interior walls and ceilings, toys, cribs, and other furniture where children lived and played. To reach this conclusion, the group relied on various theoretical calculations that estimated how much lead a toddler needed to ingest to produce poisoning and how many square inches of dried paint a child with pica needed to consume daily to reach this dangerous level.[22] One percent appeared to meet these theoretical requirements, but one member, representing the American Medical Association, was concerned that multiple coats of 1 percent paint might still be unsafe. The AMA later withdrew its objection.[23]

The standard was proposed in November 1954 and adopted in early 1955. The 1 percent limit accomplished the removal of lead pigment from interior paint. Only a small amount of lead remained, in paint's "driers." The 1 percent standard became the centerpiece of all state and local laws and regulations on the content of lead in paint until the 1970s, when pediatricians, government-sponsored researchers, and several federal regulatory agencies began to question the safety of even 1 percent lead paint.

New York City

Between 1953 and 1955 New York City, which had only lately mobilized against childhood lead poisoning, faced the problem of what to do until the AAP/ASA committee, on which it had membership, hashed out a consensus. There were groups in New York City that advocated that the city go it alone, others who urged that the city wait and join the national standard, and still others who wanted a warning label on cans of paint containing more than 1 percent lead.[24] By looking closely at New York City's evolving actions, we can gain an appreciation of how the lead-paint hazard was understood.

In the early 1950s, New York City experienced the increase in childhood lead poisoning cases that had hit Baltimore a few years earlier. Between 1951 and 1952, the Health Department investigated thirty-five cases.[25] These cases provoked an internal debate within the department over whether the public should be warned about the danger of chewing lead paint.[26] On March 29, 1953, John Mahoney, commissioner of health, decided that the time had arrived and issued a news release.[27]

As would be expected, New York City consulted with officials at Baltimore's Health Department before striking out on its own with a warning label.[28] By the summer of 1953, the New York City Health Department had a draft proposal: "WARNING: Contains Lead. Not to be Used for Painting Toys, Furniture or Interior of Dwelling."[29]

On September 24, 1953, George Wheatley wrote to William Sauer of the Bureau of Sanitary Inspections in New York City and detailed the history of the AAP/ASA committee and its goals. Wheatley credited Manfred Bowditch with the idea and the early organizational efforts. Wheatley then explained that the American Academy of Pediatrics was working with the New York Academy of Medicine, especially with early trials with the chelating agent EDTA. Wheatley tried to persuade Sauer to wait for the ASA proposal, arguing that a national standard would have the most wide-reaching effect.[30]

The LIA and the National Paint, Varnish, and Lacquer Association (NPVLA) participated in New York City's debates. Both organizations supported the thrust of the effort but objected to two points. First, both trade organizations wanted a uniform national standard rather than many different state and city regulations. From their point of view, a uniform standard simplified the marketing and distribution of paints. Second, both organizations opposed the use of the word "poison" on the label.[31]

The word "poison" on legally mandated labels had a history in the early 1950s. In discussing the content of warning labels, the Manufacturing Chemists' Association had also taken a position against the use of the word "poison": "The commonly accepted meaning of 'Poison' refers to single dose oral toxicity. It covers inadequately, in a quantitative sense, the hazards from acute and chronic exposure, ingestion, skin absorption and inhalation. Therefore, in most cases the use of a signal word such as 'DANGER,' 'WARNING,' or 'CAUTION' with a statement of the hazard present is much more informative."[32] Lead in paint, of course, did not conform to the "commonly accepted meaning" of "poison." Children became poisoned not from a single dose, but from nibbling paint flakes over time. Robert E. Mellins, an epidemiologist with the U.S. Public Health Service who was working with the Chicago Board of Health on childhood lead poisoning, urged Jerome Trichter, assistant commissioner for environmental sanitation of the New York Board of Health, to abandon the "poison" designation.[33] Trichter accepted this advice.

On August 10, 1954, Trichter presented three additional proposed wordings at the commissioner's staff meeting. They shared some elements but differed on others:

American Standards Association: "This product conforms with the American Standard Z66.1 for materials safe for the use on children's furniture toys, etc., or surfaces which may be chewed by children." [Paints containing more than 1 percent would not carry this approval, but would not be required to designate a warning.]

National Paint, Varnish, and Lacquer Association: "This paint is warranted to contain not more than 1 percent lead, including pigment and drier. Suitable for any interior painting, including children's furniture and articles."

"This paint contains more than 1 percent lead and is NOT suitable for interior painting, including children's furniture and toys."

New York City Health Department: "WARNING—This Paint Contains More than 1 Percent of lead. POISONOUS—and should not be used for interior painting or for children's toys or furniture."

Each organization accepted the 1 percent standard, but each warning contained subtle differences. The ASA label covered only paints with less than 1 percent lead; the NPVLA label made separate designations for paints with less than or more than 1 percent lead; and the Health Department would label only those paints that exceeded the safe level. In addition, the Health Department proposal included a "poison" label.[34]

The following day, the ASA considered a modified interior phrasing that clearly indicated: "A liquid coating to be deemed suitable from a health standpoint for use on article[s] such as furniture, toys, etc. or for interior use in dwelling units where it might be chewed by children."[35] The NPVLA, meeting the next day, discussed the various proposals.[36]

The New York City Health Department considered the pros and cons of a "poison" label and ultimately rejected the idea. The label it approved on October 29, 1954, conformed with the 1 percent guideline proposed by the AAP/ASA committee: "Contains lead. Harmful if eaten. Do not apply on toys, furniture, or interior surfaces which might be chewed by children."[37]

New York City—with the support of the LIA and NPVLA—eventually settled on language that included "chewing." Certainly this choice of words addressed children who gnawed on cribs, toys, and woodwork. But as some pointed out, how would a child "chew" a wall? The newly perceived danger included not only gnawing but also swallowing paint flakes lying on the floor. All parties understood this new hazard, and their choice of "chew" encompassed both the older concern of gnawing on objects and the newer concern of swallowing flakes of paint. In 1959 the Board of Health spelled out its reasons for the phrasing:

The board thought that the language implying that children chew walls was not the most desirable. The representative of the New York Paint,

Varnish, and Lacquer Association requested that the Board refrain from changing the wording, even though not desirable, because the Association at some cost had already recommended to some 4000 members that such a warning be used. . . . Since [the regulation] has been in effect for several years, and manufacturers have prepared labels in accordance with its provisions at considerable cost, it would be undesirable now, without convincing evidence of the inadequacy of the present warning, to change the required wording. Furthermore, as Dr. Harold Jacobziner advised the Board at the October, 1954 meeting . . . to the extent that children chew on window sills and eat fallen pieces of paint and plaster, they do chew interior surfaces.[38]

What did the removal of lead from pigments accomplish? It did not eliminate old lead paint already applied to walls. Application of 1 percent paint over high-lead paint cut down on peeling and flaking, especially if the repainted wall or ceiling was properly scraped and sanded. For new construction, the 1 percent standard eliminated household lead poisoning. For example, in Cleveland, a comparison of old and new public housing revealed only a few cases of childhood lead poisoning in the new buildings, and these involved children who had been cared for in older housing.[39] A similar conclusion was reached in New York City. Harold Jacobziner, an official of the New York Department of Health, observed: "Lead paint poisoning is inextricably linked with old, dilapidated housing. No cases are being reported among children living in newly constructed housing projects even in the districts of highest incidence."[40] Pediatricians and Health Department officials reported no cases of childhood lead poisoning, as understood in the 1950s and 1960s, attributed to the consumption of 1 percent paint. Edmund Bradley, a pediatrician who had been active in Baltimore's campaign against lead poisoning, summarized the state of events for a broad audience in *Parade*: "It is true that builders and reputable manufacturers now avoid using lead paint wherever children can come in contact with it. Furthermore, lead paint now costs more than other kinds; this gives builders a reason for using it only on outside work, for its weathering qualities. . . . The fight against lead poisoning is being waged on several fronts. One is the development of EDTA. Another is through law and the cooperation of progressive paint manufacturers."[41]

Chapter 11	Urban Lead Programs of the 1950s and 1960s

CHANGED ECOLOGICAL CIRCUMSTANCES of childhood lead poisoning combined with effective therapy to goad urban public health departments to develop programs to identify, prevent, and treat lead-poisoned children. Baltimore, with its long-standing concern over domestic lead poisoning coupled with its central role in discovering both ecology and treatment, led the way, followed closely by other "lead-belt" northern and midwestern cities: New York, Boston, Philadelphia, Cincinnati, Cleveland, St. Louis, and Chicago. The story in each municipality was a part of the politics of coming to grips with the "inner city." As such, each story was unique. But the imperatives of ecology and treatment dictated that each urban program have common elements.

Children were not equally at risk, so public health authorities needed to identify those who lived in older, deteriorating housing. City health departments had to perfect methods for quickly and inexpensively screening targeted children—by questioning parents about pica, testing urine for porphyrin, or, in a few cases, determining blood lead. Children found to have dangerously high levels of lead needed to be admitted to a hospital for chelation therapy. Once discharged, they needed close observation to monitor whether they reencountered lead and whether they had suffered permanent neurological consequences. Home health visitors assessed homes and apartments to discover the source of lead; once it was identified, landlords or parents needed to make repairs, or the family needed to move. These measures were expensive, and each city had to find the funds.

Prevention was frustrating. All families living in blighted housing needed constant educating about the dangers of peeling and flaking lead paint; landlords had to be urged to repair walls and either to remove lead paint or cover it with less toxic materials; home repainters had to select paints that met the 1 percent safe standard advocated by the American Standards Association. Each of these preventive measures faced daunting challenges.

Many cities passed restrictive bans on the use of lead paints for interiors, and many communities required labels that specified the lead content of paints. Although the wording of bans and labels differed slightly from city to city, all essentially conformed to the 1 percent ASA standard.

Baltimore

Even though alerted to the rising number of lead-poisoned children, the Baltimore Health Department was still surprised by the "shockingly high record" of 77 cases and 9 deaths in 1951.[1] There were 110 deaths from all causes in 1951 among Baltimore's children aged one to four years: lead ranked fourth behind pneumonia, tuberculosis, and congenital malformations.[2] Forty-six children had blood lead levels higher than 100 micrograms/dl. Once a case was identified— usually in one of the city's emergency rooms—Margaret Galbreath, a nurse on loan from the Health Department's Bureau of Industrial Hygiene, visited the child's home. In 1951 Galbreath made 399 home visits.[3] There she educated parents, investigated suspicious paint, and obtained scrapings to confirm the existence of lead, which was demonstrated in 56 percent of samples.[4] The Health Department mounted a traveling exhibit to alert physicians, and it flooded Baltimore with information in newspapers, television,[5] radio ("Death at the Window Sill, A Radio Play"),[6] and in pamphlets—"Lead Paint Poisoning in Children: A Disease You Can Prevent"—handed out during well-child visits. These pamphlets explained both the older worries (cribs, toys, woodwork) and the new ecology of flaking and peeling paint.[7] Officials were heartened when the cases declined in 1952 to 29 with 5 deaths.[8]

As soon as the Baltimore Health Department understood the new ecology of childhood lead poisoning, Huntington Williams issued a ban on the use of lead-based paints for interiors. He could do this because Baltimore had given the Health Department authority to monitor the health aspects of housing. Such congruent jurisdiction did not always occur in other cities.[9] In August 1951, lead paint officially became part of the Baltimore Plan for rejuvenating urban housing.[10]

During the early 1950s cases held fairly steady, but blood samples doubled as did the number of home visits. The Health Department had difficulty hiring enough home nurses and, when the Salk polio vaccine became available, needed to shift resources to provide enough personnel to administer injections. Despite limitations on resources, fatalities from lead poisoning declined to one in 1955, which officials attributed to parent education, to early detection, and to the availability of successful treatment.[11]

In May 1956 Julian Chisholm completed his detailed investigation of the Baltimore cases, a study that had been instigated by Manfred Bowditch and the Lead Industries Association and acknowledged by the Maryland legislature when it repealed the "Toxic Finishes" law six years earlier. This investigation became a landmark in the history of childhood lead poisoning. Chisholm and his collaborator, Harold Harrison, studied 197 children, including 89 with encephalopathy. Chisholm and Harrison divided their patients into categories, which included lead-poisoned children who did not have symptoms of brain disease. This was one of the first indications that pediatricians were concerned about children who had lead in their bodies but not enough to cause symptoms of encephalopathy.

Chisholm and Harrison investigated the location of lead paint and found that most came from windowsills and frames. Most paint came from interiors. They also noted that some children had been poisoned from eating exterior paint. Most of the offending paint—interior and exterior—had been applied many years earlier and contained far more lead than the ASA 1 percent standard. Virtually all children who had suffered from severe encephalopathy tested in the retarded range afterward; if these children returned with another episode of severe encephalopathy, all suffered severe mental handicaps.

Chisholm and Harrison reaffirmed the new ecology, but they made an important additional observation: "If it is conceded that no mother can reasonably be expected to prevent this type of ingestion in the face of crumbling paint and plaster, it will be recognized that proper maintenance of both interior and exterior painted surfaces is probably the most important environmental factor in the long-term aspect of prevention of childhood lead intoxication." Until this point, prevention had focused on parents' knowing that lead paint was hazardous if chewed from toys, cribs, or woodwork and keeping children from gnawing on such painted surfaces. Chisholm and Harrison recognized that the abundance of chips falling continually on floors in poorly maintained slum housing changed the complexity of the hazard altogether.[12]

Huntington Williams was frustrated by the city's failure to eliminate the problem, so in August 1956 he appointed a committee of Health Department officials to suggest further action.[13] The backgrounds of the membership of this task force—the Baltimore Lead Paint Poisoning Prevention Committee—indicates the bureaucratic complexity that Williams believed necessary for a successful program: members came from the Health Department's divisions of housing, industrial hygiene, laboratories, communicable diseases, health education, occupational diseases, environmental hygiene, sanitation, statistics, and medical care research.[14] Over the next year, this committee discussed additional educational programs, tying lead-poisoning prevention to diphtheria immunization in order to reach the parent of nearly every infant, and a law mandating removal of lead paint from homes in which a child had become lead-poisoned.

What particularly distressed the task force was a recent discovery that 35 percent of the families who lived in blighted housing had moved to Baltimore within the last five years.[15] Most were African Americans who had moved from the South, where knowledge of domestic lead poisoning had been scanty.[16] This knowledge brought home the futility of any single educational campaign: all Health Department educational programs would have to be repeated continually in order to reach newcomers. In addition, many of these families moved frequently, making any saturation educational program difficult.[17] A transient population also meant that making one apartment safe did not ensure that a family's next home would be safe. To meet these challenges, the Health Department targeted high-risk areas for an "all-out" program. Over 4,000 children were visited at home, parents educated, and paint samples taken. After the home visit, Huntington Williams sent a letter to the parents underscoring his concern for lead paint safety.[18] Despite all, the Health Department did not believe that this massive campaign had identified many cases that would not have come to its attention with less intensive canvassing.

One action that the committee advocated was a vigorous enforcement of the city's 1951 ban on lead paints for interiors. Although this restriction applied to all apartments,[19] the Health Department limited enforcement to landlords of housing where toddlers had been poisoned.[20] In 1957 a survey conducted by the Health Department and the Baltimore Urban Renewal and Housing Agency indicated that over 60 percent of apartments in blighted areas had significant peeling and flaking.[21] The Health Department developed rapid screening methods for inspectors to determine whether peeling and flaking paint contained lead pigment.[22] Landlords who received notices to remove old, flaking and peeling paint sought counsel from the Health Department on how to comply. In 1960 the Health Department issued guidelines: lead paint on walls up to a height of four feet had to be either removed completely or covered over with Masonite or plywood. Above four feet, the wall required sanding and repainting with paints that did not include lead pigments.[23]

The Health Department did not want children to return home until landlords had complied with paint removal or covering. Even though most landlords eventually responded, delays were common, placing a strain on hospitals in Baltimore that housed treated children who awaited a safe home. In November 1960 officials of the Health Department, the city's hospitals, and the Social Services Department met and arranged for expeditious assessment of apartments and for swift compliance of the landlord. If a treated child was ready for discharge prior to the removal or covering of lead paint, the child's family would be moved into another apartment, or, if one was unavailable, the child would go into temporary foster care.[24]

After considerable debate, the Lead Paint Poisoning Prevention Committee decided that Baltimore needed a warning label on paint cans to help with enforcement of the earlier regulation banning lead-based paint on interior surfaces. In 1954 New York City had approved a label that closely followed the ASA standard, and Baltimore considered adopting its wording. After discussion, Williams and the task force believed that the wording of the New York label placed too much emphasis on toys and furniture. In contrast, they wanted the Baltimore label to underscore the dangers of lead paint on walls, ceilings, and woodwork. Additionally, Williams observed that many cases had occurred when paint had flaked from ceiling heating pipes. To prevent this danger, he included a phrase that was more all-encompassing.[25] Mayor Thomas D'Alesandro signed the ordinance on June 9, 1958: "WARNING—Contains Lead. Harmful if Eaten. Do not apply on any interior surfaces of a dwelling, or of a place used for the care of children, or on window sills, toys, cribs, or other furniture."[26]

In 1958 Baltimore experienced another jump in childhood cases: 133 children with 10 deaths. The Health Department attributed the increase to "improvement in the recognition of the disease, the continued influx of migrants into the city particularly from the southern states, and the lack of parental supervision due, at least in part, to mothers working in order to supplement their spouse's income."[27] Huntington Williams increased his already sizable personal involvement. In one of these efforts, he was photographed under a "stalactite" ceiling of peeling lead paint.[28] Williams also sent a letter to paint dealers in Baltimore urging them to educate parents about the dangers of using lead paint for interiors.[29]

Putting warning labels on paint cans required ongoing negotiations between paint companies and the Health Department. In most cases, the companies sent proposed labels to the Health Department for approval.[30] In some instances, paint manufacturers wanted to substitute the warning label that was already in effect for New York City, arguing that multiple labels in different jurisdictions complicated marketing. Williams rejected these arguments, insisting on the precise language of Baltimore's warning label.[31] Every company complied.[32] Just how large the warning label needed to be was another point for negotiation. Some proposed lettering was so small that the warning could be easily overlooked.[33] In early 1959 Williams met with representatives of major paint companies to provide them with guidelines for acceptable warning labels.[34] What came of these negotiations was the requirement for lid labels 3 inches in diameter, with "Warning" in large boldface type.[35]

More than half of Baltimore's cases occurred in the Druid district, home to predominantly African Americans.[36] With so many cases coming from "lead alley," officials targeted the district. Nurses visited every home where a one-year-old child lived, swamped the area with educational materials, and included the subject in all well-baby visits.[37] To bring home the seriousness of the danger, the Health Department passed out a pamphlet with the banner headline

LEAD PAINT KILLS CHILDREN!
GET THE LEAD PAINT OUT OF YOUR HOME![38]

In 1959 Druid had over 30 cases with 2 deaths; a year later there were 10 cases and no deaths.[39]

In January 1962 Huntington Williams reconvened the Lead Paint Poisoning Prevention Committee. Dr. Maceo Williams, health director of the Druid district, chaired the new panel. The January and February meetings were sparked by debate between Huntington Williams, who believed that progress was being made, and George Schucker, from the city Bureau of Environmental Diseases, who thought that the Health Department was not doing enough and that landlords were being uncooperative.[40] Ignited by this debate, the Health Department embarked on an expanded campaign in a program called "Hard Sell."

The committee also debated what blood level should be considered abnormal, a point that had considerable public health implications. Julian Chisholm, a consultant to the group, suggested a level of 60 micrograms/dl.[41] Charles Couchman placed the level of concern at over 100 micrograms/dl.[42] Huntington Williams thought that 65 micrograms/dl was the upper limit of normal.[43] Robert Farber, who succeeded Williams as commissioner of health, defined a case of lead poisoning as over 100 micrograms/dl when accompanied by two or more symptoms.[44] To some, this higher level made considerable sense. Baltimore had recorded only two deaths in children who had blood lead levels below 100 micrograms/dl; most deaths occurred at levels above 200 micrograms/dl.[45] Of note, public health officials in Washington, D.C., considered a blood lead level between 60 and 80 micrograms/dl "suspicious" and above 80 micrograms/dl "toxic."[46] Physicians and policymakers would debate the blood lead level deemed dangerous over the coming decades, continually redefining it at lower and lower levels.

In 1965 there were no deaths from lead poisoning among children in Baltimore.[47] A year later, there was only 1.[48] In the late 1960s identified cases fell as well, so that in 1971 Baltimore had only 11 lead-poisoned children.[49]

Baltimore in Perspective

Baltimore officials were pleased with their program, because cases and deaths declined. Until the early 1970s, they—like all health departments—defined cases in terms of children with symptoms. This form of lead poisoning disappeared from Baltimore, and elsewhere, as the result of urban public health programs and the reduction of lead in interior paint. Lest officials rest on their laurels, it was precisely at this moment that researchers began to worry about the long-term effects of children with lead exposure that did not result in symptoms. Out of this new concern came a rebirth of lead poisoning, a "silent epidemic." In sharp contrast to the older lead poisoning, where cases were numbered in the hundreds for the country, the new lead poisoning encompassed hundreds of thousands—perhaps millions—and some believed it included every child who lived in the inner cities of the nation.

Although Baltimore officials were pleased with the decline in cases and deaths, one insight from the Hard Sell program chastened them: old lead paint was everywhere. With the continued aging of older apartments, the flakes and chips could only escalate. By 1965 it was clear that monitoring every inner-city dwelling for chips of deteriorating paint would exhaust the resources of a local health department.[50]

In 1962 Huntington Williams retired from the Health Department. His successor, Robert Farber, continued an interest in lead poisoning, but with time Baltimore would recede from leadership.[51]

New York City

Unlike Baltimore, other cities did not have a twenty-year track record with lead poisoning when the upsurge of cases began in the late 1940s. For these communities, the public health response had to start from scratch. Fortunately, Baltimore's experience often served as a template. Manfred Bowditch of the LIA also served as a clearinghouse of information for many of the urban health departments. In addition to studies in Baltimore, the LIA funded Randolph Byers's research efforts in Boston, and these studies were published in 1954, 1955, and 1959, adding insights to the new ecology of childhood lead poisoning that were helpful to cities planning lead programs.[52]

New York was one city where there was a great deal of catching up to do.[53] The city experienced a surge in cases four years after Baltimore. In 1950 there had been only 2 cases of childhood lead poisoning.[54] The following year there were 18 cases, 4 fatal.[55] What caught the attention of the New York Health Department were 11 deaths, in just 20 cases, in 1952.[56] Cases more than quadrupled two years later.[57] When Mary Culhane McLaughlin—who would later become commissioner of health—analyzed New York's 143 cases with 39 deaths to 1954, she found that all clustered in blighted areas among the poor. With the city lagging in means of rapid diagnosis, McLaughlin informed child health workers that pica might be the "only ready clue" of lead poisoning. Convinced of the value of pica as a means of identifying cases, in 1955 the Health Department embarked on a program using questions about eating behavior as a screening tool. This tactic alone doubled the number of identified cases.[58] In the early 1960s, New York City jumped from about 150 to 500 lead-poisoned children each year.[59]

Yet using pica as a screening test for lead poisoning failed to uncover most victims. Vincent Guinee, director of the Health Department's Bureau of Lead Poisoning Control, later explained: "Almost all cases of lead poisoning in children result from pica . . . and yet paradoxically, when a history of pica has been used as a case-finding method more cases were lost than found. Since a number of cases had been uncovered by eliciting this history, it was easy to see how this gradually became accepted as a good screening method. What was not appreciated was the large number of 'false negatives'—children with lead poisoning but whose mothers did not or would not volunteer a history of pica in their children."[60] Unfortunately, many mothers interpreted the question as a criticism of their effectiveness as parents in keeping children out of harm's way.

In 1968 the Health Department changed the screening question to: "Do you have a young child who is exposed to a deteriorating housing environment?" After the switch from pica to a dangerous environment, detected cases rose from 727 in 1969 to 2,649 in 1970.[61]

Citizen groups were not pleased with the Health Department's pace.[62] They suspected that New York had far more lead-poisoned children and were appalled to learn how little New York spent compared with other cities. In particular, they were outraged that the city had screened only 5,000 children in 1968, a small number when compared with Chicago's record.[63] In 1969 a number of events occurred that galvanized the city into action. Mary McLaughlin became commissioner of health. Her early concern for lead poisoning moved the issue up on the public agenda. She requested and obtained funding for blood lead testing, paving the way for a major screening program.[64] Community groups—going door-to-door in selected neighborhoods—also identified cases.[65] Some activist groups performed home urinary screening tests.[66] Writing with passion in the *Village Voice* in 1969, Jack Newfield helped to catalyze the city and its Health Department to action. Newfield was critical not only of the Health Department but also of the lack of concern of the NAACP and the United Federation of Teachers.[67] Vincent Guinee, who had spearheaded the vaccine program for rubella in New York City, was appointed to the new post of director of the Bureau of Lead Poisoning Control.[68]

St. Louis

St. Louis was the only other city to provide blood lead levels. Beginning in 1946, the Health Department performed this service for the city's hospitals. Designed primarily as an aid for uncovering industrial cases of lead poisoning, the diagnostic test was also offered for children. When a child demonstrated excess lead, the Health Department visited the home seeking to find the source. Providing this service allowed St. Louis officials to realize that, between 1949 and 1951, children poisoned at home equaled the number of occupational cases (53 occupational, 50 children). All of the children were between eight months and seven years of age. St. Louis officials did not publish the sources of lead for these children. During these years, blood lead values in cases considered to have a "definite diagnosis" ranged from 78 to 540 micrograms/dl.[69]

Cincinnati

From the mid-1930s, Robert Kehoe and the Kettering Laboratory at the University of Cincinnati on occasion provided laboratory support for pediatricians who wished to determine the blood lead level of seriously ill children. At the end of World War II, the Health Department reorganized its child health section and opened a pediatric clinic.[70] In 1948 the department turned its attention to the health problems of the developing slums in its inner city, particularly focusing on sanitation, sewerage, elimination of outside toilets, and provision of adequate light and ventilation.[71] Over the next years, the Board of Health became "vitally interested in housing and slum elimination."[72] In 1950 the Health Department carried out a survey of 6,500 urban dwellings using the checklist of the American Public Health Association.[73] Paint was not included in this survey.

In 1950-51, Manfred Bowditch engaged Robert Kehoe, the pediatricians in the University of Cincinnati Hospital, and Health Department officials in a dialogue about the upswing in cases that was occurring locally and in several other cities. In Cincinnati, the upturn occurred in 1949 and 1950. Out of this cooperative effort, the Health Department added childhood lead poisoning to its agenda: "Bureau inspectors cooperated with physicians from Kettering Laboratories and Children's Hospital in an effort to evaluate some of the causative factors of cases of lead poisoning in children. This involved the careful inspection of all homes in which lead poisoning had occurred, in an effort to find the cause and to prescribe definite methods of elimination and control."[74] In Cincinnati the child lead program became an amalgam of university and city hospitals (treatment), Kettering Laboratory (laboratory support), and Health Department (home investigation by visiting nurses). By 1953 the Health Department concluded that childhood lead poisoning was a "growing public health problem."[75] Five years later, nurses brought up lead poisoning during every home visit. When lead poisoning was the reason for the home investigation, the nurses obtained paint scrapings from the dwelling. Kettering Laboratory analyzed both scrapings and the child's blood for lead.[76] In 1959, Cincinnati—paralleling a similar explosion in Baltimore—suffered a dramatic increase in the number of cases: 68 children compared with approximately 10–12 cases per year before.[77]

Philadelphia

For Philadelphia too there was an upsurge in cases in 1958. As elsewhere the public health response included home inspections, targeted areas where older homes and apartments were likely to have pre–World War II paint, extensive education, and a requirement that every case be reported to the Health Department.[78] Epidemiological spot maps pinpointed the location of cases permitting the marshaling of efforts where most cases occurred.[79] Emil Tiboni, chief of the Accident Control Section, provided a blueprint for urban childhood lead programs:

> Detection—screening targeted populations of children, education of health professionals to recognize cases, official reporting of cases, inclusion of lead poisoning screening as part of all well-baby clinics, screening of siblings of all cases.
> Environmental investigation—home investigation of every case; selective home surveys in high-risk neighborhoods.
> Education—professionals, public at large, at-risk populations.
> Legal controls—prohibitions of paint with more than 1 percent lead, removal of old paint, labeling.
> Services—diagnostic tests, tests of paint samples, social work for finding safer housing.
> Treatment

Tiboni also detailed Philadelphia's efforts to engage landlords and religious organizations in paint removal.[80]

Chicago

In Chicago, cases jumped to 13 per year in 1953 compared with a fourteen-year average of less than 2 per year. Home visits were begun that year to identify the sources of paint. The Health Department provided the laboratory back-up (mostly urine tests), and the Children's Memorial Hospital admitted children for treatment with EDTA.[81] Robert Mellins, whom we met in our discussion of neurological outcomes, was involved in the home investigations of these children. Cases jumped again in 1959, with 142 children diagnosed at Cook County

Children's Hospital alone, 42 of whom had lead encephalopathy.[82] Chicago's program caught the attention of *Time* in 1963.[83] The Poison Control Center recorded that during a three-year period, 1959–1961, Chicago had 9,853 accidental poisonings; lead was the cause of 429, or 4.7 percent. There were 85 deaths during this same period, 67 due to lead, or 79 percent of the total.[84] Most deaths occurred in just a few districts, and the Health Department targeted these for a screening test with urinary coproporphyrin. In one high-risk district 18 percent had a positive urine test; of these, nearly one-half were diagnosed as suffering lead poisoning. These startlingly high numbers led to additional large screening surveys. The results would both alert and frighten the nation.[85]

Seasonality

Urban studies explored additional epidemiological aspects of childhood lead poisoning. One was seasonality.[86] For decades, many observers had noted that children most often became poisoned during warm weather, whether in the extreme temperatures of Queensland or during the summers of Baltimore, Boston, or New York. Many of the educational programs sponsored by the Baltimore Health Department reflected this distinct seasonal risk. Why would a hazard, which in the 1930s and 1940s consisted of exposure to painted cribs and toys or in the 1950s to peeling and flaking interior paints, vary with the seasons? Anna Baetjer, who worked in Baltimore, believed that hot weather produced dehydration that enhanced the effects of lead in the system. Julian Chisholm, reviving Joseph Aub's metabolic studies linking calcium and lead, thought that sunlight and vitamin D mobilized lead that had been stored in a child's bones.[87]

Air Pollution

In the early 1960s researchers investigated atmospheric lead from the exhausts of internal combustion engines. There was considerable lead in the air that every American breathed, and investigators began to determine how much lead from the air made its way into each citizen.[88] Some studies of adults revealed that air pollution accounted for a blood level of about 20 micrograms/dl of lead, a value that other researchers questioned. Although children were not evaluated, presumably infants and toddlers received a similar dose of atmospheric lead.[89] For pediatricians concerned about children living in decaying cities, the worry was the potential additive danger of deteriorating lead paint and tetraethyl lead.

Household Poisonings

How did lead compare with other household poisonings at mid-century? Katherine Bain, a physician at the U.S. Children's Bureau, concluded that lead was a significant, but certainly not the most common, household poison in children.[90] Bain found that the most common poison was kerosene, followed by aspirin and other drugs. Lead and corrosives came next in frequency, followed by arsenic and other pesticides. When she considered childhood deaths from accidental household poisonings, lead trailed drugs and kerosene.[91] A similar conclusion came from New York City. From 1955 to 1963, about 3 percent of cases reported to the New York City Poison Control Center were the result of lead, following in frequency drugs, pesticides, and household chemicals.[92] Paint was not the only household source of lead. Other sources in the 1960s included ceramic glazes, home remedies, gasoline sniffing, and untaxed whiskey.[93]

American Academy of Pediatrics

In 1961 the Subcommittee on Accidental Poisonings of the American Academy of Pediatrics issued its first statement on childhood lead poisoning. Its review provided one mirror of how child health professionals viewed the disease. The AAP identified the source and setting of the lead:

> With rare exceptions children exhibiting clinical lead intoxication reside in the older sections of urban areas where they may have ready access to crumbling, peeling or easily chipped paint. Lead pigment paints were widely used for indoor painting until approximately 25 years ago. Lead pigments are still found in exterior paints, particularly those specified as mildew suppressants. . . . Old tenements or other dwellings that might have been painted and repainted over 15 or 20 years ago may be the frequent sources of lead poisoning.[94]

The children at risk were those with pica who "must nibble upon these flakes for several months before a quantity of lead sufficient to produce toxic manifestations is absorbed into the body."[95] The AAP considered a blood level of greater than 60 micrograms/dl to be elevated and concluded that "in severely ill patients blood lead concentrations are usually greater than 100 micrograms/dl."[96] A child with lead poisoning needed admission to a hospital for chelation therapy to prevent death and neurological complications. While the child was in the hospital, "steps should be taken in conjunction with the Social Service Department and the Public Health Department to locate and identify the sources of lead and to remove them from the home environment before the patient is discharged. Since this requires time, temporary placement in [a] foster home, convalescent home or home of a relative may be necessary. The prevention of re-exposure to lead is one of the most important factors in the management of childhood lead poisoning."[97] The AAP statement thus mirrored the experience of many American cities throughout the 1950s and early 1960s. As cities mobilized to find those affected by lead and treat them and their environment, some observers returned to the question of how much, if any, lead in a child's surroundings was safe.

Chapter 12

Children and Lead, 1960–1965

IN THE 1960s, some scientists questioned whether *any* amount of lead in a child's environment posed a hazard. This concern contrasted sharply with the view over the previous three decades that considered small amounts of lead as simply a normal constituent of the everyday environment. Between these polar views were pediatricians, child psychologists, and public health administrators who sought to determine how much lead a child could consume without permanent neurological detriment. In these discussions, Robert Kehoe and Clair Patterson represented the contrasting positions; Julian Chisholm negotiated the center.

Robert Kehoe

Kehoe, who retired from the directorship of the Kettering Laboratory in 1965, summarized in 1960 the state of knowledge about lead metabolism as he saw it in the Harben Lectures presented to the Royal Institute of Public Health and Hygiene in London. Kehoe believed that the amount of lead taken in from the normal diet had remained virtually the same as when he first determined it in the 1930s. There was great variation (100 to 2000 micrograms/day), but Kehoe thought that the average citizen ate approximately 300 micrograms/day. The lead content of air had risen since the 1930s, as a consequence of tetraethyl lead in gasoline, so that a citizen absorbed between 10 and 90 micrograms each day from the atmosphere. Combining sources, Kehoe thought the average daily consumption of lead was around 400 micrograms. This ingestion did not concern him, because he was able to measure nearly equivalent amounts leaving the body each day in stool and urine:

It appears from the foregoing facts, that an equilibrium is established at an early age between the human organism and its usual environment in the United States, whereby the stream of lead absorbed into the body from the environment is balanced by a counter stream of lead issuing forth from tissues and from the body via excretory routes. . . . [I]t may be that some slight accumulation of lead occurs in the tissues (or in specific tissues) of the human body during life. Thus far, any such phenomenon has been too small to detect, and it seems likely, in view of the variability referred to, and the minuteness of the quantities represented therein daily, that this will continue to be the case.[1]

Kehoe determined that, on average, an American had a blood lead level of 27 micrograms/dl. Although most of Kehoe's research over the preceding decades had centered on adults, it is safe to assume that toddlers took in approximately as much lead from food and the atmosphere as adults. The blood lead level for infants and toddlers was nearly identical to that of adults when measured in Philadelphia in 1958.[2] Around 30 micrograms/dl might be the average value in the early 1960s, but most pediatricians believed that the normal range for blood lead in children extended to at least 60 micrograms/dl.[3]

Where "normal" ended and disease began was also debated. Kehoe firmly argued that he had never seen a case of either adult or child lead poisoning where the blood lead level was below 80 micrograms/dl.[4] This was the point at which most pediatricians elected to treat a child, unless the child had symptoms at a lower level, a rare event.

Clair Patterson

In 1965 Clair Patterson, a geochemist at the Massachusetts Institute of Technology, challenged Kehoe's view that human consumption of environmental lead in the twentieth century was harmless.[5] Patterson did not dispute Kehoe's calculations; in fact he used them and others, agreeing with Kehoe's estimated daily lead intake of around 400 micrograms.[6] What struck Patterson was evidence—produced from tree rings and other sources—that this amount of lead was about one hundred times the amount taken in by humans before the Industrial Revolution. Patterson argued that the atmosphere in the Northern Hemisphere contained as much as one thousand times more lead as centuries earlier. In his view, the blood lead level of 27 micrograms/dl was one hundred times the "natural" level.[7]

Anne Minot

Although Patterson was neither a biologist nor a physician, he also attacked the view that the daily intake of lead was harmless to humans simply because it did not produce symptoms. Patterson's view that lead in doses less than those that produced symptoms might be harmful was not entirely new. Nearly thirty years earlier, Anne Minot, who had worked with Joseph Aub in the 1920s, had raised this issue. In 1938 Minot tried to pinpoint what amount of lead, absorbed daily, produced symptoms. Blood lead determinations had been introduced only a few years earlier, and Minot looked to this new technology for precision. Unfortunately, it did not help her: "While there is considerable lack of agreement in the concentrations of lead found in normal blood, where sufficiently complete data are available, there is a reassuring difference in the amounts found in the blood of normal persons and in those with early signs of lead poisoning. . . . One can conclude from the data available that the daily lead intake of the average individual at present is considerably less than the intake which has been generally found to be dangerous."[8] Minot did express a concern that scientists in 1938 simply did not know exactly how much lead was safe to absorb each day or what daily dose produced symptoms. With so much unknown, Minot speculated that amounts of lead that did not yield symptoms might be harmful. To support this idea, she cited literature on tadpoles and seedlings and roots as well as the animal studies of Aub and others on the effect of lead in the test tube. What Minot discovered in the literature worried her:

> From the entire foregoing discussion it is apparent that the recognition of the harm done by the small amounts of lead absorbed by the average individual is bound to be difficult. The investigations which give evidence of the marked influence of lead in great dilution on various isolated tissues incline one to the view that the continuous absorption of any amount of lead must result in less than optimal conditions for the organism as a whole. At present, however, we do not know what to look for in the average individual as subjective or objective manifestations of this slightly unfavorable condition.[9]

Minot's speculation brought a swift response from Robert Kehoe. Minot had no quarrel with Kehoe's data. Indeed, she cited eight of his papers. In a letter to Minot in 1938, Kehoe objected to her speculation, arguing that his painstaking studies of lead workers indicated that no harm occurred unless symptoms developed.[10]

USPHS Symposium, 1965

During a symposium sponsored by the U.S. Public Health Service in December 1965, Kehoe clashed openly with Patterson's just-published ideas. Although Patterson was not an invited participant, nearly all speakers mentioned his findings; some embraced them.[11] Kehoe presented a summary of his Harben Lectures. On two points he was adamant. First, "with respect to whether the concentration of lead in the tissues of people . . . constitute[s] a risk—the risk of intoxication by lead in any form known to physicians, physiologists, and pathologists—the answer is in the negative."[12] Second, Kehoe was equally firm on his view that blood levels below 80 micrograms/dl posed no health risk:

> [80 micrograms/dl] is the lowest concentration that has occurred, in the experience of the Kettering Laboratory, in association with the onset of lead poisoning in a child or adult. . . . This value is not, as some ill-informed persons have believed, the critical level above which one may properly conclude that the person concerned is suffering from lead poisoning. It is rather . . . the level below which no case of poisoning induced by inorganic lead, however mild, has been found in our nearly thirty years of extensive experience with all types of lead poisoning.[13]

Kehoe translated his beliefs into public policy: as long as the average person consumed no more than 600 micrograms of lead each day and inhaled no more than 90 micrograms of lead from the atmosphere, there was no public health risk.[14]

Harriet Hardy, an occupational physician at the Massachusetts Institute of Technology who had worked with Alice Hamilton, took issue with Kehoe. Likening the absorption of small amounts of lead to dangers from ionizing radiation, Hardy argued, citing Patterson: "Prevention of diagnosable lead poisoning in healthy male workers is important but not enough in our society. There is a wealth of knowledge of the biologic effects of lead and its compounds at hand. There is no available evidence that lead is useful to the body."[15] On the final day of the conference, Kehoe felt besieged. One proposed summary of the conference did not adopt Kehoe's view, an entirely new experience for him, and, in fact, had misinterpreted some of the data he had presented. He commented: "I seem to be a bit under the gun. . . . I made a very grave mistake in trying to present to this audience, even representing as it does a good many experts, information gathered by very careful, minute attention to detail over a period of twenty or thirty years and then condensing this into twenty minutes of speech."[16] At one point, the moderator intervened: "It's obvious that this whole question has become overladen with certain emotional responses on the part of the people involved, and I think this is natural. I don't think we should avoid these. It's perhaps a little unusual that the emotional bias of the individuals involved come to the surface in a meeting of this kind so readily. Perhaps it's because the trigger, Dr. Patterson's article, is so obviously an emotional article."[17] Kehoe insisted that a summary of his views be appended to the final report of the symposium.[18]

Harriet Hardy took issue with Kehoe directly, arguing that "there is lead damage even though the man isn't ill." This was no small point: it went to the heart of Kehoe's view that lead caused bodily harm only when it produced symptoms.[19]

Kehoe did not let the matter drop. In an exchange of letters with Hardy, Kehoe disputed Patterson's views in general and Hardy's symposium comments in particular. He also indicated that the ground under him had given way and that many experts were beginning to move away from his point of view, a development that he described to Hardy as his "downfall."[20]

Patterson's concern about the potential toxicity of small amounts of lead reflected a burgeoning awareness of environmental toxins, a worry that spread into many aspects of life. For example, home safety advocates added household lead to a list of household problems: "[Former] microbiological agents are being replaced by an increasing number of new mechanical agents of death and disability such as those associated with the automobile, the airplane, and the motor boat, plus physical agents like ionizing radiations from x-rays and radioactive isotopes and the chemical agents such as carcinogens and vast numbers of potential poisons [among them lead]."[21]

J. Julian Chisholm, Jr.

Infants exposed to peeling and flaking walls had far more lead in their environments than did the average citizen. In 1965 Julian Chisholm assessed the danger to toddlers. Chisholm, who corresponded with Kehoe in the mid-1960s, accepted the older physician's calculations of the amount of lead in food and water. Chisholm also conceded that Kehoe's views about the lack of harm to industrial workers might well be accurate. In contrast, Chisholm's focus was on children and especially on the child's developing nervous system. In essence, Chisholm argued that development itself created a special vulnerability. He agreed with Kehoe that "ample supporting evidence of a dangerous body burden of lead can always be found when the blood-lead exceeds 80 to 100 micrograms of whole blood." Chisholm worried, "but what is the toxicologic significance of values between 40 and 80 micrograms?" Physicians understood that lead inhibited the formation of heme, a constituent of hemoglobin, at blood lead levels less than those required to produce neurological symptoms. Indeed, this phenomenon had resulted in urinary diagnostic tests, coproporphyrin (CPP) and delta-aminolevulinic acid (ALA), that enjoyed some popularity before being rejected at the end of the 1960s. Some physicians pondered whether similar blood lead levels that interfered with heme formation also injured the nervous system.[22] These were speculative essays, not research studies,[23] and prominent workers in the field recognized that proof lay in the future. For example, Hardy suggested that even though children over 60 microgram/dl were often asymptomatic, "logic forces the question whether damage to" the nervous system might still occur;[24] and Chisholm acknowledged, "it may logically be asked whether long-sustained minor elevation in blood lead concentration is associated with continuing toxicity to the brain despite our present inability to demonstrate this objectively."[25] Six years later, Chisholm still believed that the "biological consequences [of blood lead levels between 50 and 80 micrograms/dl] were unclear."[26]

Patterson had sown the seeds for another rebirth of childhood lead poisoning. Smaller amounts of lead were possibly dangerous, especially for young children; exposure to lead in adequate quantities to produce these lower levels of concern was clearly a probability as inner cities continued to crumble; early urban programs counted a high percentage of children who had reached this new, lower, threshold of concern.

Part V

The New Ecology

Chapter 13

A "Submerged"
National Epidemic

IN THE LATE 1960s childhood lead poisoning exploded as a major national epidemic. Until then, cases of lead-poisoned children had numbered in the hundreds, most clustered in a few northern and midwestern cities. Now every urban toddler was viewed as a potential victim of lead poisoning. This new perception of a far larger epidemic came from a number of sources, key among them an awareness of lead-afflicted children who suffered no symptoms.

Urban lead programs of the fifties and sixties, which targeted blighted inner-city neighborhoods with house-to-house surveys, identified few children with symptomatic lead poisoning. Those children found their way to emergency rooms. What the small-scale surveys discovered was many children with blood lead concentrations that, though short of causing seizures or coma, nevertheless were considered in excess of normal. The public health concern was obvious: these children had sources of lead in their intimate environments that, if not identified and eliminated, might push the level of lead to the danger point. This worrisome group of children had a condition that public health officials called "undue lead absorption." Over the next decade, as symptomatic lead poisoning essentially disappeared, undue lead absorption became the "new" lead poisoning. What pediatricians considered "undue" rapidly changed, with warning levels in the late 1990s one-sixth those of the late 1960s.

Undue Lead Absorption

Small-scale, targeted screening surveys revealed that symptomatic lead poisoning was only the tip of the iceberg—"the small visible portion represents the children with encephalopathy, and the larger, submerged portion represents the children with asymptomatic lead poisoning."[1] The public health question was how many children lay "submerged" in the undue lead absorption group. The first hints that these children numbered in the hundreds of thousands—perhaps millions—came in large-scale screening surveys in Chicago and New York City.

In 1966 the Chicago Board of Health began a mass-screening program that employed a new technology—atomic absorption spectroscopy—to measure blood lead levels. This method allowed a single technician to determine the lead content of nine hundred blood samples in eight hours. In two years, 68,744 children between the ages of one and six years were screened. The Board of Health chose 50 micrograms/dl and above as the level of concern. During the first year of the survey, 8.5 percent of children exhibited this level. The following year, 3.8 percent did. When officials combined the results of both years, they found that 4,000 children, or nearly 6 percent, had elevated levels of lead. They also noted that the number of identified children fell markedly in the second year, for reasons that were not immediately apparent. Of note, Chicago's mass-screening project measured far more blood samples than did the Baltimore Health Department from 1935 to 1968.[2]

Chicago public health officials treated 1,155 of these children, most with blood levels above 70 micrograms/dl. Many were treated on an outpatient basis; only those with moderate or severe encephalopathy were admitted to a hospital. Physicians noted that only 3 children suffered from seizures, all with blood lead levels above 200 micrograms/dl. Only 8.9 percent had any cerebral symptoms that might be attributable to excess lead, such as drowsiness, irritability, or vomiting.[3]

Two years later New York City, under mounting pressure from angry civic groups and employing atomic absorption spectroscopy, began mass screening. In 1970 nearly 80,000 children were screened, and 2,500 children were identified with an elevated blood lead level. Public health officials in New York City defined a "case" as a blood lead level of over 60 micrograms/dl. Vincent Guinee, director of the Bureau of Lead Poisoning Control of the New York City Health Department, was acutely aware of the "vagaries of definition": "The study of lead poisoning has been hampered by, and obscured by, semantics. When we speak of a case of lead poisoning, 'case' has the connotation of symptoms and 'poisoning' has a connotation of damage. Neither is necessarily true."[4] Guinee noted that Chicago had chosen 50 micrograms/dl as a "case." Had New York City picked the same level, the rate of lead poisoning would have been nearly 11 percent, or twice the identification rate of Chicago. At the higher level, New York City had a rate of 5.2 percent, or approximately the same rate as the Windy City. In both cities, public health authorities were attempting to identify children "at risk" for later symptoms if they were not separated from sources of lead.[5]

Chicago pediatricians assessed the long-term damage to children identified in the screening program. In 1966 Meyer Perlstein and Ramzy Attala studied the neurological outcomes of 435 children treated for lead poisoning. Perlstein and Attala did not include blood lead values in their published account, but they stated that most of these children were admitted to the hospital. Because Chicago public officials treated all but the most severely encephalopathic children on an outpatient basis, we can assume that many, if not most, of these children were in this severely affected category. Perlstein and Attala divided the children into six groups. The first three groups showed definite brain symptoms at the time of treatment: (1) coma; (2) seizures; (3) ataxia (loss of balance and coordination). The fourth group included children with mixed symptoms that included mild encephalopathy (vomiting) and non-neurological complaints such as abdominal pain or anemia. The fifth group presented with fever (not a manifestation of lead), and the sixth group was asymptomatic with undue lead absorption. This last group of children had been identified because a sibling had previously developed symptoms. All the children in the study were evaluated after treatment. Sixty-one percent were thought to be normal. The degree of impairment of the remaining 39 percent closely followed the seriousness of the initial poisoning: coma (82 percent had persistent symptoms), seizures (67 percent), ataxia (59 percent), mild encephalopathy (31 percent), fever (15 percent), and asymptomatic (9 percent).

In one sense, Perlstein and Attala confirmed the findings reached by Byers and Lord a quarter of a century earlier: children who suffered from lead encephalopathy often had intellectual problems when they entered school. In another sense, the Chicago study raised a new specter: some children who did not suffer lead encephalopathy and, in fact, were entirely asymptomatic, nevertheless were left with measurable impairments. Perlstein and Attala were not certain how to interpret their findings. For example, they did not know the level of intellectual functioning of these children prior to the detection of excess lead in their system. Moreover, they were not certain how far they could rely on the recall of the children's parents.[6] Measuring the pre-exposure neurological functioning was just one methodological issue that would plague research on the long-term effects of lead over the next two decades.

The mass screening in Chicago and New York City brought into sharp relief the fact that most children with excess lead were entirely asymptomatic to their parents, or even to a trained observer. Even if only a small percentage of this large group was permanently hurt by lead, it would represent a very large number. Lead poisoning morphed into an epidemic.

This concern for asymptomatic children dovetailed with Clair Patterson's observation about the greatly increased amount of lead in the environment. In 1966 Harriet Hardy, the physician at the Massachusetts Institute of Technology who had long been interested in lead poisoning, connected the two streams of thought, concluding: "If, as seems likely from the accumulated and growing evidence, growing tissue is more vulnerable to lead than adult tissue, far smaller doses than those required to produce diagnosable lead poisoning in a healthy adult male worker become important."[7] Five years later Hardy, after studying the results of the Chicago mass screening, speculated: "Lack of untreated controls [in the Chicago study] . . . makes it impossible to be certain about the ensuing permanent disability. Logic, however, forces the question of whether cellular damage in the central nervous system, kidneys, and reproductive system from this enzymatic poison [lead] may not result in significantly impaired function even when the symptoms of physical disability are not brought to medical attention and correctly assessed as due to lead."[8] In Britain, D. Bryce-Smith, a professor of organic chemistry, posed a similar question: "One most vital question is not yet clearly answered. Is an asymptomatic child with elevated blood lead at risk of long-term brain damage, even if overt clinical symptoms of lead poisoning do not subsequently appear? . . . If exposure to lead can damage the child's brain without necessarily producing conventional clinical symptoms of poisoning, the implications are grave."[9]

Gerald Wiener, a professor in the Johns Hopkins School of Hygiene and Public Health, addressed the same issue. Wiener carefully reviewed published and unpublished studies and found serious methodological problems with each, concluding:

> All but two of the preceding studies reported some degree of mental impairment caused by lead poisoning. Yet it seemed clear that none of the studies provided a definitive answer to the question: is mental deficiency associated with lead ingestion which is asymptomatic or which produces symptoms less severe than encephalitis? Those reports which claimed positive findings had either used too few cases from which to generalize or had not provided for controls for relevant variables such as social class, pica, or premorbid status. A rigorous and experimental approach has been conspicuously absent. Further, the variations in diagnostic procedures and definitions led to unclear conclusions regarding the degree of lead ingestion which may or may not be important for later development.[10]

At the end of the 1960s there were converging lines of evidence that a new form of lead poisoning was looming, asymptomatic, and widespread, which might leave damaging marks on the brain. Still, prominent researchers held widely divergent views. As physicians from Dartmouth observed in 1968:

> One school of thought [Kehoe] holds that present exposures are safe, that lead does not accumulate in human tissues with age at these levels,

that there is no such entity as subclinical lead toxicity [there being a well-defined threshold for toxicity], and that man can exist in a healthy state under present conditions unless overt additional exposures occur. Another viewpoint implies that the present body burden of lead is approximately 100 times "natural" levels [Patterson], that this burden is harmful in some unknown and undefined manner [perhaps manifesting itself by a chronic disease or by increased mortality], that lead is a cumulative poison, and that the threshold for innate adverse effects has already been or will soon be exceeded.[11]

A National Program

Hordes of asymptomatic children with "undue lead absorption" threatened to overwhelm communities. In response, the focus of childhood lead poisoning shifted to the national level.

In 1969 the American Academy of Pediatrics took the lead in setting the national agenda, building on the experience of many urban programs—especially Baltimore's—and on the careful research of Julian Chisholm. Chisholm and Eugene Kaplan best summed up the constellation of social and cultural events leading to the causes of childhood lead poisoning: "It results from the impact upon the urban slum child, in particular, of a variety of causative factors—pica and environmental exposure to lead, cultural and behavioral patterns of parents, and certain aspects of lead metabolism."[12] Chisholm and Kaplan described the aggressive eating behaviors of lead-poisoned children who had come from rural environments where pica was considered normal as a "habitual, purposeful, and compulsive search for and ingestion of . . . unnatural food substances."[13] In fact, the children's mothers often displayed pica behaviors.[14] In addition, these children were inadequately supervised, because their mothers:

> may be absent in order to earn a living outside the home, and there may be no father to share the domestic responsibilities. . . . She may be overwhelmed by too many children to care for and thus be deficient in her caring role for the toddler. . . . Another pattern encountered is the mother who is not aware of the child's pica. This may reflect a basic ignorance that ingestion of these materials could be harmful, or she may be absent from the home for much of the day and not realize that the persons who care for her child allow or support his pica activity.[15]

Chisholm and Kaplan described the environment where childhood lead poisoning occurred: "deteriorating urban housing; the interior woodwork, painted wallpaper, and painted plaster of houses built prior to 1940 and still in use may contain layers of lead-pigment paints which have never been removed."[16]

Exterior Paint

From their experience in Baltimore, Chisholm and Kaplan knew that deteriorating exterior paints could also present a problem.[17] In the 1960s these paints contained far more lead because of their need to withstand the vagaries of weather. When home health visitors searched for a source of lead inside a child's home, occasionally they were unable to discover one. As Edmund Bradley and Samuel Bessman explained in 1958: "The majority of the children apparently swallowed paint from indoor surfaces. However, others may have eaten paint which had peeled from exterior walls. The interior of the home of one child with lead poisoning did not have toxic amounts of lead on its painted surfaces, but it was learned that the child sat on the stoop outside and ate particles of paint fallen from the exterior walls."[18] That same year, a widely distributed pamphlet—sponsored by the National Paint, Lacquer, and Varnish Association, the U.S. Public Health Service, the Food and Drug Administration, and the Children's Bureau—made parents aware "that outdoor things are important, too, such as painted steps, porches, railings, benches, swings, fences, and other painted surfaces."[19] A year later, Randolph Byers explained to a pediatric audience in Boston: "Over one half of our cases have their onset in July; the mechanism of this is probably due to three things: first, outdoor paint is more likely to contain lead than indoor paint so that children playing outdoors are exposed to lead more readily."[20] Evelyn Hartman illustrated similar circumstances in Minneapolis.[21] A physician in Cleveland, Ohio, raised a similar worry. "Outdoor paint may still contain a high percentage of lead because of its excellent weather resistance. Thus, flaking outdoor paint may also present a definite hazard if found in a youngster's favored playing corner."[22] In Philadelphia Emil Tiboni, chief of the Accident Control Section of the Department of Health, thought the exterior hazard extended only to porches. As he explained:

> Interior paints used before 1940 usually contained lead in an amount substantially greater than the level of 1 percent by weight, which is regarded as the safe limit. The interior of homes in older neighborhoods may contain many layers of leaded paint. Paint containing lead may also be found in exterior appurtenances of homes. Except for porches, the hazard to children in these locations is usually less serious, however, because a small child seldom has access to them for prolonged periods of time.[23]

"Safe" Daily Amounts of Lead

Chisholm and Kaplan identified the tension in conflicting views about the dangers of "normal" amounts of lead in the environment. They called attention to "the meticulous long-term balance studies of Kehoe in human adult volunteers [which indicated] that the average adult in the United States today ingests about 0.3 milligrams [of lead] daily in food and beverage." In addition, urban dwellers inhaled an additional 30 to 40 micrograms daily from polluted air. These combined "normal" sources of lead resulted in blood concentrations between 15 and 40 micrograms/dl. Although fully aware of Patterson,[24] Chisholm and Kaplan concluded, "no untoward effect of this 'normal' exposure has been demonstrated."[25] Chisholm and Kaplan also captured the debate over the long-term effects of lead in children who were not symptomatic: "Whether children without overt encephalopathy sustain significant CNS injury as a result of plumbism in early childhood is not clear. Although the usual psychometric tests and performance in school indicate deficiencies in comparison with norms derived from more privileged groups of children, it has not been shown that they differ greatly from other underprivileged children not known to have had plumbism who also reside in deprived urban areas."[26] Chisholm and Kaplan explained how Baltimore managed children with undue lead absorption, offering it as a model for the nation: hospitalization of all such children—as much for protection from further absorption of lead as for medical treatment; investigation of the home by the Health Department; identification of lead source and cleanup of the hazard; evaluation of other children in the home; parental education by a social worker to provide information about the dangers of pica and how best to supervise children; foster home or convalescent hospital to provide a safe haven so that a child with undue lead absorption would not return to the same leaden environment.[27]

In 1967 the Children's Bureau published an educational pamphlet, written by Jane S. Lin-Fu, which was based on the same materials and reached the same conclusions. The Lead Industries Association republished this pamphlet, packaged it with the LIA's "Facts about Lead Poisoning and Pediatrics," and distributed it widely.[28] The Government Printing Office sold 12,600 copies; the LIA distributed 65,000 free copies to physicians, health departments, poison control centers, and child care centers.[29] In the 1970s Jane Lin-Fu would become one of the federal government's most respected advocates for public health measures to contain childhood lead poisoning.[30]

American Academy of Pediatrics

In 1969 the American Academy of Pediatrics used Chisholm and Kaplan's template as the basis for a policy statement. Chisholm consulted with Robert Kehoe to gain his advice on the most accurate screening tests and the blood level at which a child needed treatment.[31] The AAP statement incorporated the first reports from the mass screenings in Chicago and New York City: "Prospective surveys in various cities indicate that 10 to 25 percent of such children [living in deteriorating pre–World War II urban housing] have absorbed potentially dangerous quantities of lead and that 2 to 5 percent have clinical symptoms compatible with those of acute intoxication."[32] And the AAP called attention to a study from Cleveland that dramatically demonstrated that lead poisoning did not occur in public housing painted with 1 percent lead paint. The AAP identified interior paint as the most common source of paint, but urged pediatricians to look outside the home when investigation of the inside of the house yielded no source.

The AAP focused on the identification and treatment of symptomatic children. In this first report, it did not address the issue of the long-term consequences of asymptomatic exposure. In doing so, the AAP followed Kehoe's view of the importance of symptoms and Kehoe's recommendation that treatment should be reserved for children with blood lead levels above 80 micrograms/dl.[33] The AAP differed from Kehoe in recommending treatment for children with lower levels if they had symptoms or if they showed abnormalities in heme synthesis. It seems likely that the AAP avoided the issue of asymptomatic children in this policy statement because it wished to focus attention on the critical danger posed to symptomatic children and because it did not want its warning to be diluted with elements that most researchers believed were still in question.[34] The AAP urged the establishment of large-scale screening programs in municipalities with identified crumbling inner cities. The AAP recommended a "community-centered" approach that largely mirrored Baltimore's program.

The AAP statement thus summarized the lessons of the previous two decades. It became the guidepost for pediatricians in practice throughout the country, serving as the script for local programs. The AAP also became a leading advocate for federal assistance.

U.S. Public Health Service

In 1970 the surgeon general issued a policy statement that closely followed the AAP recommendations.[35] The surgeon general did, however, refine some aspects of the AAP report. The pediatric group had defined the "normal" level of lead in the blood as between 15 and 40 micrograms/dl. It left the range of 40–60 micrograms/dl undesignated, but identified 60–80 micrograms/dl as the lowest point where problems were likely to arise. In contrast, the Public Health Service (USPHS) defined blood lead levels over 40 micrograms/dl as "evidence suggestive of undue absorption of lead."[36] In designating this amount of lead as potentially dangerous, the USPHS greatly increased the number of children deemed at risk.[37] In cities so overwhelmed, the USPHS suggested investigating only those children with levels higher than 50 micrograms/dl, which had been Chicago's guideline. The surgeon general, rejecting urine tests for lacking sensi-

tivity, recommended screening children with blood lead determinations. In doing so, the USPHS followed the example of Chicago and New York City. The
Public Health Service also suggested treating children with blood lead levels
above 80 micrograms/dl.

Jane Lin-Fu was quick to point out the gap in the surgeon general's warning,
criticizing the identification of 40 micrograms/dl as "undue" while not recommending intervention at this level.[38] In redefining the hazard from lead at this
lower level, the USPHS recognized that it was describing a health menace that
outstripped the resources of local communities, paving the way for federal programs.

Public Law 91-695

In the summer and fall of 1970, the U.S. House of Representatives and Senate
held hearings on childhood lead poisoning and debated a new federal statute.
Once enacted, Public Law 91-695 provided federal funds for mass screening,
treatment, education, and research on how to lessen the hazard.[39] The act also
mandated that federally funded public housing meet the 1 percent paint standard. The hearings, which included testimony from pediatricians, urban public
health officials, industry leaders, politicians, and citizens, provided a rich source
of information about childhood lead poisoning.[40]

What members of Congress heard from all witnesses was that an epidemic
was afflicting millions of poor children, most of them black or Hispanic, who
lived in the decaying inner city. Representatives and senators learned that public health officials identified the hazard in pre–World War II housing, and they
heard praise of the American Standards Association's 1 percent voluntary standard. They listened to various strategies of screening children for lead poisoning, particularly about the emerging consensus that blood lead tests, while
expensive and still technically difficult—both in obtaining samples and in per-
forming the determination—were the best means of diagnosis. From many pediatricians, they also learned that there was no precise blood level that was
considered dangerous in all cases and that pediatricians were investigating the
long-term effects of asymptomatic levels of lead in the blood. New York's Vincent
Guinee pointed out to the members of Congress that a "case" of lead poisoning
differed from city to city, and he estimated the cost of "deleading" an apartment
in his city at $1,263. A vice president of the National Paint, Varnish, and Lac-
quer Association testified in support of the law.

P.L. 91-695 in Practice

The federal law had the greatest influence on mass screening. One issue the federal mandate forced was the choice of a method for screening. Urinary tests,

which employed either coproporphyrin or delta-aminolevulinic acid, were cheap, and samples were easy to obtain from toddlers. After considerable comparison testing from Chicago and New York City, however, pediatricians concluded that urinary tests simply missed too many children in the "undue lead absorption" range, which was becoming the major area of public health concern.[41] Jane Lin-Fu and others argued for mass screening with blood lead, calling attention to the programs in Chicago and New York City.[42] Others described the difficulty in obtaining blood samples from toddlers.[43]

Another test, free erythrocyte protoporphyrin (FEP)—also based on lead's effect on heme synthesis—had the benefit of higher accuracy in the undue lead absorption range. Significantly, it could be performed with a finger-prick sample.[44] Julian Chisholm became an early advocate.[45] Of course FEP was not the same as a blood lead level, and pediatricians and chemists had to develop charts to interpret FEP values in terms of blood lead.[46] In 1974 Chisholm was able to claim that the FEP could identify 95 percent of children who had blood levels of 50 micrograms/dl or above.[47] In the mid-1970s the FEP became the screening test favored by most clinics and health departments.

Measuring blood lead by a "micro" method also became available in the 1970s. This permitted the most accurate testing with the ease of a finger prick. Special concerns emerged about the chemistry of the test and particularly about errors that occurred when children had lead dust on the pricked finger, but by 1980, many health departments had switched to microlead determinations.[48]

Between 1972 and 1975, the federally assisted screening projects tested over one million children in thirty-three states and the District of Columbia. This represented about one-third of the nation's children believed to be at risk. In 1973, 11 percent of screened children had blood lead concentrations above 40 micrograms/dl, roughly twice the percentage for 1974 and 1975. Of these, about one-sixth had blood lead levels high enough (above 80 micrograms/dl) to receive chelation therapy. Of one million screened, 10,000 were treated.[49]

The federal government also sponsored spot-screening in twenty-seven cities that were not yet conducting systematic screening surveys. These less-intensive studies also revealed that about one child in six under the age of six years had blood lead levels greater than 40 micrograms/dl.[50] In addition, screening programs demonstrated that many more urban than rural children had blood lead levels over 40 micrograms/dl (23 percent versus 9 percent).[51]

The Federal Program Redefines Lead Poisoning in Baltimore

In Baltimore, it is possible to see how the federal program redefined childhood lead poisoning on a local level. Between 1968 and 1971, the Baltimore Health Department was quite pleased that symptomatic lead poisoning was at its lowest point in over twenty years. In 1972 Baltimore received a federal grant of $150,000 for screening blighted areas. The federal level of concern—following the recommendations of the U.S. Public Health Service—was 40 micrograms/ dl. Until 1972, the Baltimore Health Department had reported only symptomatic cases. After that, it reported blood lead levels, because virtually all children identified in the federally assisted program were not "cases" in the older sense because they had no symptoms. The screening program and the new concern for "undue lead absorption" transformed a program previously considered "successful" into an effort with much work left to do. For example, in 1972 the Health Department identified 8 children with symptomatic lead poisoning. In addition there were 37 children with blood lead levels above 60 micrograms/dl; 55 between 50 and 59 micrograms/dl; and 131 between 40 and 49 micrograms/ dl. Thus, by past reckoning, Baltimore had 8 cases of lead poisoning; by new standards, it had 8 cases of lead poisoning *and* 223 children with worrisome undue lead absorption. The following year, screening yielded 865 children with undue lead absorption.[52]

Health ordinances in many cities mandated that the peeling and flaking paint from the walls and ceilings in a home where a child had been found with an elevated blood lead level be checked for lead content. Visiting nurses in Baltimore had obtained scrapings for years. The nurses brought the scrapings back with them to the Health Department for analysis in its laboratories. In the early 1970s, portable devices became commercially available so that home visitors could ascertain the lead content of paint on walls while making the visit. Baltimore was one of the first cities to use these aids.[53]

Lead Industries Association

The Lead Industries Association joined in the national campaigns to get the word out. In 1972 and 1973 the LIA and the American Academy of Pediatrics sponsored large regional meetings in Chicago,[54] Delaware,[55] and Washington, D.C.[56] In each of these conferences, national figures, such as Julian Chisholm, joined local leaders on the platform. The LIA also assisted cities such as Philadelphia in crafting local ordinances to promote lead safety at home.[57]

Calls for Abatement

The American Academy of Pediatrics and the surgeon general learned from Baltimore's experience in dealing with landlords and unsafe housing:

> The first precept is: *no child ever returns to a leaded house.* This aspect of therapy requires the coordinated efforts of public health authorities to

effect the removal of hazardous lead sources; assistance for the mother in her quest for safe housing, and, increasingly, mobilization of the community itself.

Hopefully, the elimination or proper rehabilitation of substandard housing, and the rebuilding of the inner core of our cities, will eliminate childhood lead poisoning as it is now seen.[58]

The U.S. Public Health Service recommended: "Dwellings identified in screening programs as potential sources of lead hazards should be brought promptly to the attention of the local government agency responsible for enforcing housing codes and regulations so that proper corrective action may be taken."[59] Other observers thought that abatement was a distant goal. First, the extent of crumbling lead paint was enormous. Second, there was no consensus on what constituted adequate abatement. Some thought that sanding roughened old paint and repainting with 1 percent paint was sufficient. Others believed it necessary to cover old paint with boards. Still others thought that all old paint needed to be removed. Jane Lin-Fu pointed out that landlords balked at the expense and were more likely to evict tenants than to abate old paint.[60]

Rhetoric

Many child health professionals in the late 1960s and early 1970s altered their rhetoric when describing childhood lead poisoning. In many accounts, the large number of asymptomatic children was termed the "silent epidemic." The intimate connection between lead poisoning and the deteriorating inner city was phrased "a preventable disease of the slums," a "crisis of conscience," or a "social crime."[61] The fervor that infused medical writing can be seen in an article that appeared in the *American Journal of Public Health* in 1970: "For the community, [lead poisoning] represents just one more of the many burdens it must bear, react to, and fight against in order to survive the hell of impoverishment."[62]

Chapter 14

Air Pollution and an Epidemic Redefined

IN THE 1970s major changes occurred in the public's perception of the danger that lead posed to all humans. In large measure, this change coincided with a more general concern over environmental pollution, especially over the safety of air, water, and soil. In this larger arena, atmospheric lead figured almost as prominently as flaking lead paint.

Congressional hearings in 1970 reflected the consensus on where the hazard that lead posed to children lay: in the peeling and flaking interior paint of pre–World War II, inner-city housing that had been poorly maintained. Those who testified at the hearings supported the American Standards Association's 1 percent standard and wanted it extended by law to federal housing. The children most at risk were those who had symptoms and blood lead levels in excess of 80 micrograms/dl.

By 1978 the lead hazard calculus had shifted. Air, household dust, and playground dirt were new dangers. Exterior paints came under closer scrutiny. Even the hand-to-mouth behavior of toddlers with sticky fingers posed a danger to health that was described, not in terms of symptoms, but entirely in terms of alterations in biochemical and psychological tests. One percent paint was no longer considered safe, and a blood lead level of 30 micrograms/dl was alarming. Some called for the abatement of all lead paint.

Tetraethyl Lead

The federal government had a long-standing concern about atmospheric lead dating from the 1920s, when tetraethyl lead was added to gasoline to increase engine efficiency.[1] In 1958, manufacturers of tetraethyl lead asked the U.S. Public Health Service about the health consequences of increasing the concentration of the additive from 3 milliliters per gallon to 4 milliliters per gallon. The surgeon general convened a conference to discuss the implications of the change. It concluded that the increase would not significantly alter the lead content of the atmosphere. The surgeon general directed the Public Health Service and the petroleum industry to monitor atmospheric lead.

In 1963 Congress passed the Clean Air Act, assigning responsibility for monitoring air quality to the Environmental Protection Agency (EPA). Two years later, the Public Health Service published its *Survey of Lead in the Atmosphere of Three Urban Communities* (Cincinnati, Los Angeles, and Philadelphia).[2] This report found that drivers of cars in Cincinnati had blood lead levels on average of 33 micrograms/dl; after the increase in tetraethyl lead the value actually declined slightly, to 31 micrograms/dl.[3] In Los Angeles the average blood lead level was lower than in Cincinnati, about 20 micrograms/dl.[4] In Philadelphia the average blood lead level was still lower.[5]

Even though this study did not concern the dangers of lead paint, its results directly pertained to the issue of children poisoned at home. The measurements in the Three-City Study came from adults, often municipal employees on the job. These firemen, policemen, postmen, and others did not chew paint flakes either at home or in the workplace. Yet they had considerable lead in their bodies, presumably from breathing atmospheric lead. Although the levels did not appear to be increasing because of the additional tetraethyl lead in gasoline, the report argued that atmospheric lead was responsible for much, if not most, of this amount.

In the 1930s, Robert Kehoe had argued that food was responsible for most of the lead consumed by adults who were not employed in a lead industry. In the mid-1960s, most of the lead in food came from atmospheric fallout and no longer from agricultural pesticides. Toddlers, of course, ate the same foods and breathed the same air as adults. It was reasonable to conclude that atmospheric lead was responsible for blood lead levels of about 20 micrograms/dl, or about half of what the surgeon general considered to be an unacceptable concentration. From this perspective, atmospheric lead provided a substantial "foundation" upon which consumption of paint chips built. This recognition fused the histories of air pollution and childhood lead-paint poisoning. The main environmental battlefield was over tetraethyl lead, but for inner-city children the skirmish that counted most was over lead paint.[6]

Congress broadened the EPA's mandate with the passage of the Clean Air Amendments of 1970. To help in assessing the danger of lead in the atmosphere, the EPA asked the National Academy of Sciences (NAS) to investigate the state of air pollution. The resulting report, *Lead: Airborne Lead in Perspective*, was issued in 1972.[7] The NAS empaneled a group of experts from industry and the public health community. As the mandate indicated, the focus was atmospheric lead, but the committee also considered the hazard to children from crumbling paint. Anna Baetjer, J. Julian Chisholm, Jr., Harriet Hardy, Robert Kehoe, and Jane Lin-Fu joined the deliberations. Also included was a large contingent of experts from industry, a decision that drew comment and criticism—especially in the absence of an "identifiable 'environmentalist.'"[8]

Tetraethyl lead was responsible for 98 percent of atmospheric lead.[9] In addition, most of the lead found in street dust and surface dirt fell from the air.[10] In 1947 Paul Reznikoff, who had worked in Joseph Aub's laboratory at Harvard in the 1920s, coauthored a study that first called attention to the increasing amount of lead in street dust following the introduction of tetraethyl lead to gasoline. He found that street dust in New York City had 50 percent more lead in 1934 than in 1924, the year when tetraethyl lead was first added to gasoline.[11] In 1946 Robert Kehoe's laboratory in Cincinnati began measuring the lead content of air and soil;[12] in 1949 a similar study was conducted in Detroit, Michigan, and Windsor, Ontario.[13] By 1968 Americans consumed forty-five times as much lead in the form of gasoline additives as in white lead carbonate in paint.[14]

Urban street dust contained so much lead in 1970 that just one gram contained more than ten times the amount of lead normally consumed in food each day: "Although the available data on the distribution of blood lead concentration and other epidemiological data clearly indicate that this *alone* does not account for clinical lead poisoning in children, the swallowing of lead-contaminated dusts may well account, in large part, for the higher mean blood lead content in urban children and the rather large fraction whose blood lead content falls in the range of 40–60 micrograms/dl of whole blood."[15] Urban adults had blood lead levels that ranged between 11 and 31 micrograms/dl. In the view of the NAS group, lead-paint chips were the major source of lead in poisoned children, with atmospheric lead and lead in street dust having a "significant additive effect."

The panel also discussed the controversy over the long-range neurological effects of "undue lead absorption," concluding: "The damaging effects of lead poisoning associated with frank encephalopathy seem well substantiated, but an intriguing question remains: whether excessive lead ingestion in young children produces permanent central nervous system and behavioral deficits if the magnitude of ingestion is not sufficient to result in demonstrable encephalopathy."[16]

The NAS committee also estimated the cost for treating lead-poisoned children: $1,500–$2,000 for a child without symptoms of encephalopathy; $18,000 in additional funds for a child with encephalopathy to cover the costs of special schooling; and $245,000 for institutional care for children who survived severe encephalopathy. The committee additionally reported on the costs of "deleading" an apartment: $150–$1,200 in Baltimore; $1,263 in New York City. The cumulative costs for the nation were not calculated. In its summation, the NAS panel raised the possibility that atmospheric lead—inhaled or swallowed street dust—posed a most significant hazard for children, especially those living in congested cities.[17]

Maximum Daily Permissible Intake

In 1971 a broadly based committee of public health, government, and academic physicians recommended that a toddler consume daily not more than 300 micrograms of lead from all sources. The committee members based this estimate on several assumptions: (1) daily consumption of lead should not permit an accumulation sufficient to yield a blood lead concentration of more than 40 micrograms/dl (U.S. Public Health Service recommendation); (2) children absorbed lead at the same rate as adults (10 percent, based on Kehoe's balance studies of lead workers in the 1930s and Aub's animal studies in the 1920s); (3) a child's diet contained about 165 micrograms of lead (Kehoe estimate, Harben Lectures); and (4) that a child inhaled about 6 micrograms of lead from the atmosphere (Kehoe estimate, Harben Lectures). The committee selected 300 micrograms on the basis of Kehoe's experimental work, which had demonstrated that a worker could consume that much each day with no net increase in the total amount of body lead. The committee also reviewed more recent data that estimated the daily amount of dietary and atmospheric lead at somewhat lower levels than Kehoe's older studies (112 micrograms from the diet, 6 micrograms from the air). These considerations left about 200 micrograms of lead each day to come from "all other sources." Over the next decade much policy would be based on this calculation. It is important to realize that these numbers represented theoretical levels of consumption, absorption, retention, and the point where damage occurred. They were not based on measurements in any particular group of children.[18] Although the committee did take atmospheric lead into account, it did not consider lead in street dust.

One Percent Standard Revisited

Between 1972 and 1978 a national consensus was reached that lowered the lead content of all household paints—for both interiors and exteriors—from 1 percent to 0.06 percent. This change resulted from the interplay of newly acquired scientific information; recommendations from the American Academy of Pediatrics, the Center for Disease Control (CDC), and the Department of Housing and Urban Development (HUD); two reviews of the issue of childhood lead poisoning by the National Academy of Sciences; several congressional hearings; and regulatory actions by the Food and Drug Administration (FDA) and the Consumer Product Safety Commission (CPSC).

The AAP recommendation that the daily consumption of 200 micrograms of lead from nonfood sources called into question whether the American Standards Association's 1 percent standard for newly applied paint provided an adequate margin of safety. In 1971 the Food and Drug Administration (which had been given regulatory authority for the content of lead paint) solicited opinions on whether the 1 percent standard (adopted by Congress for use in federal housing) should be lowered. The American Academy of Pediatrics, which had been a partner in the ASA standard, was quick to advise that the standard should be lowered. The two proposed levels were 0.5 percent and 0.06 percent; the AAP argued for the lower level. The AAP accepted the 300-microgram limit for daily safe consumption. Translating 200 micrograms from "all other sources" into the percentage of lead in paint required some estimate of how much paint a child with pica consumed, how much paint was in a coat, and how many layers of paint were on the wall. The AAP made educated guesses. It thought that a toddler might consume one square inch daily. Six layers of 1 percent paint would contain 2400 micrograms, clearly in excess of the 200-microgram recommended amount. Half that much (0.5 percent) would still contain more than the recommended amount. Six layers of 0.06 percent paint would contain 125 micrograms, which was less than what was deemed the limit. These assumptions were guesses.[19] In fact, there was no published case in the medical literature that implicated 1 percent paint in any case of childhood lead poisoning. Although the AAP committee cited the NAS's, *Lead: Airborne Lead in Perspective*, that panel had not included street dust in its calculation.

In March 1972, the Food and Drug Administration banned paint with an excess of 0.5 percent lead from interstate commerce under provisions of the Federal Hazardous Substances Act.[20] This order ended the use of 1 percent lead paint for housing. This FDA action, and the petitions, hearings, and rulings it provoked, eventually led to the removal of all lead from all paint, both for interiors and for exteriors.

The AAP endorsement and the 300-microgram maximum daily intake prompted a new round of congressional hearings.[21] Congressmen heard from federal health officials, leading pediatricians, and public health administrators. All abandoned the 1 percent standard, not on the basis of cases of lead-poisoned children, but rather on the basis of concern over adding to future problems as the layers of 1 percent paint accumulated.[22] The lead-paint industry, which had supported P.L. 91-695 and acquiesced to the subsequent lowering to 0.5 percent, objected to the proposed lowering to 0.06 percent for household paints because there was "no sound toxicological basis" for the new level.[23] The congressional committee learned of only a few cases, all unpublished, of children poisoned from consuming paint that met the original ASA standard. In one case the child had eaten a hole measuring 26 inches by 32 inches in the kitchen wall.[24] The committee also heard from witnesses who estimated that "one-third or more of the lead in city dwelling Americans comes from inhalation of airborne lead from automobiles."[25]

The hearings opened new ground in two areas. One was limiting the lead content for exterior paints.[26] The other was an estimate on how much it would cost to remove lead paint from urban housing. Preliminary calculations ranged from $14 billion to $70 billion.[27]

The AAP recommendation itself began to carry weight, and a few months later the Consumer Product Safety Commission, which now had jurisdiction over paint, asked the National Academy of Sciences to determine whether there was sufficient scientific data to merit lowering the limit to 0.06 percent.[28] The NAS committee reviewed the AAP document and the 300-microgram recommended maximum daily intake. In addition, its members considered the biochemical data that indicated that lower levels of lead interfered with body chemistry and the growing psychological literature that was beginning to implicate lead as a source of neurological damage at lower levels.[29] The National Academy of Sciences concluded that there was insufficient evidence in 1973 to justify lowering the mandated amount of lead to 0.06 percent. Their judgment was based on the uncertainties involved with each of the AAP's assumptions. In particular, the NAS concluded:

> The only statement in the literature that deals with [the lowest concentration of lead in paint that has been associated with lead intoxication] was published 17 years ago and stated that no case of lead intoxication had been found where the only source of lead contained less than 1 percent of lead in the dried paint surface. Although this conclusion has not since been refuted, the Committee is unable to conclude that subtle but nevertheless significant forms of lead intoxication that may have escaped clinical detection have not occurred from exposure to paint films with lead concentrations lower than 1 percent.[30]

Consumer Product Safety Commission

In 1974 Congress asked the Consumer Product Safety Commission to assess the danger of multiple layers of paint and to determine a "safe" amount of the lead in paint.[31] To answer these questions, the CPSC funded research on baboons that concluded that 100 micrograms/kg/day failed to raise the blood level above 40 micrograms/dl. For a 10-kilogram toddler, this would translate to 1000 micrograms per day, or more than three times the level recommended by the American Academy of Pediatrics. On this calculation, 0.5 percent lead in paint was "safe."[32] Physicians at the Center for Disease Control took issue with this conclusion, arguing that baboons differed from human toddlers and that human dietary intake of lead from all sources was far more variable than the AAP realized.[33] Despite CDC objections, the Consumer Product Safety Commission held its ground at 0.5 percent.[34]

In 1975 the Senate held hearings on the CPSC ruling. Herbert Needleman, a pediatrician who was finding neurological deficits in children with undue lead absorption, and Ellen Silbergeld, a fellow in neurosciences at Johns Hopkins, attacked the baboon study and questioned whether even the 0.06 percent limit ensured safety.[35]

The matter was once again referred to the National Academy of Sciences.[36] Now, in 1976, the NAS reversed its prior conclusion. In the interim since its report in 1973, two important events had occurred. First, there was some evidence that children absorbed lead at rates higher than that of adults (10 percent, based on Aub and Kehoe's studies of animals and adult lead workers), perhaps as high as 40–50 percent.[37] Second, the Public Health Service had lowered its level of concern to blood lead levels of 30 micrograms/dl.[38] These two findings lowered the recommendation for maximum intake of lead to 6 micrograms/kg/day. For a 10-kg toddler, this would translate to 60 micrograms instead of 300.[39] The NAS also used a different estimate of the quantity of paint consumed by a child with pica. Relying on an X-ray study from Chicago, the NAS believed that a child might consume as much as 1–3 grams of paint each week. For 0.5 percent paint, this would mean 29 micrograms/kg/day, or nearly five times the new recommendations. A similar calculation with 0.06 percent lead paint did not reach a danger point. In 1977 the Consumer Product Safety Commission adopted the 0.06 recommendation of the AAP and NAS.[40]

Exterior Paint

The federal regulatory response in the 1970s also extended restrictions on the use of lead-based paints to include both interiors and exteriors. Regulations under the Lead Paint Poisoning Prevention Act adopted by HEW and HUD in 1972 and 1976 barred the use of lead-containing paint in federally assisted housing and required abatement of existing lead paints from federal housing for interior surfaces and for those exterior surfaces "which are readily accessible to children."[41] In regulating paint sold through interstate commerce, however, the Food and Drug Administration in 1972 and the Consumer Product Safety Commission thereafter proposed lowering the lead content of all lead-containing paints intended for use "in or around the household" to 0.06 percent.[42] In modifying "readily accessible to children" to "in or around the household," the FDA and CPSC sought to extend what had been a restriction for interior paints and paints for porches to a restriction on all paints used for household purposes.

The FDA and CPSC solicited comments from the paint manufacturers about their proposal to extend the lower permissible content of lead to all paints. The National Paint and Coatings Association (NPCA), successor to the National Paint, Lacquer, and Varnish Association, urged the CPSC to exempt eight painting categories:

1. Refinish coatings for automobiles and machinery
2. Industrial maintenance paints, including traffic and safety marking paints
3. Graphic arts paints for billboards and road signs
4. Touch-up paints for automobiles, lawn and garden equipment
5. Exterior marine paints for small craft
6. Exterior rubber-based roof coatings
7. "Exterior primer paints for wood siding containing extractives (products marketed solely for application on redwood and cedar)"
8. Radio controlled model aircraft paints (added in 1977)[43]

Of these, only the request for an exemption for a primer coat for exterior sidings provoked a strong response from the public health community. The NPCA claimed:

> Continued manufacture and sale of exterior staining wood primers of this type which contain lead is necessary for this limited purpose. We do not believe that the use of this product poses a reasonably foreseeable lead hazard to children for each of the following reasons: 1. a lead-containing primer need only be used once, and thus, there is no buildup of layers of lead-containing paint, which is recognized as a primary cause of lead poisoning; 2. exterior house siding is not readily accessible to children in the sense that porch railings and ornamental surfaces are accessible; 3. staining, as distinguished from non-staining woods are not widely used for siding; and 4. some of the primer penetrates the wood substrate and thus, should the coating peel, little, if any, of the primer peels with it.[44]

Between 1972 and 1977, these proposed exemptions remained acceptable to the CPSC.

After the 1976 report of the National Academy of Sciences, the CPSC reopened the issue. The National Paint and Coatings Association renewed its plea for exemptions. Taking issue with the NPCA's request, the Consumers Union argued: "Young children play in dirt, frequently put their dirty hands into their mouths and, thus, the lead-bearing exterior coating finds this indirect path into children's systems. . . . Additionally, the CPSC cannot control end use. The leftover of paints purchased by owners of residential property for exterior application, common experience shows, will sometimes be used for interior application. This greatly increases the danger to a child with paint pica of ingesting such paint."[45] These concerns were echoed by several prominent health departments.[46] After gathering comments, the Consumer Product Safety Commission rejected the proposed exemption for external priming coats, resulting in the reduction of lead to 0.06 percent for paints in 1978. The extension of the new limit to all household paint was based on the view that reliance on precautionary labeling against particular uses of lead paint was impractical.[47] The extension also reflected the concern of some public health officials that the weathering of outside paints generated hazardous contamination of the soil around the home.[48] Complementing federal regulations were a few state and city ordinances that also extended the lower limit on the use of lead-based paint to all house paint.[49] In these regulations most local and state governments continued to specify only interior surfaces and those exterior surfaces readily accessible to children.[50]

The Consumer Product Safety Commission also pointed out that several agencies of the federal government were issuing guidelines, regulations, and rulings that were duplicative and conflicting.[51] In addition to the CPSC and the FDA, the Environmental Protection Agency, the Center for Disease Control, and the Department of Housing and Urban Development all had policies on childhood lead poisoning.

An example of conflicting strategies within the federal government was the Department of Health, Education, and Welfare's "health approach" to childhood lead poisoning that stressed screening and treating and the Department of Housing and Urban Development's mandate of abatement.[52] Officials at HUD complained that there had been very little funding for abatement despite the congressional mandate that HUD remove dangerous levels of lead paint from housing. HUD officials argued that the experience in New York City suggested that widespread abatement might not be necessary. Mean blood lead levels fell from 31 micrograms/dl (African American children) and 26 micrograms/dl (white and Hispanic children) in 1970 to 22 micrograms/dl (African American children) and 19 micrograms/dl (white and Hispanic children) in 1976. By 1976 there were far fewer children in New York City with blood lead levels in the treatment range. During the first years of the screening program, public health officials had identified about 3 percent of children with blood lead levels in excess of 60 micrograms/dl; in 1976 there were between 0.2 and 0.5 percent.[53] Similar declines occurred in Newark, New Jersey, and Chicago.[54]

HUD experts saw no clear relationship between lead paint in a child's home and lead in a child's body. These encouraging signs called into question whether the unfunded congressional mandate to abate lead paint made sense.[55] HUD officials estimated that the average cost to abate an apartment was $1,000. However, the nation's bill depended on what degree of abatement was believed necessary:

$2.1 billion for removal of peeling and flaking paint in apartments housing young children; $20 billion for removal of paint with greater than 1 percent lead; and $55 billion for the removal of all lead paint.[56] These officials complained that a proper cost-benefit analysis could not be carried out because "too little is known and too little data are available on the relative contributions of the different sources of lead."[57] Complicating the question of abatement was a lack of consensus on how best to accomplish paint removal without creating new environmental health hazards.[58] Clearly, HUD officials looked at the problem of childhood lead poisoning and reached conclusions different from those of pediatricians, the CDC, and Congress.

In contrast, the Center for Disease Control in 1978 focused on data showing "a growing body of knowledge indicat[ing] that subtle effects of lead may be expressed in altered neuropsychological behavior of considerable significance, especially in the growing child."[59] The CDC lowered its definition of "undue lead absorption" to 30 micrograms/dl and in doing so greatly increased the number of children deemed at risk: "Large scale screening studies of children without symptoms have demonstrated that the number of children with undue lead absorption is greater than previously thought."[60] In 1978 the CDC still identified lead-based paint on interior and exterior surfaces as the single most important source of lead in severely poisoned children. But the CDC also stressed that air, dust, and dirt were additional sources of lead.[61]

The CDC, which did not have responsibility for abatement, nonetheless had definite ideas on how to accomplish it. CDC officials urged the immediate scraping of peeling and flaking areas and covering them with adhesive-backed paper. While this work was being accomplished, the CDC recommended that children leave the premises. Families should be taught "housekeeping techniques such as thorough sweeping and wet mopping floors to remove dust."[62] The CDC then urged a more permanent abatement. Of the possible methods, public health officials thought that wall coverings were safe, effective, and relatively inexpensive. Burning, while effective, produced hazardous fumes. Scraping and sanding was effective but labor intensive and expensive. Liquid paint removers were dangerous to workers. The CDC did not estimate costs.[63]

Local and state governments also passed ordinances requiring the removal or covering of hazardous lead-painted surfaces.[64] On the federal level, the 1973 Amendments to the Lead-Based Paint Poisoning Prevention Act directed HUD to "eliminate as far as practicable" the hazards of existing lead paint in federally assisted housing. HUD interpreted the law to address only peeling and flaking paint, reflecting the view that intact paint on well-maintained walls or woodwork did not present a danger to toddlers.[65]

Conflicting regulations were one result of agencies' efforts to manage an epidemic of ever-increasing scope. Concern over lead in the air intensified while paint came under new scrutiny as the level of lead deemed acceptable in the human body, particularly in children, was steadily lowered.

Chapter 15

Dust, Dirt, and Mouthing in 1980

ALTHOUGH SOME PUBLIC HEALTH officials were enthusiastic about the decline in the number of symptomatic cases of childhood lead poisoning and in the decline in the average blood lead levels even within inner-city neighborhoods, new worries about the effects of lead continued to surface as the 1970s progressed. Pediatricians queried whether lead's interference with heme formation might represent a template for other vital bodily reactions. Neurologists and psychologists uncovered subtle, but statistically significant, deficits in intellectual, neurological, and behavioral functioning. Although housing and public health officials continued to direct the nation's attention to the dangers of old peeling and flaking paint, overall lower blood levels indicated that children had less access to this source of lead.

Additional worries came from a number of places. Further investigations into air pollution discovered that atmospheric lead accounted for a significant foundation of around 20 micrograms/dl. With the Center for Disease Control's identification of the danger point as 40 micrograms/dl (until 1975) and later 30 micrograms/dl (in 1978), atmospheric lead figured more prominently. Not only was inhaled air of concern, but also the dust and dirt where air pollution settled. Alarming as well were studies that pointed out that infants absorbed a higher percentage of ingested lead than did adults.[1] As the point of concern—as determined by blood lead levels—lowered, suburbs, where more white children lived, were also seen to pose dangers to children.[2] When middle-class home renovators scraped and sanded old paint from walls and woodwork, they created dust, posing a risk.[3]

House Dust

House dust joined paint flakes and street dust as a hazard for children. Home visits, pioneered in Baltimore, had identified peeling and flaking paint. But by 1970, perhaps half of visited homes no longer had evidence of this deterioration. Where was the lead coming from?[4] Julian Chisholm—citing the National Academy of Sciences' *Lead: Airborne Lead in Perspective*—pointed to atmospheric lead and to street dust: "It is likely that the degree of lead absorption which this range [30–50 micrograms] reflects can be attributed, in large measure, to overall environmental pollution, other factors, and in urban areas, particularly to dust."[5] It was also proposed that toddlers' sticky hands attracted sufficient lead from both street dust and household dust to elevate blood lead levels during normal hand-to-mouth behaviors: "Lead in street dirt in Boston and Washington has been measured in concentrations exceeding 0.5 percent, and Boston house dust has been found to contain 0.1 to 0.2 percent of lead. Ingestion of 1/24 of a teaspoon of dust can exceed the daily permissible intake of 300 micrograms of lead."[6] In just months, a group of pediatricians in Rochester, New York, measured house dust on children's hands and from household surfaces; they concluded that there was enough lead to raise the blood level if the hands were licked and sucked over time.[7] They did not actually measure the lead intake of any particular child, and they did not determine the source of lead in house dust, other than to suggest air pollution and decaying paint.

The "dust hypothesis" caught on quickly. By 1974 it had been mentioned in several prominent reviews of childhood lead poisoning.[8] Members of the Rochester group amplified their views that same year: "The theory implies that the lead on children's hands is then ingested and absorbed in sufficient quantities to result in an elevated blood level. At present, there is no direct evidence to support this idea. However, if only 50 percent of the average hand contamination is transferred into the mouth and swallowed several times per day, the daily permissible intake may be easily exceeded, especially since the intestinal lead absorption has been found much higher at young ages than in adults."[9]

In 1975 a group of researchers from Connecticut measured the amount of lead in household air, household dust, and outside dust. They reached similar conclusions about the theoretical possibility of ingesting enough lead from licking household dust from sticky fingers. Of note, the concentration of lead in household air was about 3 micrograms/cubic meter, or less than 1 percent the level measured in factories by Thomas Legge in the first years of the century.[10] Values from the Connecticut study found their way into various calculations of the daily intake of lead.[11]

Researchers debated the source of lead in house dust and outside dust.[12] Some believed that pulverized lead paint contributed the most lead;[13] others thought air pollution.[14] Proximity to heavily trafficked roads elevated the blood lead levels.[15] In one of the best studies, the Rochester group documented that most lead appeared to enter households through ill-fitting windows, a finding that pointed to air pollution as the major source of lead.[16] By 1980 atmospheric lead, proximity to heavily traveled roads, and household dustiness were the best predictors of which children were likely to become lead-poisoned.[17]

Mouthing

For fifty years, pediatricians had believed that children with aggressive eating behaviors—children who literally stripped porch railings, cribs, and other furniture bare of paint or chewed large holes into walls—were most at risk for lead poisoning. Their actions differed from the normal hand-to-mouth behavior that all children display.[18] But in the 1970s this normal mouthing activity became seen as a risky behavior, because the amount of lead that a toddler licked from dusty hands contained enough lead to raise blood lead levels to the new level of concern. The small number of children with pica were still at greatest risk, but nearly all toddlers had dust-covered sticky fingers.[19] When parents made concerted efforts to wet-mop floors and walls and to wash toddlers' hands frequently, blood lead levels declined.[20] The Rochester pediatricians summarized:

> More recent studies have led to new concerns. These studies suggest that the paint chip ingestion we so commonly saw among children suffering from lead encephalopathy, though still the major lead source, may be only one of a number of environmental risks. These risks are probably additive and may combine to explain the source of environmental lead in a child who does not appear to have pica and whose home may not contain obvious chipping paint. Milk, polluted air, the use of ceramic drinking vessels, and dust are now under careful study. Dust present on household surfaces (floor, window sills, and walls) has been shown to contain substantially higher amounts of lead in old inner city homes than in suburban homes. Similarly, lead can be found on the hands of children living in inner city homes in higher amounts than on the hands of their counterparts living in suburban homes. The suggestion was made that daily ingestion of this hand surface lead by normal hand-to-mouth activity may play a substantial role in childhood lead exposure.[21]

Neurological, Psychological, and Behavioral Consequences

Air, dust, dirt, and sticky fingers changed the ecology of childhood lead poisoning: *all* American children were potentially at risk.[22] In the 1970s investigators measured lead's toll in terms of damage to the nervous system. For decades, workers in the field had agreed that symptomatic children were at risk. Before the 1970s, only two studies had attempted to assess the intellectual and emotional outcome of asymptomatic children. In 1963, Hugo Smith compared the outcome of exposed children who had blood lead levels above 60 micrograms/ dl who were symptomatic with those who were asymptomatic. Only those with symptoms suffered neurological consequences.[23] The other study came from Chicago's mass-screening project.

Meyer Perlstein and Ramzy Attala tested 425 children identified in some of the city's worst slums.[24] Perlstein and Attala understood that they had no objective measure of the children's intellectual and emotional functioning prior to lead exposure; they relied solely on parental recollections. And they did not attempt to sort out what many researchers termed the "complex of adverse health, social, educational, and economic factors" that encompassed the lives of lead-exposed children.[25] Although the majority of children showed no long-term effects from lead exposure, most of the children who had symptoms prior to treatment were left with handicaps, a conclusion, while not new, that Chisholm included in his testimony before a Senate hearing in 1970. Perlstein and Attala added to the discussion in their finding that some asymptomatic children also suffered long-range neurological problems.[26]

Public health guidelines reflected the general state of medical thought about the neurological consequences of lead exposure. In 1969 the American Academy of Pediatrics issued its "Prevention, Diagnosis, and Treatment of Lead Poisoning in Childhood."[27] The following year, the surgeon general issued "Medical Aspects of Childhood Lead Poisoning."[28] As consensus reports based on a wide range of expert opinion, both were important in illustrating how physicians thought about the relationship between lead exposure and neurological damage. Both reports tied concern for neurological outcome to overt symptoms of encephalopathy, pegged at a blood lead level of greater than 80 micrograms/dl; and both reports were concerned at lower blood lead levels, roughly 50–79 micrograms/dl, only if the child also had symptoms. These were the children who required prompt treatment to prevent permanent neurological damage. Blood lead levels in the 50–79 micrograms/dl range, but without symptoms, were worrisome only because the levels indicated that the children lived in environments containing a source of lead that, if not eliminated, might eventually drive up the blood lead to symptomatic (in excess of 80 micrograms/dl) levels. Significantly, neither report stated that a blood lead level below 80 micrograms/dl, without symptoms, was likely to cause permanent neurological damage.

In the early 1970s, many researchers attempted to address questions about the potential neurological danger of lead exposure at levels lower than those known to result in symptoms. These studies reached different conclusions. In part, this disparity stemmed from methodological difficulties.

In Boston, Siegfried Pueschel performed psychological and neurological testing on children screened for lead. About one-fourth of those with a blood lead
level of 50 micrograms/dl or higher demonstrated "minor neurological dysfunction" at the time of screening, eighteen months later,[29] and upon retesting three
years after initial screening, findings that suggested that these asymptomatic lead
levels resulted in a "subtle" handicap.[30] Selecting a "screened" population, of
course, meant that many of these children most likely came from impoverished
backgrounds, doubtless also contributing to lower scores on psychological tests.
In Richmond, Brigette de la Burdé determined that lead-exposed children had
slight impairment in fine motor behaviors[31] and measurable deficits in global
IQ.[32] Both studies were marred by a failure to obtain blood lead levels for control children and by selecting control children from backgrounds distinctly different from those of the lead-exposed test subjects. In New Haven, David Kotok
compared children identified in a screening survey, who had an average blood
lead level of 83 micrograms/dl, with a "normal" control group of children, who
had an average blood lead level of 38 micrograms/dl. He found no differences
in neurological or developmental testing between the two groups. Rather, he
discovered that both groups were equally delayed, a finding that he interpreted
as the effect of poverty, not exposure to lead.[33] Some commentators criticized
Kotok's conclusions, claiming that the "normal" group of children also had significant lead exposure so that they could not serve as "controls."[34] Julian
Chisholm, commenting on the same study, concluded that it demonstrated the
difficulty in finding adequate control groups for sorting out the relative importance of lead exposure in children with "multiple adverse environmental factors."[35] Using psychometric tests, R. E. Albert found significant impairments
in children with blood lead levels above 80 micrograms/dl, but no handicap at
40 micrograms/dl. Children with levels between 40 and 80 micrograms/dl demonstrated mixed results.[36] One researcher suggested that all studies were marred
because the psychometric tests that were employed failed to take into account
socioeconomic factors.[37]

In 1975 Philip Landrigan measured psychological functioning in children
with blood lead levels between 40 and 68 micrograms/dl (but without symptoms)
and compared them with children with blood lead levels below 40 micrograms/
dl. He found a "subtle but statistically significant impairment in the non-verbal
cognitive and perceptual motor skills." Despite the findings, Landrigan concluded
that the "biological and developmental significance of our findings is not clear."[38]
Some researchers argued that children evaluated and treated for hyperactivity
had slightly higher levels of lead in their blood.[39]

Other studies were not as conclusive. Robert Baloh measured a degree of
hyperactivity in children with blood lead levels in excess of 50 micrograms/dl
but could demonstrate no abnormalities on quantitative psychological tests,

leading him to conclude that "there is still uncertainty about the neuropsycho-logical effects of asymptomatic increased lead absorption in children."[40] This was a conclusion also reached in one British study.[41]

Midway through the 1970s, there was a suspicion among some researchers that lead exposure at asymptomatic levels resulted in "subtle" neurological im-pairments. But most researchers tempered this suspicion with the understand-ing that the jury was still out on the subject. For example, Chisholm stated that there was "no clear evidence whether this lower level of increased absorption [50–80 micrograms/dl] is associated with neurological impairment."[42] Herbert Needleman, who would become an adamant advocate for neurological damage at lower blood levels, also recognized the deficiency in knowledge: "Whether subclinical exposure to lead produces significant neuropsychiatric impairment is a critical question . . . and [is] recognized as crucial to the setting and proper standards for both treatment and environmental prevention of exposure."[43] Another researcher expressed doubt on the subject: "There is very little clinical evidence that children who have even very high blood lead levels but do not develop overt encephalopathy suffer any important temporary or permanent ill effects from their lead exposure."[44] The editors at Lancet and the British Medi-cal Journal also concluded that studies were inconclusive whether low-level lead exposure resulted in intellectual handicaps.[45]

Public health pronouncements reflected this cautious view. For example, the U.S. Public Health Service (Center for Disease Control) issued revised guide-lines in 1975. Symptomatic lead poisoning remained the major worry; treatment was targeted for children who had blood lead levels above 80 micrograms/dl and lower (50–79 micrograms/dl) if symptoms occurred. The upper limits of what was considered a normal blood lead level was lowered to 30 micrograms/dl (from 40 micrograms/dl in 1970). The area between 30 and 80 micrograms/dl remained hazy, especially at the upper end, but the CDC did not conclude that children in this range were at risk to sustain neurological injury.[46]

In the years after 1975, several studies added evidence that children with lead exposures that produced blood lead levels in the "hazy" area suffered from measurable, and statistically significant, impairments. Nevertheless the studies conflicted, often on methodological grounds. Four studies published in 1979 dem-onstrated the spectrum of opinion. Herbert Needleman, comparing psychologi-cal testing in children with the highest 10 percent of dentine lead compared with children with the lowest 10 percent of dentine lead, found that the higher-lead group had a lower full-scale IQ (102.1 versus 106.6).[47] Needleman's study received quick praise from some,[48] but other researchers were critical of his se-lection of control groups.[49] In contrast, R. Lansdown in the United Kingdom could demonstrate no psychological impairments in children with blood lead levels in the range of 25–60 micrograms/dl. He explained his findings by arguing that children who lived in areas with considerable access to lead were also exposed to many adverse socioeconomic conditions: he could demonstrate no effect uniquely due to lead.[50] In Chicago, Henrietta Sachs also failed to demonstrate statistically significant neurological or psychological impairments in asymptomatic children who had blood lead levels from 40 to 471 micrograms/ dl. Both her test group and controls had lower-than-average IQ (87), which she attributed to growing up in an inner-city environment.[51] Needleman immediately called attention to four methodological shortcomings that he perceived in Sachs's study design;[52] Philip Landrigan joined Needleman in his criticism.[53] In a fourth study published in 1979, Judith Rummo measured differences in neurological examinations, developmental testing, and degree of hyperactivity in children she studied with blood lead levels over 40 micrograms/dl, but she conceded that these differences were too small to achieve statistical significance.[54]

In 1980 two lengthy analyses appeared that attempted to sift through the many studies. Both detailed the methodological problems that plagued most of them. The authors reached slightly different conclusions. Michael Rutter, aware of Landrigan and Needleman's work among others, thought that sufficient evidence existed to conclude that children with a blood lead level in excess of 60 micrograms/dl suffered a reduction in IQ of 3–4 points on average. He thought that the evidence for neurological impairment was inconclusive in children whose blood lead levels fell between 40 and 60 micrograms/dl.[55] Robert Bornschein, reading much the same literature, reached similar conclusions about the methodological shortcomings. But he found "no clear trend indicating that moderate lead exposure caused any abnormalities in behavioral development . . . nor was there compelling evidence which suggested that this was not the case."[56] In less all-encompassing reviews, two additional reassessments reached conclusions similar to those of Rutter.[57]

In 1979 Julian Chisholm and Donald Barltrop pooled their experiences in the United States and Britain. Much of their attention was directed toward the continuing issue of the long-term effects of asymptomatic levels of lead:

> There is no longer any reasonable doubt that acute lead encephalopathy and recurrent symptomatic plumbism in children can, in a big percentage of cases, result in severe residual CNS injury, including seizures, mental retardation, severely handicapping behavioural disorders and, in rare cases, blindness and hemiparesis. In asymptomatic or mildly symptomatic plumbism, clinical studies have given conflicting results. There is some evidence, however, that a sustained [blood lead level greater than] 50–60 micrograms/dl during early childhood carries significant risk of subtle neurobehavioural impairment, but not for the serious sequelae associated with symptomatic lead poisoning. Such subtle deficits do not become evident until later in childhood.[58]

Public health guidelines reflected concerns about the effects of lower levels of lead on children's nervous systems. For example, the CDC modified its recommendations again in 1978, recommending treatment at blood lead levels of 70 micrograms/dl and at lower blood lead levels if symptoms existed. The upper range of normal remained 30 micrograms/dl. For blood lead levels in the middle range, the CDC warned for the first time that "subtle effects may be expressed in altered neuropsychological behavior of considerable significance."[59] Despite this conclusion, the CDC did not advocate treatment for children whose blood lead levels fell in the 30–70 micrograms/dl range.

How to manage children with blood lead levels between 30 and 70 micrograms/dl was a debated issue. These children, identified in screening programs, were clearly at risk. But what was the prudent approach? Some urged chelation therapy for children in order to prevent subtle neurological damage. The introduction of an effective oral chelating drug, D-penicillamine, made this course safe and attractive. Others argued that chelation did not prevent these problems. Still others thought removal of the child from the leaden environment was "all" that was needed.[60]

Epilogue

In 1978, THE year when tetraethyl lead was removed from gasoline and virtually all lead from all household paints, the Center for Disease Control issued a new set of guidelines for the diagnosis and management of childhood lead poisoning. The CDC defined three categories of concern: "elevated lead level," greater than 30 micrograms/dl; "undue lead absorption," 30–69 micrograms/dl; and "lead poisoning," 70 micrograms/dl, or lower if symptoms existed.[1] The CDC's focus was the "undue lead absorption" group: "Because of the large number of children involved, these adverse effects ['altered neuropsychological behavior'] would appear to be the main cause for societal concern."[2] Children with blood lead levels of 70 micrograms/dl were rare; those with higher levels and symptoms, rarer still. The CDC considered children with blood lead levels below 30 micrograms/dl "low risk" and stated that they "are usually not given other diagnostic tests."[3]

The contrast between this CDC report and the ones of 1970 and 1975 was stark. Earlier statements had alerted pediatricians and health departments to symptoms. By 1978 virtually all children, even in the "lead-poisoning" group, looked entirely well both to parents and to doctors. In less than a decade, the public health target had shifted from preventing death and devastating brain damage to preventing subtle behaviors that "impair[ed] progress in school."[4] What accounts for this switch of emphasis? It was not that pediatricians no longer worried about symptomatic children, but they were, in fact, largely gone. Coupled with the disappearance of symptomatic cases was mounting evidence of small, but measurable, neurological injury. Before 1970, such evidence did not exist.

By the early 1990s, the CDC's 1978 "undue lead absorption" category had also largely disappeared. One measure of this public health triumph was the

Table 1
Blood Lead Levels (μg/dl) in U.S. Children by Race and Age, 1976–1980

Race and age	Mean Pb-B	Median Pb-B	Prevalence of Pb-B at μg/dl Levels of			
			<20	20–29	30–39	≥40
White						
0.5–2 yr	15.0	14.0	80.2	17.3	2.2	0.3
3–5 yr	14.9	14.0	82.7	15.4	1.6	0.3
Black						
0.5–2 yr	20.9	19.0	50.5	34.2	13.0	2.3
3–5 yr	20.8	20.0	46.3	43.3	8.5	1.9

SOURCE: "The Nature and Extent of Lead Poisoning in Children in the United States: A Report to Congress," U.S. Department of Health and Human Services, July 1988, V-32.

decline in blood lead concentration. In the late 1970s the mean blood lead level for white children between six months and five years of age was 15 micrograms/dl; for African American children, 21 micrograms/dl, indicating that the spectacular decline in blood lead levels was not universally shared. (See table 1.)[5] Ten years later, in the early 1990s, mean blood lead levels for children under five years of age fell to 2.7 micrograms/dl. By then the CDC was concerned about children with levels over 10 micrograms/dl, so its report in *Morbidity and Mortality Weekly Report* divided children into those above and below this new threshold. Only 4.4 percent had blood lead levels above 10 micrograms/dl. The racial gradient persisted at this lower level: for African American children, 11.2 percent had levels above 10 micrograms/dl; for Mexican American children, 4.0 percent; for white children, 2.3 percent.[6] In other words, the children who worried the CDC in 1978 were largely gone by 1994, just as the children who concerned the surgeon general in 1970 had mostly disappeared by 1978. The emergence and disappearance of lead poisoning and undue lead absorption as defined in the 1970s, I believe, are just recent examples of what has happened over and again in the history of childhood lead poisoning during the course of the twentieth century.

Although the numbers were sparse, in the 1940s, the average blood lead level for children in Baltimore who did not have pica was about 30 micrograms/dl. In the early 1970s, adults in Rochester, New York, had blood lead levels of 20 micrograms/dl. The decline to 2.7 micrograms/dl in 1990 from 30 micrograms/dl roughly a half century earlier, a drop of over 90 percent, resulted from the existence of far less lead in the child's environment. What happened? It is important not to jump to facile conclusions. For example, even though many communities had adopted strict abatement laws, the Centers for Disease Control concluded in 1991: "Lead-based paint is rarely completely abated in many of the largest childhood lead prevention programs. Instead, various degrees of incomplete abatement—designed to eliminate the worst hazards and prevent near-term exposures—are conducted."[7] But even though much—perhaps as much as three million tons—of the old paint, which contains the highest concentration of lead, remained on the walls of houses and apartments, children did not consume sufficient lead either to experience symptoms or even to reach the blood levels that pediatricians defined as hazardous as late as 1978 or, for that matter, 1994.

The several emergences and disappearances of childhood lead poisoning in twentieth-century America represent complicated intersections: exposures to environmental lead from sources that changed over the course of the century; the intimate surroundings of toddlers; the perceptions of physicians, public health officials, and psychologists about the nature of the lead menace and how children encountered it; chemical diagnostic technologies; the increasing sophistication of psychological testing that permitted researchers and clinicians to measure the effects of lead more precisely; and the effectiveness of public health responses crafted to meet the lead hazard as understood at the time.

Childhood lead poisoning was rare in the first decades of the twentieth century because few toddlers consumed enough lead to produce the symptoms that would allow pediatricians to make a diagnosis. This is not to say that there were no children poisoned from lead paint before Henry Thomas and Kenneth Blackfan encountered their first patient in 1914. That this boy had to return several times to the Harriet Lane Home before his physicians even thought of the possibility of lead poisoning speaks to its rarity. Even when pediatricians were alerted to consider a diagnosis of lead poisoning in children with seizures who did not have brain infections, there were few diagnoses until the 1930s. How did toddlers get enough lead into their bodies during the first decades of the century? Certainly insecticide-drenched foods played a role; in fact, Robert Kehoe believed this was how most Americans—children and adults—encountered lead when he investigated the average diet in the 1930s. But diet alone would not raise the level of lead high enough for a toddler to lapse into coma. Casual chewing of a crib or toy was probably not enough either. Cribs might be repainted over and over again, but if a toddler chewed on only one or two spots, it is unlikely that the infant would consume enough lead to produce symptoms.

Parents, home health visitors, and pediatricians did not witness casual gnawing. Instead, they described chewing that stripped every bit of paint off cribs, toys, or porch railings. This was not normal hand-to-mouth behavior; this was pica. Cribs, toys, other furniture, and woodwork were the observed sources of lead, but were they the only ones? Could these toddlers have just as easily attacked the walls or ceilings, or collected peeling or flaking paint from the apartment floor? The historical record indicates that no home health visitors observed this until the late 1940s. Even Baltimore Health Department officials, who were a repository of the nation's experience with this disease, did not witness children chewing on walls or consuming paint flakes until late 1948. Huntington Williams, who in 1941 aggressively acquired for the Health Department responsibility for housing health hazards, did not add lead paint to the Baltimore Plan until 1951.

It is likely that the dozens of lead-poisoned children whom pediatricians diagnosed before the great upsurge in the late 1940s ingested sufficient lead in just the manner that their parents described: by aggressively chewing all the paint from the surfaces of their intimate surroundings. This could go on for months, in some cases years, before symptoms developed.

The public health response to this hazard made sense: alerting parents to pica, to the dangers of chewing on painted cribs and toys, and to the need for selecting nonleaded paints when it came time to repaint. Crib and toy manufacturers responded to the hazard by decorating new cribs and toys with paints that did not contain lead pigments. Pediatricians, health departments, toy and crib manufacturers, and the Lead Industries Association thus all understood the hazard and the public health response in the same way. They were successful in their efforts. In the 1940s, few believed that toys, cribs, or other children's furniture were dangerous to children unless improperly repainted with lead-containing paint.

Then the lead environment altered. Lead insecticides contaminated foods less, but tetraethyl lead polluted the atmosphere. Atmospheric lead slowly increased, providing a base that no American could escape. Lead paint spread on walls earlier in the century aged, flaked, and peeled. In the imploding inner city, walls that had once been repainted and kept in good repair were allowed to deteriorate.

Paint chips and flakes, lying everywhere about the tenements, were not understood as a problem until home health visitors—those in Boston and Baltimore—journeyed into the slums after World War II. They did not observe an occasional flake or chip. They described walls and ceilings where the paint hung in "stalactites." Surrounded by this state of decay—with old lead paint strewn everywhere—toddlers could obtain sufficient lead to reach levels capable of producing coma. Children with pica were still at greatest risk, but all toddlers living in this type of environment might be poisoned. Lead poisoning cases jumped in the 1950s and 1960s because lead in the American child's environment greatly increased.

Public health officials, pediatricians, and lead industry leaders met this hazard head on. First, they warned the public that paint chips and flakes were dangerous and could not remain on floors where toddlers played. "Intact" surfaces—

ones that had been scraped, sanded, repainted, or covered—became the goal of local health and housing departments in the 1950s and 1960s and the focus of federally sponsored programs in the 1970s. All public health officials identified old paint as the problem, most of it applied before World War II. In fact, paint with the highest concentrations of lead had been applied in the first decades of the century and was now buried under coats of paint with less lead or with zinc-based or titanium-based pigments. Landlords and public housing officials learned that the paint on walls needed to be in good repair. In 1955 leaders of public health organizations, government, pediatricians, and industry supported the 1 percent voluntary standard so that paints with lead pigments would no longer be used on interior walls. For newly constructed buildings, 1 percent paint was the only paint applied. As the experience with Cleveland public housing demonstrated, few, if any, children became lead-poisoned living in new public housing.

At the end of the 1960s, what had been thought of as a hazard affecting thousands of children expanded into an epidemic that threatened hundreds of thousands, perhaps millions, of American children. Mass-screening technologies, such as free erythrocyte protoporphyrin (FEP) and microlead—unavailable until the 1970s—played a role in quantifying this epidemic. Pervasive concerns for environmental and atmospheric pollution in general and worries about subtle injuries of asymptomatic "undue lead absorption" joined forces to focus public health efforts on lower and lower levels of lead. As neuropsychological tests pinpointed the dangers at less and less exposure to lead, the specter of risk altered.

In the early 1970s, home visitors reported that many homes where poisoned children resided no longer had obvious sources of decaying lead paint—itself a public health triumph. Street dust contaminated by atmospheric lead emerged as a new menace. By the mid-1970s, house dust collected on sticky fingers created anguish for parents and physicians. The history of childhood lead paint poisoning has been a story of changing dangers and a constantly evolving calculus of risk.

It is the shift in public health thinking, which eventually identified any amount of lead exposure as hazardous because it might result in measurable neurological damage, that provides the key for understanding childhood lead poisoning and its history over time. By 1980, pediatricians looked beyond physically apparent symptoms, pica, and considerable lead consumption. Any child was at risk. Public health solutions that made sense when a small amount of lead was thought permissible both in the environment and in the child yielded to a world where any amount of lead was considered hazardous. Nevertheless, a child health worker of 1900 or, for that matter, of 1980 would judge the reduction of lead in a child's environment as the new millennium began a public health triumph.

Notes

Preface

1. American Academy of Pediatrics, Subcommittee on Accidental Poisoning, "Prevention, Diagnosis, and Treatment of Lead Poisoning in Childhood," *Pediatrics* (1969), 44: 291–298; anonymous, "Medical Aspects of Childhood Lead Poisoning," *Pediatrics* (1971), 48: 464–468; and Lead-Based Paint Poisoning Prevention Act, P.L. 91–695.
2. Huntington Williams, Emanuel Kaplan, Charles E. Couchman, and R. R. Sayers, "Lead Poisoning in Young Children," *Public Health Reports* (1952), 67: 230–236.
3. (Boston) Randolph K. Byers, Clarence A. Maloof, and Margaret Cushman, "Urinary Excretion of Lead in Children: Diagnostic Application," *American Journal of Diseases of Children* (1954), 87: 548–558; Byers and Maloof, "Edathamil Calcium–Disodium (Versenate) in Treatment of Lead Poisoning in Children," *American Journal of Diseases of Children* (1954), 87: 559–569; (New York City) Harold Jacobziner and Harry W. Raybin, "Lead Poisoning in Young Children—Fatal and Nonfatal," *New York State Journal of Medicine* (1960), 60: 273–277; (Philadelphia) Emil Tiboni and Raymond L. Tyler, "Childhood Lead Poisoning in Philadelphia," *Philadelphia Medicine* (1960), 56: 668–669; (Cincinnati) Hugo Dunlap Smith, "Lead Poisoning in Children and Its Therapy with EDTA," *Industrial Medicine and Surgery* (1959), 28: 148–155; Smith, "Pediatric Lead Poisoning," *Archives of Environmental Health* (1961), 3: 256–261; and (Cleveland) Robert C. Griggs, Irving Sunshine, Vaun A. Newill, Burritt W. Newton, Stuart Buchanan, and Cleo A. Rasch, "Environmental Factors in Childhood Lead Poisoning," *Journal of the American Medical Association* (1964), 187: 703–707.
4. Peter C. English, *Rheumatic Fever in America and Britain: A Biological, Epidemiological, and Medical History* (New Brunswick, N.J.: Rutgers University Press, 1999).
5. Charles E. Rosenberg and Janet Golden, eds., *Framing Disease: Studies in Cultural History* (New Brunswick, N.J.: Rutgers University Press, 1992).
6. Peter C. English, "Therapeutic Strategies to Combat Pneumococcal Disease: Repeated Failure of Physicians to Adopt Pneumococcal Vaccine, 1900–1945," *Perspectives in Biology and Medicine* (1987), 30: 170–185.
7. Henry A. Gardner, *Papers on Paint and Varnish, and the Material Used in Their Manufacture* (Washington, D.C.: Paint and Varnish Manufacturers Association, 1920), 401–402.

8. Jack Newfield, "Lead Poisoning: Silent Epidemic in the Slums," *Village Voice* (September 18, 1969), 1.

9. Anonymous, "American Academy of Pediatrics Committee on Environmental Health. Lead Poisoning: From Screening to Primary Prevention," *Pediatrics* (1993), 92: 176. See also Centers for Disease Control, *Preventing Lead Poisoning in Young Children* (Atlanta: U.S. Department of Health and Human Services, 1991), 7; and National Research Council, *Measuring Lead Exposure in Infants, Children, and Other Sensitive Populations* (Washington, D.C.: National Academy Press, 1993), 254.

Prologue

1. Robert A. Kehoe, Frederick Thamann, and Jacob Cholak, "On the Normal Absorption and Excretion of Lead. II. Lead Absorption and Lead Excretion in Modern American Life," *Journal of Industrial Hygiene* (1933), 15: 273–288.

2. Joint FAO/WHO Expert Committee on Food Additives, *Evaluation of Certain Food Additives and the Contaminants Mercury, Lead, and Cadmium*, World Health Organization Technical Report Series, no. 505 (Geneva: World Health Organization, 1972), 19.

3. Joint FAO/WHO Expert Committee on Food Additives, *Evaluation of Certain Food Additives and Contaminants*, World Health Organization Technical Report Series, no. 696 (Geneva: World Health Organization, 1993), 32–35.

4. M. A. Adams, "FDA Total Diet Study: Dietary Intakes of Lead and Other Chemicals," *Chemical Speciation and Bioavailability* (1991), 3: 40; and see also Kathryn R. Mahaffey, "Quantities of Lead Producing Health Effects in Humans: Sources and Bioavailability," *Environmental Health Perspectives* (1977), 19: 285–295.

5. Joint FAO/WHO Expert Committee on Food Additives, *Evaluation of Certain Food Additives and Contaminants*, no. 696, 32–35.

6. Robert A. Kehoe, Frederick Thamann, and Jacob Cholak, "On the Normal Absorption and Excretion of Lead. III. The Sources of Normal Lead Absorption," *Journal of Industrial Hygiene* (1933), 15: 290–300.

7. Joint FAO/WHO Expert Committee on Food Additives, *Evaluation of Certain Food Additives and the Contaminants Mercury, Lead, and Cadmium*, no. 505, 17.

8. Joint FAO/WHO Expert Committee on Food Additives, *Evaluation of Certain Food Additives and Contaminants*, no. 696, 34.

9. J. J. Bloomfield and H. S. Isbell, "The Presence of Lead Dust and Fumes in the Air of Streets, Automobile Repair Shops, and Industrial Establishments of Large Cities," *Journal of Industrial Hygiene* (1933), 15: 144-149.

10. U.S. Public Health Service, Advisory Committee on Tetraethyl Lead to the Surgeon General of Public Health Service, *Public Health Aspects of Increasing Tetraethyl Lead Content in Motor Fuel* (Washington, D.C.: U.S. Public Health Service, Government Printing Office, 1959), 11.

11. Working Group on Lead Contamination, *Survey of Lead in the Atmosphere of Three Urban Communities* (Washington, D.C.: U.S. Department of Health, Education and Welfare, Government Printing Office, 1965), 46.

12. Joint FAO/WHO Expert Committee on Food Additives, *Evaluation of Certain Food Additives and the Contaminants Mercury, Lead, and Cadmium*, no. 505, 16–17.

13. John M. McDonald and Emanuel Kaplan, "Incidence of Lead Poisoning in the City of Baltimore," *Journal of the American Medical Association* (1942), 119: 871.

14. Anonymous, "Update: Blood Lead Levels—United States, and Selected States, 1996–1999," *Morbidity and Mortality Weekly Report* (2000), 49: 1133–1137.

15. Centers for Disease Control, *Preventing Lead Poisoning in Young Children* (Atlanta: U.S. Department of Health and Human Services, 1991), 18–19.

16. J. S. Lin-Fu, "Undue Lead Absorption and Lead Poisoning in Children—An Over-

view," in *International Conference on Heavy Metals in the Environment*, ed. T. C. Hutchinson (Toronto: University of Toronto, 1975), 29–52; Jane S. Lin-Fu, "Modern History of Lead Poisoning: A Century of Discovery and Rediscovery," in *Human Lead Exposure*, ed. Herbert L. Needleman (Boca Raton: CRC Press, 1992), 23–43; Jane S. Lin-Fu, "Lead Poisoning and Undue Lead Exposure in Children: History and Current Status," in *Low Level Lead Exposure: The Clinical Implications of Current Research*, ed. H. L. Needleman (New York: Raven Press, 1980), 7; J. Julian Chisholm, Jr., "Interrelationships among the Lead in Paint, House Dust, and Soil in Childhood Lead Poisoning: The Baltimore Experience," in *Lead in Soil: Issues and Guidelines*, ed. Brian E. Davies and Bobby G. Wixson, (n.p.: Science Reviews, 1988), 185–193; Harold H. Sandstead, "A Brief History of the Influence of Trace Elements on Brain Function," *American Journal of Clinical Nutrition* (1986), 43: 293–298; Richard Rabin, "Warnings Unheeded: A History of Child Lead Poisoning," *American Journal of Public Health* (1989), 79: 1668–1674; and Raymond R. Suskind, "Kettering Laboratory: A Pioneer in Lead Research," *American Journal of Public Health* (1990), 80: 1001–1002.

17. Barbara Berney, "Round and Round It Goes: The Epidemiology of Child Lead Poisoning, 1950–1990," *Milbank Quarterly* (1993), 71: 3–39; Samuel P. Hays, "The Role of Values in Science and Policy: The Case of Lead," in *Human Lead Exposure*, ed. Herbert L. Needleman (Boca Raton: CRC Press, 1992), 267–283; Theodore H. Tsoukalas, "Science, Socioenvironmental Inequality, and Childhood Lead Poisoning," *Society and Natural Resources* (1998), 11: 743–754; John C. Burnham, "How the Discovery of Accidental Childhood Poisoning Contributed to the Development of Environmentalism in the United States," *Environmental History Review* (1995), 19: 57–81; Burnham, "Why Did the Infants and Toddlers Die? Shifts in Americans' Ideas of Responsibility for Accidents—From Blaming Mom to Engineering," *Journal of Social History* (1996), 29: 817–837; Burnham, "Biomedical Communication and the Reaction to the Queensland Childhood Lead Poisoning Cases Elsewhere in the World," *Medical History* (1999), 43: 155–172; Christian Warren, "The Silenced Epidemic: A Social History of Lead Poisoning in the United States since 1900" (Ph.D. diss., Brandeis University, 1997); Jacquelyn K. Corn, "Historical Perspective to a Current Controversy on the Clinical Spectrum of Plumbism," *Milbank Memorial Fund Quarterly* (1975), 53: 93–114; Elizabeth Fee, "Public Health in Practice: An Early Confrontation with the 'Silent Epidemic' of Childhood Lead Paint Poisoning," *Journal of the History of Medicine and Allied Sciences* (1990), 45: 570–606; and Robert S. Broadhead, "Officer UGG, Mr. Yuk, Uncle Barf . . . Ad Nausea: Controlling Poison Control, 1950–1985," *Social Problems* (1986), 33: 424–437.

18. Christian Warren, *Brush with Death: A Social History of Lead Poisoning* (Baltimore: Johns Hopkins University Press, 2000); Gerald Markowitz and David Rosner, "'Cater to the Children': The Role of the Lead Industry in a Public Health Tragedy, 1900–1955," *American Journal of Public Health* (2000), 90: 36–46.

Chapter 1   Children and Lead before 1920

1. Henry M. Thomas and Kenneth D. Blackfan, "Recurrent Meningitis, Due to Lead, in a Child of Five Years," *American Journal of Diseases of Children* (1914), 8: 377–380.

2. Kenneth D. Blackfan, "Lead Poisoning in Children, with Especial Reference to Lead as a Cause of Convulsions," *American Journal of the Medical Sciences* (1917), 153: 885.

3. Henry Burton, "A Remarkable Effect upon the Human Gums Produced by the Absorption of Lead," *Medico-Chirurgical Transactions* (London) (1840), 23: 63–79; James Alderson, "On the Effects of Lead upon the System," *Lancet* (1852), 2: 73–75 and 95–98; John Bacon, "Elimination of Lead from the System," *Boston Medical and Surgical Journal* (1859), 60: 429–431; J. M. Da Costa, "Series of Cases of Lead-Poisoning,"

Medical and Surgical Reporter (1867), 17: 51–54; James G. Kiernan, "Psychoses Produced by Lead," *Journal of Nervous and Mental Diseases* (1881), 8: 454–460; Edward D. Fisher, "Lead Poisoning with Special Reference to the Spinal Cord and Peripheral Nerve Lesions," *American Journal of the Medical Sciences* (1892), 104: 51–54; J. W. Courtney, "A Case of Multiple Cerebral Hemorrhages from Chronic Lead Poisoning, with Necropsy," *Boston Medical and Surgical Journal* (1900), 142: 136–138; and William G. Spiller, "The Pathological Changes in the Nervous System in a Case of Lead Poisoning," *Journal of Medical Research* (1903), 10: 142–152.

4. Blackfan, "Lead Poisoning in Children with Especial Reference to Lead as a Cause of Convulsions," 878.

5. David Dennison Stewart, "Notes on Some Obscure Cases of Poisoning by Lead Chromate; Manifested Chiefly by Encephalopathy," *Medical News* (1887), 50: 676–681.

6. William Glenn, "Chrome Yellow Considered as a Poison," *Science* (1889), 13: 347–349.

7. D. D. Stewart, "Lead Convulsions: A Study of Sixteen Cases," *American Journal of the Medical Sciences* (1895), 109: 288–306.

8. John Deering and William Shearman, "History of Fatal Effects from the Accidental Use of White Lead," *Transactions of the Medical Society of London* (1810), 1: 64–77.

9. W.A.A., "Poisoning with Lead" (letter to the editor), *Boston Medical and Surgical Journal* (1837), 16: 239–240.

10. A. B. Shipman, "Poisoning with Lead," *American Journal of the Medical Sciences* (1843), 6: 89–90.

11. Thomas Bancks, "Wholesale Poisoning by the Acetate of Lead," *Provincial Medical and Surgical Journal* (1849): 266–267.

12. T.A.O. Earle, "Lead Poisoning; Eight Persons Victims of Colica Pictonum," *American Journal of the Medical Sciences* (1874), 67: 279–280.

13. William E. Magruder, "Lead-Poisoning from Canned Food," *Medical News* (1883), 43: 261–263.

14. Fallon Percy Wightwick, "Canned Vegetables and Lead Poisoning," *Lancet* (1888), 2: 1121–1122.

15. Henry M. Thomas, "A Case of Generalized Lead Paralysis, with a Review of the Cases of Lead Palsy Seen in the Hospital," *Johns Hopkins Hospital Bulletin* (1904), 15: 209–212.

16. James Harvey Young, *Pure Food: Securing the Federal Food and Drugs Act of 1906* (Princeton, N.J.: Princeton University Press, 1989), 110.

17. Thomas Thomson, "Observations on Poisoning by Water Passed through Leaden Tubes, and Retained in Leaden Cisterns," *Medical Times* (1848), 19: 193–196.

18. E. D. Fenner, "Special Report on Lead-Poisoning in the City of New Orleans," *Southern Medical Reports* (1850), 2: 247–280.

19. James Robertson, "An Account of Cases of Chronic Lead Poisoning, Caused by Drinking Water Kept in a Leaden Cistern," *Lancet* (1851), 1: 202.

20. Jacob Bigelow, "Report on the Action of Cochituate Water on Leaden Pipes, and the Influence of the Same on Health," *American Journal of the Medical Sciences* (1852), 24: 98–100.

21. John Brown, "Unsuspected Lead Poisoning in Children," *British Medical Journal* (1890), 1: 177.

22. T. D. Haigh, "Lead Poisoning in an Infant from Dalley's Salve," *North Carolina Medical Journal* (1888), 21: 79–80; N. R. Norton, "A Case of Chronic Lead Poisoning with Encephalitis," *International Clinics* (1922), 4: 231–233; and Stafford McLean, "Diseases of Children (Lead Poisoning in Infancy)," *Progressive Medicine* (1924), 1: 220–222.

23. Frederick W. M. Stephenson, "Lead Poisoning in an Infant Four Weeks Old," *Lancet* (1898), 2: 1473.

24. T. Suzuki and J. Kaneko, "Serous Meningitis in Infants Caused by Lead Poisoning from White Powders," *Journal of Oriental Medicine* (1924), 2: 55–66; and M. Fukusima and H. Matumoto, "Statistics of 298 Cases of Infantile Lead-Poisoning," *Oriental Journal of Diseases in Infants* (1928), 3: 27–31.
25. L. R. Sante, "Lead Neuritis from Cosmetics: With Report of Two Cases," *Journal of the American Medical Association* (1915), 64: 1573–1574; and Moses Barron and Harold C. Habein, "Lead Poisoning, with Special Reference to Poisoning from Lead Cosmetics: Report of Four Fatal Cases of Encephalopathia Saturnina Occurring in One Family," *American Journal of the Medical Sciences* (1921), 162: 833–862.
26. Shipman, "Poisoning with Lead."
27. Henry D. Chapin, "Lead Paralysis in Children," *Medical Record* (1884), 25: 546-547.
28. Wharton Sinkler, "On Lead-Palsy in Children; with a Report of Three Cases," *Medical News* (1894), 65: 88.
29. "Lead Poisoning," in John M. Keating, *Cyclopaedia of the Diseases of Children: Medical and Surgical* (Philadelphia: J. B. Lippincott Co., 1890), 4: 615–642; see also J. J. Putnam, "On the Distribution of the Paralysis in the Lead-Poisoning of Children," *Boston Medical and Surgical Journal* (1893), 128: 187–188.
30. "It is probable, therefore, that children are not so liable to lead-poisoning as adults; and this is no doubt due to the fact of their possessing more active powers of elimination; their greater bodily activity, and the greater energy of all of their secretions, causing the ready elimination of the lead from the system." Sinkler, "On Lead-Palsy in Children; with a Report of Three Cases," 85.
31. Ibid., 85.
32. Leo Newmark, "Lead Palsy in Children," *Medical News* (1895), 66: 505–507.
33. R. Abrahams, "Acute Lead Poisoning in an Infant, with Report of Two Other Interesting Cases," *American Medico-Surgical Bulletin* (1896), 10: 531.
34. W. F. Hamilton, "Lead Poisoning: A Study of Forty Cases," *Montreal Medical Journal* (1905), 34: 732.
35. H. W. Wright, "A Case of Lead Poisoning," *Archives of Pediatrics* (1909), 26: 131–132.

Chapter 2   The Queensland Epidemic

1. D. C. Fison, "The History of Royal Children's Hospital, Brisbane," *Medical Journal of Australia* (1969), 1: 417–422.
2. See John C. Burnham, "Biomedical Communication and the Reaction to the Queensland Childhood Lead Poisoning Cases Elsewhere in the World," *Medical History* (1999), 43: 155–172; and Christian Warren, *Brush with Death: A Social History of Lead Poisoning* (Baltimore: Johns Hopkins University Press, 2000), 29, 42.
3. Ross Fitzgerald, *From the Dreaming to 1915: A History of Queensland* (Queensland: University of Queensland Press, 1982), pt. 2. See also Geoffrey Curgenven Bolton, *A Thousand Miles Away: A History of North Queensland to 1920* (Brisbane: Jacaranda Press, in association with the Australian National University, 1963).
4. L. J. Jarvis Nye, *Chronic Nephritis and Lead Poisoning* (Sydney: Angus and Robertson, 1933), chart opp. p. 98.
5. Thomas Neville Bonner, *American Doctors and German Universities: A Chapter in International Intellectual Relations, 1870–1914* (Lincoln: University of Nebraska Press, 1963).
6. Anonymous, "John Lockhart Gibson, M.D.," *Queensland 1900: A Narrative of Her Past, Together with Biographies of Her Leading Men* (Brisbane: Alcazar Press, 1900), 63–64 (biography section).
7. J. Lockhart Gibson, Wilton Love, David Hardie, Peter Bancroft, and A. Jefferis Turner, "Notes of Lead Poisoning as Observed among Children in Brisbane," *Trans-*

actions of the Intercolonial Medical Congress of Australia (1892), 3: 76–83. In the article the authors mentioned an additional case in 1890 (treated by Turner), also with foot-drop and wrist-drop, which they now believed was the result of lead but which went unrecognized earlier.

8. A. Jefferis Turner, "Lead Poisoning among Queensland Children," *Australasian Medical Gazette* (1897), 16: 475–479; and J. Lockhart Gibson, "Optic Neuritis, Simulating Basal Meningitis—Plumbism," *Australasian Medical Gazette* (1897), 16: 479.

9. T. E. Green, "Some Unusual Forms of Lead Poisoning," *Australasian Medical Gazette* (1897), 16: 483–484.

10. J. Lockhart Gibson, "A Plea for Painted Railings and Painted Walls of Rooms as the Source of Lead Poisoning amongst Queensland Children," *Australasian Medical Gazette* (1904), 23: 149–153.

11. Nye, *Chronic Nephritis and Lead Poisoning*, 103.

12. R. Elliott Murray, *Plumbism and Chronic Nephritis in Young People in Queensland* (Sydney: University of Sydney School of Public Health, 1939), table 7, 84.

13. James W. Sayre, Evan Charney, Jaroslav Vostal, and I. Barry Pless, "House and Hand Dust as a Potential Source of Childhood Lead Exposure," *American Journal of Diseases of Children* (1974), 127: 167–170 (Figure 2, 169).

14. J. Macdonald Gill, "Peripheral Neuritis due to Lead Poisoning in Children," *Australasian Medical Gazette* (1907), 26: 278.

15. J. Lockhart Gibson, "Plumbic Ocular Neuritis in Queensland Children," *British Medical Journal* (1908), 2: 1488.

16. A. Jefferis Turner, "On Lead Poisoning in Childhood," *British Medical Journal* (1909), 1: 895.

17. Ibid., 897.

18. J. Lockhart Gibson, "The Importance of Lumbar Puncture in the Plumbic Ocular Neuritis of Children," *Transactions of the Australasian Medical Congress* (1911), 2: 750–755; and Gibson, "The Diagnosis, Prophylaxis and Treatment of Plumbic Ocular Neuritis amongst Queensland Children," *Medical Journal of Australia* (1917) 2: 201–204.

19. A. Breinl and W. J. Young, "The Occurrence of Lead Poisoning amongst North Queensland Children," *Annals of Tropical Medicine and Parasitology* (1914), 8: 589.

20. E. S. Littlejohn, "Three Cases of Lead Poisoning in Children," *Medical Journal of Australia* (1922), 2: 63-64.

21. David L. Edsall, in "Chronic Lead Poisoning," in *Modern Medicine: Its Theory and Practice*, ed. William Osler (Philadelphia: Lea Bros., 1907), notes, "Cerebral symptoms, convulsions have been noted by the largest number of observers [in Europe and America], but there is a very suggestive interest in the reports of Gibson and Turner of twenty-four instances in which the chief symptoms were prolonged rigidity of the neck, retraction of the head, and ocular symptoms" (1: 108). (Edsall then went on to describe these peculiar eye findings.)

22. Ibid., 87. For discussions of the rare eye findings in lead poisoning, see Jonathan Hutchinson, "On Lead-Poisoning as a Cause of Optic Neuritis," *Royal London Ophthalmic Hospital Reports* (1871–1873), 7: 6–13; M. Landesberg, "Affections of the Eye Consequent upon Lead Poisoning," *Medical Bulletin (Philadelphia)* (1880), 2: 108–110; and E. W. Alexander, "Eye Changes in Chronic Lead Poisoning, with Report of a Case," *Ophthalmology* (1909) 5: 634–636.

23. Edsall, "Chronic Lead Poisoning," 92.

24. Henry M. Thomas and Kenneth D. Blackfan, "Recurrent Meningitis, Due to Lead, in a Child of Five Years," *American Journal of Diseases of Children* (1914), 8: 377–380.

25. Kenneth D. Blackfan, "Lead Poisoning in Children, with Especial Reference to Lead as a Cause of Convulsions," *American Journal of the Medical Sciences* (1917), 153: 879-880.

26. Nye, *Chronic Nephritis and Lead Poisoning*, 122–127.

27. Blackfan, "Lead Poisoning in Children, with Especial Reference to Lead as a Cause of Convulsions," 877–878.
28. Ibid.
29. "Poisoning by lead is a rare occurrence in early life, and is, therefore, seldom considered as a diagnostic possibility in young children. Although much has been written on the subject as it concerns older children, particularly in Australia, the condition is very rare in infants." L. Emmett Holt, Jr., "Lead Poisoning in Infancy," *American Journal of Diseases of Children* (1923), 25: 229.
30. "In these cases, there was a great variety in the sources of the lead. In only one was the poison introduced by inhalation of dust which contained lead. In the others it was introduced by mouth, in paint from toys, in buns and candies colored with lead chromate; in printers' type, ointment of lead oxide (litharge), water and milk which had stood in lead receptacles. Improper medication was responsible for two cases. In three cases, the child obtained the poison from the mother: one by sucking paint from the mother's face, and two . . . by nursing following the use of a lead ointment on the mother's breast" (ibid., 232).
31. L. Emmett Holt and John Howland, *The Diseases of Infancy and Childhood* (New York: D. Appleton and Co., 1926), 542.
32. John C. Ruddock, "Lead Poisoning in Children: With Special Reference to Pica," *Journal of the American Medical Association* (1924), 82: 1683.
33. Charles F. McKhann, "Lead Poisoning in Children, with Notes on Therapy," *American Journal of Diseases of Children* (1926), 32: 387.
34. Joseph C. Aub, Lawrence T. Fairhall, A. S. Minot, and Paul Reznikoff, *Lead Poisoning, with a Chapter on the Prevalence of Industrial Lead Poisoning in the United States by Alice Hamilton* (Baltimore: Williams and Wilkins, 1926), 213.
35. Carl Vernon Weller, "Some Clinical Aspects of Lead Meningo-Encephalopathy, *Annals of Clinical Medicine* (1924–1925), 3: 607.
36. Queensland Branch of the British Medical Association, "An Historical Account of the Occurrence and Causation of Lead Poisoning among Queensland Children," *Medical Journal of Australia* (1922), 1: 152.
37. Acts of the Parliament of Queensland, Session of 1922 (Brisbane: Anthony James Cumming, Government Printer), vol. 12, pt. 1, sect. 29: 10023.
38. J. Lockhart Gibson, "Ocular Plumbism in Children," *British Journal of Ophthalmology* (1931), 15: 638.
39. International Labour Office, *White Lead* (Geneva, 1927), 40.
40. Gibson, "Ocular Plumbism in Children," 637.
41. Nye, *Chronic Nephritis and Lead Poisoning*, 114.
42. "The children whose environment has predisposed them to the greatest risks of lead poisoning, are those of poorer women who not infrequently have been compelled to spend most of the day earning a living. Such children have been left often to amuse themselves for hours at a time, day after day, confined to the verandas where they could be in the fresh air yet safe from the dangers of the street" (ibid., 117). See also S. F. McDonald, "Looking Backward: A Quarter-Century of Paediatrics. III: Juvenile Lead Poisoning," *Medical Journal of Australia* (1946), 2: 373–374.
43. L. J. Jarvis Nye, "Further Observations on Chronic Nephritis and Lead Poisoning in Queensland, with Comments on the Federal Official Inquiry," *Medical Journal of Australia* (1933), 2: 241. Nye first called attention to the possible connection between Queensland childhood lead poisoning and adult nephritis in Nye, "An Investigation of the Extraordinary Incidence of Chronic Nephritis in Young People in Queensland," *Medical Journal of Australia* (1929), 2: 145–159.
44. The conclusions of the inquiry Commonwealth Department of Health (1932) were reprinted in Murray, *Plumbism and Chronic Nephritis in Young People in Queensland*: "Lead paint is very generally distributed, and while this renders it the most acces-

sible source of lead in poisonous quantities, it serves also to cast doubt upon its ab-
solute significance, owing to the strict limitation of lead poisoning to certain areas
within the wide range of [lead paint's] general distribution, and this disparity is also
emphasized by its rarity outside Brisbane, Queensland. . . . On the other hand, a very
strong chain of circumstantial evidence incriminating white lead paint is recorded
from the special series of cases dealt with, while indications in any other direction
are extremely few" (31).

45. Quoted in Murray, *Plumbism and Chronic Nephritis in Young People in Queensland*: "In
Brisbane, where such predispositions exist, the concurrent ingestion of infinitesimal
doses of lead appears in a large proportion of cases to precipitate the fatal issue many
years earlier than would otherwise be the case, weeding out the great mass of chronic
nephritics before they attain the age of 40" (30).

46. Nye, *Chronic Nephritis and Lead Poisoning*.

47. Keith D. Fairley, "A Review of the Evidence Relating to Lead as an Aetiological
Agent in Chronic Nephritis in Queensland," *Medical Journal of Australia* (1934), 1:
600–606.

48. Murray, *Plumbism and Chronic Nephritis in Young People in Queensland*, 47.

49. "Plumbism and Chronic Nephritis," *Journal of the American Medical Association* (1939),
113: 1503.

50. "Juvenile Nephritis and Lead Poisoning" (editorial), *Journal of the American Medical
Association* (1940), 114: 1753.

51. Jarvis Nye to Robert Kehoe, November 25, 1946; Kehoe to Nye, March 1, 1947;
and Nye to Kehoe, March 17, 1947, Kehoe Papers, Robert A. Kehoe Archives, Cincinnati Medical Heritage Center, University of Cincinnati Medical Center.

52. Felix Wormser to Robert Kehoe, November 27, 1945, Kehoe Papers.

53. For discussions, see Lloyd B. Tepper, "Renal Function Subsequent to Childhood Plumbism," *Archives of Environmental Health* (1963), 7: 76–85; and Robert A. Goyer, "Lead
and the Kidney," *Current Topics in Pathology* (1971), 55: 147–176.

54. J. Julian Chisholm, Jr., letter in response to "Chelating Agents in Treatment of Lead
Intoxication," *Journal of Pediatrics* (1969), 74: 323.

55. D. A. Henderson, "A Follow-up of Cases of Plumbism in Children," *Australasian Annals of Medicine* (1954), 3: 219–224; and Henderson, "The Aetiology of Chronic Nephritis in Queensland," *Medical Journal of Australia* (1958), 1: 377–386.

56. For a more recent account of childhood lead poisoning in Australia, see Ronald Free-
man, "Chronic Lead Poisoning in Children: A Review of 90 Children Diagnosed in
Sydney, 1948–1967: 1. Epidemiological Aspects," *Medical Journal of Australia* (1970),
1: 640–647. See also J. A. Inglis, D. A. Henderson, and B. T. Emmerson, "The Pathology and Pathogenesis of Chronic Lead Nephropathy Occurring in Queensland,"
Journal of Pathology (1978), 124: 65–76.

57. Jane S. Lin-Fu, "Modern History of Lead Poisoning: A Century of Discovery and
Rediscovery," in *Human Lead Exposure*, ed. Herbert L. Needleman (Boca Raton: CRC
Press, 1992), 27.

58. Ibid.

59. Jane S. Lin-Fu, "Lead Poisoning and Undue Lead Exposure in Children: History and
Current Status," in *Low Level Lead Exposure: The Clinical Implications of Current Research*, ed. H. L. Needleman (New York: Raven Press, 1980), 7.

60. J. Julian Chisholm, Jr., "Interrelationships among the Lead in Paint, Housedust, and
Soil in Childhood Lead Poisoning: The Baltimore Experience," in *Lead in Soil: Issues and Guidelines*, ed. Brian E. Davies and Bobby G. Wixson (n.p.: Science Reviews, 1988), 186.

61. Recent historians have also incorrectly judged the significance of the Queensland
epidemic for contemporary pediatricians. See, for example, Gerald Markowitz and
David Rosner, "'Cater to the Children': The Role of the Lead Industry in a Public

Health Tragedy, 1900–1955," *American Journal of Public Health* (2000), 90: 36–37.

Chapter 3   The Scientific Study of the American Workplace

1. Alice Hamilton, *Recent Changes in the Painters' Trade*, United States Division of Labor Standards Bulletin no. 7 (Washington, D.C: Government Printing Office, 1936).
2. Alice Hamilton, *Exploring the Dangerous Trades: The Autobiography of Alice Hamilton*, with a foreword by Barbara Sicherman (Boston: Northeastern University Press, 1985 [1943]), 18–56.
3. Regina Markell Morantz-Sanchez, *Sympathy and Science: Women Physicians in American Medicine* (New York: Oxford University Press, 1985); and Rima D. Apple, ed., *Women, Health, and Medicine in America: A Historical Handbook* (New Brunswick, N.J.: Rutgers University Press, 1992 [1990]).
4. Hamilton, *Exploring the Dangerous Trades*, 57-94.
5. Lewis J. Amster, "Gentlewoman Explorer in the Dangerous Trades (Alice Hamilton)," *Hospital Practice* (1986), 21: 206–254.
6. Hamilton, *Exploring the Dangerous Trades*, 114–127.
7. Angela Nugent Young, "Interpreting the Dangerous Trades: Workers' Health in America and the Career of Alice Hamilton, 1910–1935" (Ph.D. diss., Brown University, 1983), 20–35.
8. Wilma Ruth Slaight, "Alice Hamilton: First Lady of Industrial Medicine" (Ph.D. diss., Case Western Reserve University, 1974).
9. Alice Hamilton, "Lead Poisoning in Illinois," *Journal of the American Medical Association* (1911), 56: 1240–1244.
10. "We have found such great difference in the conditions in factories doing the same kinds of work that it would be impossible to make any general statement as to the precautions taken in Illinois to protect the workers in lead. Two factories belonging to the same company will be found at the two extremes as regards cleanliness, use of machinery, solicitude for the health of the men." Alice Hamilton, "Lead Poisoning in Illinois," *Proceedings of the First Conference on Industrial Diseases* (New York: American Association of Labor Legislation, 1910), 30.
11. Ibid., 31.
12. "It is, of course, far better that the improvements should come in response to the demands of economic management, not of philanthropy, for they are on a much surer basis, and it is to be hoped that there will be a growing recognition of the value of what one manufacturer calls 'experienced, unskilled labor' so that it will be recognized as worth the effort to keep a steady force of workmen" (ibid., 33).
13. Ronald E. Lane, "The Care of the Lead Worker," *British Journal of Industrial Medicine* (1949), 6: 125–143. For example, as L. Tanquerel des Planches observed: "When we survey these various trades, and their separate processes, it is at once seen, that the liability to [lead] colic is greatest among those, who are employed in drying, packing, pulverizing, or mixing and grinding the various products. Indeed this view allows a classification of workmen: 1st, those who live and work in an atmosphere loaded with lead particles. . . . Those [types of work] most disseminating lead particles and emanations are most to be feared as causes of colic. Among these are: 1st Scraping off old paint, which diffuses lead dust. 2d. Color grinding. 3d. Painting in closed and heated apartments, or rooms where many are at the same time engaged with the paint brush." L. Tanquerel des Planches, *Lead Diseases: A Treatise, from the French. With Notes and Additions on the Use of Lead Pipe and its Substitutes*, trans. Samuel L. Dana (Boston: Tappan, Whittemore & Mason, 1850), 56, 57.
14. Thomas M. Legge and Kenneth W. Goadby, *Lead Poisoning and Lead Absorption: The Symptoms, Pathology, and Prevention, with Special Reference to Their Industrial Origin, and an Account of the Principal Processes Involving Risk* (London: E. Arnold, 1912), 7

(light measurement), 9 (quotation).

15. Sir Thomas Oliver, *Lead Poisoning: From the Industrial, Medical, and Social Points of View* (New York: Paul B. Hoeber, 1914), 38–39.

16. Alice Hamilton, "The Hygiene of the Lead Industry," address at the Meeting of Superintendents, National Lead Company, Chicago, December 7, 1910 (Booklet of the Manufacturing Committee).

17. Hamilton, *Exploring the Dangerous Trades*, 127-160.

18. Young, "Interpreting the Dangerous Trades," 43.

19. Alice Hamilton, *Lead Poisoning in Potteries, Tile Works, and Porcelain Enameled Sanitary Ware Factories*, Bulletin of the United States Bureau of Labor Statistics, no. 104 (Washington, D.C.: Government Printing Office, 1912).

20. Ibid.

21. Alice Hamilton, *Lead Poisoning in the Smelting and Refining of Lead*, Bulletin of the United States Bureau of Labor Statistics, no. 141 (Washington, D.C.: Government Printing Office, 1914): "The ground product of the mills is often discharged in such a way as to allow clouds of dust [19]. . . . the whole place was enveloped in clouds of dust [21]. . . . clouds of fume and dust fill the air surrounding the workmen [29]. . . . men working in clouds of dust at the pots or the roast and sinter machines [50]."

22. Alice Hamilton, *Lead Poisoning in the Manufacture of Storage Batteries*, Bulletin of the United States Bureau of Labor Statistics, no. 165 (Washington, D.C.: Government Printing Office, 1915): "In one plant visited the molds are dusted with very finely ground soapstone, used in such quantities that the room looks like a flour mill, while the men are powdered like millers" [9]; "it is an extremely dusty process and in spite of the protection of the glass case, there were heaps of dust all around the place in the one plant in which these plates are made [13]."

23. Tanquerel des Planches, *Lead Diseases*, 43.

24. Ruth Marjorie Hutton, *Lead Poisoning: A Compilation of Present Knowledge* (Ontario: Provincial Board of Health, 1923), 8; and Oliver, *Lead Poisoning*, 167.

25. Oliver, *Lead Poisoning*, 36, 167; and Thomas M. Legge and Kenneth W. Goadby, *Lead Poisoning and Lead Absorption* (New York: Longmans, Green & Co., 1912), 207.

26. Alice Hamilton, "Lead Poisoning in the United States," *American Journal of Public Health* (1914), 4: 478.

27. Robert A. Kehoe, Jacob Cholak, Donald M. Hubbard, Karl Bambach, Robert R. McNary, and Robert V. Story, "Experimental Studies on the Ingestion of Lead Compounds," *Journal of Industrial Hygiene and Toxicology* (1940), 22: 381–400.

28. Barry L. Johnson and Robert W. Mason, "A Review of Public Health Regulations on Lead," *Neurotoxicology* (1984), 5: 1–22.

29. Alice Hamilton, *Lead Poisoning in Potteries*, 66.

30. Alice Hamilton, *Hygiene of the Painters' Trade*, Bulletin of the United States Bureau of Labor Statistics, no. 120 (Washington, D.C.: Government Printing Office, 1913).

31. Hamilton, *Lead Poisoning in the Smelting and Refining of Lead*, 14 (factory inspection, medical inspection), 73–74 (insurance), 79 (compulsory reporting).

32. Hamilton, *Lead Poisoning in the Manufacture of Storage Batteries*.

33. Hamilton, "Lead Poisoning in the United States," 479.

34. Alice Hamilton, *Women in the Lead Industries*, Bulletin of the United States Bureau of Labor Statistics, no. 253 (Washington, D.C.: Government Printing Office, 1919).

35. Hamilton, *Exploring the Dangerous Trades*, 161–199.

36. Alice Hamilton, "Lead Poisoning in American Industry," *Journal of Industrial Hygiene* (1919), 1: 8–21.

37. Alice Hamilton to David Edsall, May 1, 1920, Papers of David Linn Edsall, Countway Library of Medicine, Harvard University; Joseph C. Aub and Ruth K. Hapgood, *Pioneer in Modern Medicine: David Linn Edsall of Harvard* (Cambridge, Mass.: Harvard

Medical Alumni Association, 1970), 260–261.

38. Hamilton, "Lead Poisoning in the United States," 480.
39. Christopher C. Sellers, *Hazards of the Job: From Industrial Disease to Environmental Health Science* (Chapel Hill: University of North Carolina Press, 1997), 69–140.
40. Aub and Hapgood, *Pioneer in Modern Medicine*, 251–252.
41. Barbara Sicherman, *Alice Hamilton: A Life in Letters* (Cambridge, Mass.: Harvard University Press, 1984), 237–310.
42. George Cheever Shattuck, "Industrial Medicine at Harvard," unpublished ms. (1919), 44. Archives, Countway Library of Medicine, Harvard University.
43. Aub and Hapgood, *Pioneer in Modern Medicine*, 158-262.
44. Shattuck, "Industrial Medicine at Harvard," 185.
45. Joseph Aub, Memoirs, Oral Transcript, Oral History Research Office, Butler Library, Columbia University, 1956, 170–184.
46. E. J. Cornish to David L. Edsall, May 12, 1921. Papers of D. L. Edsall.
47. Joseph Aub, Memoirs, Oral Transcript, 170–184.
48. For summaries of the Harvard research, see J. C. Aub, A. S. Minot, L. T. Fairhall, and Paul Reznikoff, "Recent Investigations of Absorption and Excretion of Lead in the Organism," *Journal of the American Medical Association* (1924), 83: 588–592; and Joseph C. Aub, Lawrence T. Fairhall, A. S. Minot, and Paul Reznikoff, *Lead Poisoning, with a Chapter on the Prevalence of Industrial Lead Poisoning in the United States by Alice Hamilton* (Baltimore: Williams and Wilkins, 1926).
49. William Graebner, "Hegemony through Science: Information Engineering and Lead Toxicology, 1925–1965," in *Dying for Work: Workers' Safety and Health in Twentieth-Century America*, ed. David Rosner and Gerald Markowitz (Bloomington: Indiana University Press, 1989), 140–159.
50. Sellers, *Hazards of the Job*, 161–164.
51. Joseph C. Aub, "Third Report on the Investigation of Lead Poisoning," unpublished ms., 1.
52. For a discussion, see Peter C. English, *Shock, Physiological Surgery, and George Washington Crile: Medical Innovation in the Progressive Era* (Westport, Conn.: Greenwood Press, 1980), 121–127.
53. Sellers, *Hazards of the Job*, 160-164.
54. Aub, "Third Report on the Investigation of Lead Poisoning," 1–2.
55. See J. J. Putnam, "Lead Poisoning Simulating Other Diseases" (summary of his delivered paper), *Journal of Nervous and Mental Diseases* (1883), 10: 466–469.
56. Lawrence T. Fairhall, "Lead Studies: I. The Estimation of Minute Amounts of Lead in Biological Material," *Journal of Industrial Hygiene* (1922), 4: 9–20; Fairhall, "Lead Studies: VIII. The Microchemical Detection of Lead," *Journal of Biological Chemistry* (1923), 57: 455–461; and Fairhall, "Lead Studies: IX. The Solubility of Various Lead Compounds in Blood Serum," *Journal of Biological Chemistry* (1924), 60: 481–484.
57. W. Denis and A. S. Minot, "A Method for Determination of Minute Amounts of Lead in Urine, Feces, and Tissues," *Journal of Biological Chemistry* (1919), 38: 449–452; and Minot, "Lead Studies: II. A Critical Note on the Electrolytic Determination of Lead in Biological Material," *Journal of Biological Chemistry* (1923), 55: 1–8.
58. Lawrence T. Fairhall, "Precision Methods in the Determination of the Heavy Metals," *American Journal of Public Health* (1938), 28: 826.
59. Carl Vernon Weller and Aileen Dean Christensen, "The Cerebrospinal Fluid in Lead Poisoning," *Archives of Neurology and Psychiatry* (1925), 14: 340. For an Australian appraisal see R. W. Tannahill, "A Critical Survey of the Methods for the Determination of Lead in Biological Material," *Medical Journal of Australia* (1929), 1: 194–201.
60. Robert A. Kehoe, Graham Edgar, Fred Thamann, and Lester Sanders, "The Excretion of Lead by Normal Persons," *Journal of the American Medical Association* (1926), 87:

2081–2084.

61. A. S. Minot, "Lead Studies: V. A. The Distribution of Lead in the Organism after Absorption by the Gastrointestinal Tract," *Journal of Industrial Hygiene* (1924), 6: 125–136; Minot, "Lead Studies: V. B. The Distribution of Lead in the Organism after Absorption by the Lungs and Subcutaneous Tissue," *Journal of Industrial Hygiene* (1924), 6: 137–148; and Minot and J. C. Aub, "Lead Studies: V. C. The Distribution of Lead in the Human Organism," *Journal of Industrial Hygiene* (1924), 6: 149–158. For another Harvard study on a similar topic, see Herrmann L. Blumgart, "Lead Studies: VI. Absorption of Lead by the Upper Respiratory Passages," *Journal of Industrial Hygiene* (1923), 5: 153–158.

62. Joseph C. Aub, Paul Reznikoff, and Dorothea E. Smith, "Lead Studies: III. The Effects of Lead on Red Blood Cells. Part 1. Changes in Hemolysis," *Journal of Experimental Medicine* (1924), 40: 151–172; "Part 2. Surface Phenomena and Their Physiological Explanation," *Journal of Experimental Medicine* (1924), 40: 173–187; "Part 3. A Chemical Explanation of the Reaction of Lead with Red Blood Cells," *Journal of Experimental Medicine* (1924), 40: 189–208. For another Harvard study on the effects of lead on red blood cells, see J. Albert Key, "Lead Studies: IV. Blood Changes in Lead Poisoning in Rabbits, with Especial Reference to the Stippled Cells," *American Journal of Physiology* (1924), 70: 86–99.

63. Paul Reznikoff and Joseph C. Aub, "Lead Studies: XIV. Experimental Studies of Lead Palsy," *Archives of Neurology and Psychiatry* (1927), 17: 444–465.

64. Donald Hunter and Joseph C. Aub, "Lead Studies: XV. The Effect of the Parathyroid Hormone on the Excretion of Lead and of Calcium in Patients Suffering from Lead Poisoning," *Quarterly Journal of Medicine* (1927), 20: 123–140; Walter Bauer, Aub, and Fuller Albright, "Studies of Calcium and Phosphorus Metabolism. V. A. Study of the Bone Trabeculae as a Readily Available Reserve Supply of Calcium," *Journal of Experimental Medicine* (1929), 49: 145–162; Bauer, William T. Salter, and Aub, "Studies of Calcium and Phosphorus Metabolism: The Use of Calcium Chloride to Relieve Peristaltic Pain," *Journal of the American Medical Association* (1931), 96: 1216–1217; and Aub, George P. Robb, and Elsie Rossmeisl, "Significance of Bone Trabeculae in the Treatment of Lead Poisoning: Lead Studies XVII," *American Journal of Public Health* (1932), 22: 825–830. For earlier studies on the same research agenda, see Lawrence T. Fairhall, "Lead Studies: VII. The Phosphates of Lead Equilibrium in the System Lead Oxide-Phosphoric Anhydride-Water at 25 degrees C.," *Journal of the American Chemical Society* (1924), 46: 1593–1598; and Fairhall and Charlotte P. Shaw, "Lead Studies: X. The Deposition of Lead Salts, with a Note on the Solubilities of Di-Lead Phosphate in Water at 25 degrees C. and of Di-Lead and Tri-Lead Phosphates in Lactic Acid at 25 degrees C.," *Journal of Industrial Hygiene* (1924), 6: 159–168.

65. Sellers, *Hazards of the Job*, 163.

66. E. J. Cornish to David L. Edsall, March 29, 1923. Papers of David Linn Edsall.

67. Hamilton, *Exploring the Dangerous Trades*, 252–289.

68. Alice Hamilton, *Industrial Poisons in the United States* (New York: Macmillan Co., 1925).

69. Young, "Interpreting the Dangerous Trades," 107–158.

70. Alice Hamilton, Paul Reznikoff, and Grace A. Burnham, "Tetra-ethyl Lead," *Journal of the American Medical Association* (1925), 84: 1481–1486.

71. Hamilton, *Exploring the Dangerous Trades*, 415–416; and Young, "Interpreting the Dangerous Trades," 156–174.

72. Hamilton, *Industrial Poisons in the United States*, 165.

73. Alice Hamilton, "The Prevalence and Distribution of Industrial Lead Poisoning," *Journal of the American Medical Association* (1924), 83: 583–588; and Hamilton, "The Storage Battery Industry," *Journal of Industrial Hygiene* (1927), 9: 346–369.

74. Hamilton, *Recent Changes in the Painters' Trade*.

75. S. H. Katz, E. G. Meiter, and F. H. Gibson, *Efficiencies of Painters' Respirators Filtering Lead Paint, Benzol, and Vitreous Enamel Sprays*, Public Health Bulletin, no. 177 (Washington, D.C.: Government Printing Office, 1928), 2.

Chapter 4　Leads Hazards, Lead Safety, and Alice Hamilton

1. For example, see E. D. Fenner, "Special Report on Lead-Poisoning in the City of New Orleans," *Southern Medical Reports* (1850), 2: 247–280; David Denniston Stewart, "Notes on Some Obscure Cases of Poisoning by Lead Chromate; Manifested Chiefly by Encephalopathy," *Medical News* (1887), 1: 676–681; Stewart, "Lead Convulsions, A Study of Sixteen Cases," *American Journal of the Medical Sciences* (1895), 109: 288–306; Henry M. Thomas and Kenneth D. Blackfan, "Recurrent Meningitis, Due to Lead, in a Child of Five Years," *American Journal of Diseases of Children* (1914), 8: 377–380; Kenneth D. Blackfan, "Lead Poisoning in Children, with Especial Reference to Lead as a Cause of Convulsions," *American Journal of the Medical Sciences* (1917), 153: 877–887; and L. Emmett Holt, Jr., "Lead Poisoning in Infancy," *American Journal of Diseases of Children* (1923), 25: 229–233.

2. Thomas M. Legge and Kenneth W. Goadby, *Lead Poisoning and Lead Absorption: The Symptoms, Pathology and Prevention, with Special Reference to Their Industrial Origin, and an Account of the Principal Processes Involving Risk* (London: Edward Arnold, 1912), 230–239; Sir Thomas Oliver, *Lead Poisoning: From the Industrial, Medical, and Social Points of View* (New York: Paul B. Hoeber, 1914), 203; and Alice Hamilton, *Hygiene of the Painters' Trade*, Bulletin of the United States Bureau of Labor Statistics, no. 120 (Washington, D.C.: Government Printing Office, 1913), 66.

3. Thomas Oliver, "Lead Poisoning and the Race," *British Medical Journal* (1911), 1: 1096–1098.

4. Alfred S. Taylor, "A Case of Poisoning by Lead, with Chemical Analysis, and Remarks on the Detection of Lead in the Tissues," *Guy's Hospital Reports* (1846), 4: 471–476.

5. Legge and Goadby, *Lead Poisoning and Lead Absorption*, 35–36; Oliver, *Lead Poisoning*, 203; and Alice Hamilton, "Lead-Poisoning in Illinois," *Journal of the American Medical Association* (1911), 56: 1242.

6. "Children are rarely employed in establishments where preparations of lead are used, but it is certain that they are very easily affected with lead colic. In a manufactory of fancy cards and paper in Paris, the five or six children employed there are often attacked with this disease, the adults less frequently. Children have often had to be removed immediately, because they were so frequently ill. Many master house painters have been obliged to give up taking children as apprentices, because they were so often attacked with colic. . . . Very young children being rarely placed in situations which favor the development of lead colic, it cannot be known with certainty whether they are predisposed to it or not." L. Tanquerel des Planches, *Lead Diseases: A Treatise, from the French. With Notes and Additions on the Use of Lead Pipe and Its Substitutes*, trans. Samuel L. Dana (Boston: Tappan, Whittemore & Mason, 1850), 65.

7. Ibid., 65.

8. Ibid., 272–273.

9. Legge and Goadby, *Lead Poisoning and Lead Absorption*, 35. In their discussion of "Preventive Measures against Lead Poisoning," Legge and Goadby reiterated their concern about adolescents in the workplace: "Wherever lead dust or fumes arise, whether exhaust ventilation is applied or not, persons of either sex under eighteen years of age are probably rather more susceptible to attack by reason of natural failure to appreciate the risk run. When periodical medical examination in addition to exhaust ventilation has been adopted, the age limit can safely be reduced to sixteen. Where

handling only of metallic lead and ordinary soldering with an iron are done, risk of contracting plumbism is so remote that an age limit may be unnecessary" (239).

10. Sir Thomas Oliver, *Diseases of Occupation from the Legislative, Social, and Medical Points of View* (New York: E. P. Dutton, 1908), 137, 153.

11. Alice Hamilton, "Lead Poisoning in Illinois," in *Proceedings of the First Conference on Industrial Diseases* (New York: American Association for Labor Legislation, 1910), 31; Hamilton, "Lead-Poisoning in Illinois," 1242; Alice Hamilton, "Lead Poisoning in the United States," *American Journal of Public Health* (1914), 4: 479; and Alice Hamilton, "Lead Poisoning in American Industry," *Journal of Industrial Hygiene* (1919), 1: 9.

12. Alice Hamilton, *Exploring the Dangerous Trades: The Autobiography of Alice Hamilton*, with a foreword by Barbara Sicherman (Boston: Northeastern University Press, 1985 [1943]), 161–199; Wilma Ruth Slaight, "Alice Hamilton: First Lady of Industrial Medicine" (Ph.D. diss., Case Western Reserve University, 1974), 67–99; and Angela Nugent Young, "Interpreting the Dangerous Trades: Workers' Health in America and the Career of Alice Hamilton, 1910–1935" (Ph.D. diss., Brown University, 1983), 68–106.

13. Alice Hamilton, *Women in the Lead Industries*, Bulletin of the United States Bureau of Labor Statistics, no. 253 (Washington, D.C.: Government Printing Office, 1919), 5.

14. Ibid., 11, 38.

15. Ibid., 31.

16. Ruth Marjorie Hutton, *Lead Poisoning: A Compilation of Present Knowledge* (Ontario: Provincial Board of Health, 1923), 141–276.

17. Hamilton, *Hygiene of the Painters' Trade*, 47.

18. Ibid., 64.

19. Hamilton, "Lead Poisoning in American Industry," 13.

20. Alice Hamilton, "The Prevalence and Distribution of Industrial Lead Poisoning," *Journal of the American Medical Association* (1924), 83: 585.

21. Alice Hamilton, *Industrial Poisons in the United States* (New York: Macmillan Co., 1925), 196–199.

22. Sir William Warrender Mackenzie, *Lead Paint (Protection against Poisoning) Act, 1926: Report to His Majesty's Secretary of State for the Home Department on the Draft Regulations for Preventing Danger from Lead Paint to Person Employed in or in connection with the Painting of Buildings* (London: H. M. Stationery Office, 1927), 4.

23. "The question whether white lead can be displaced by leadless paints is dealt with in an important government report. In 1911, the home secretary appointed two committees to investigate in regard to the painting of buildings and of coaches. These committees reported in 1915 and 1920, and advised that it was not practicable adequately to safeguard the health of painters by regulations, and further, that substitutes existed which could satisfactorily displace white lead for all purposes. They therefore recommended its prohibition. During the war no attempt was made to give effect to the recommendation. In 1921, owing to the serious failures of these substitutes, which had been observed in government work, a new committee was appointed to examine the matter. This committee now reports that it cannot support the recommendation that the use of lead paint for the painting of buildings be entirely prohibited, and that for outside painting and certain internal painting there is no efficient substitute for lead. . . . Since the reports of the 1911 committees were made, further research on the hygienic problems of painters has indicated preventive measures which would make their calling safer to health. A study of the whole of the scientific work done in this connection shows that the chief danger lies in the inhalation of dust produced during the dry rubbing-down process. As it is now practicable to substitute a dustless process, the former can be discontinued." "Foreign Letters: The

Prohibition of Lead in Paints," *Journal of the American Medical Association* (1923), 80: 1391–1392.

24. Hamilton, *Exploring the Dangerous Trades*, 254.
25. Ludwig Teleky, "German Literature on the White Lead Question, 1921," *Journal of Industrial Hygiene* (1922), 4: 100–105.
26. I disagree with recent scholarship that has concluded that Hamilton advocated a ban in the United States. See Gerald Markowitz and David Rosner, "'Cater to the Children': The Role of the Lead Industry in a Public Health Tragedy, 1900–1955," *American Journal of Public Health* (2000), 90: 37. Markowitz and Rosner argue that had the United States followed Hamilton's recommendation, there would have been less childhood lead poisoning.
27. Alice Hamilton, *Lead Poisoning in Potteries, Tile Works, and Porcelain Enameled Sanitary Ware Factories*, Bulletin of the United States Bureau of Labor Statistics, no. 104 (Washington, D.C.: Government Printing Office, 1912), 48–51.
28. Alice Hamilton to Charles H. Verrill, February 12, 1913, in Barbara Sicherman, *Alice Hamilton: A Life in Letters* (Cambridge, Mass.: Harvard University Press, 1984), 172.
29. Alice Hamilton, "Lead Poisoning among Journeymen Painters," OPDR (March 3, 1913), 32. Hamilton's speech to the Master Painters mirrored her views just published in *Hygiene of the Painters' Trade*. Hamilton argued that the danger from using lead-based paint came largely from lead dust created by dry sandpapering of old lead paint from interior surfaces, "Paint dust is caused chiefly by rubbing old or new paint with dry sandpaper. This process is universally recognized as the most dangerous part of the painters' trade. It could be completely done away with by the use of cheap mineral oil to wet the sandpaper and catch the dust." Hamilton, *Hygiene of the Painters' Trade*, 65.
30. In *Hygiene of the Painters' Trade*, Hamilton spelled out this special concern: "Ship painting is fraught with more dangers to the health of the painter than any other branch of the trade, according to the statements of men who have been both ship painters and house painters. This is partly because the work is of a high grade, requiring many coats of pure lead paint and turpentine, with the usual accompaniment of dry sandpapering" (40).
31. Ibid., 66.
32. Ibid.
33. Ibid., 32.
34. Ibid., 17.
35. Hamilton, *Exploring the Dangerous Trades*, 154–155.
36. Hamilton, *Hygiene of the Painters' Trade*, 11-17.
37. Ibid., 65.
38. Ibid., 66.
39. Ibid., 32–33.
40. Ibid., 34, 38, 63, 66.
41. Ibid., 35.
42. Hamilton, *Exploring the Dangerous Trades*, 161-199; and Young, "Interpreting the Dangerous Trades," 68–106.
43. Hamilton, *Exploring the Dangerous Trades*, 293–298.
44. Sir Thomas Oliver, "Industrial Hygiene: Its Rise, Progress, and Opportunities," *British Medical Journal* (1921), 2: 110.
45. "Lead paint is not often used in spraying machines; quick-drying leadless paints with petroleum or coal-tar solvents are the ones chiefly used; and many complaints of ill health are beginning to come from painters engaged in such work." Hamilton, *Industrial Poisons in the United States*, 193.
46. Hamilton, *Industrial Poisons in the United States*, 189.
47. S. H. Katz, E. G. Meiter, and F. H. Gibson, *Efficiencies of Painters' Respirators Filtering*

Lead Paint, Benzol, and Vitreous Enamel Sprays, Public Health Bulletin no. 177 (Washington, D.C.: Government Printing Office, 1928), 2.

48. Alice Hamilton, *Recent Changes in the Painters' Trade*, United States. Division of Labor Standards Bulletin no. 7 (Washington, D.C.: Government Printing Office, 1936), 1, 6, 15, 23, 28, 29, 41.

49. Hamilton, *Recent Changes in the Painters' Trade*, 3, 17–29, 43–63.

50. Tanquerel, *Lead Diseases*, 338.

51. Clement Biddle, "Some Experiments on the Alleged Poisonous Action of Lead Carbonate in Freshly Painted Rooms," *American Journal of the Medical Sciences* (1878), 76: 439–443.

52. Henry K. Armstrong and C. A. Klein, "The Behaviour of Paints under the Conditions of Practice, with Special Reference to the Aspersions Cast upon Lead Paints," *Journal of the Society of Chemical Industry* (1913), 32: 320–331.

53. Hamilton, *Hygiene of the Painters' Trade*, 9–10, 14–17.

54. Henry A. Gardner, *Paint Researches and Their Practical Application* (Washington, D.C.: Judd and Detweiler, 1917), 233.

55. Hearings before the Committee on Interstate and Foreign Commerce of the House of Representatives on H.R. 21901: Manufacture, Sales, etc., of Adulterated or Mislabeled White Lead and Mixed Paint (Washington, D.C.: Government Printing Office, 1910), 14–15.

56. Ibid., 13.

57. Ibid.

58. Ibid., 15.

59. Ibid., 12.

60. For a detailed analysis of these hearings and the ultimate rejection, see Christian Warren, "Toxic Purity: The Progressive Era Origins of America's Lead Paint Poisoning Epidemic," *Business History Review* (1999), 73: 705–736.

61. Oliver, *Lead Poisoning*, 39–55.

62. Alice Hamilton, "The Hygiene of the Lead Industry," address at Meeting of Superintendents, National Lead Company, Chicago, December 7, 1910 (Booklet of the Manufacturing Committee), 12.

63. Edward Cornish, reply to Alice Hamilton's address to the Superintendents of the National Lead Company, December 7, 1910.

64. Hamilton, *Exploring the Dangerous Trades*, 131–132.

65. Ibid., 135.

66. Slaight, "Alice Hamilton," 73.

67. Hamilton, *Exploring the Dangerous Trades*, 114–127; Slaight, "Alice Hamilton," 56–57; and Young, "Interpreting the Dangerous Trades: Workers' Health in America and the Career of Alice Hamilton, 1910–1935," 46–55.

68. Alice Hamilton, *Lead Poisoning in the Smelting and Refining of Lead*, Bulletin of the United States Bureau of Labor Statistics, no. 141 (Washington, D.C.: Government Printing Office, 1914), 58.

69. Hamilton, "Lead Poisoning in the United States," 479.

70. Hamilton, *Women in the Lead Industries*, 5–6.

71. Hamilton, "Lead Poisoning in American Industry," 12.

72. Hamilton, *Industrial Poisons in the United States*, 165.

73. Joseph C. Aub, Lawrence T. Fairhall, A. S. Minot, and Paul Reznikoff, *Lead Poisoning, with a Chapter on the Prevalence of Industrial Lead Poisoning in the United States by Alice Hamilton* (Baltimore: Williams and Wilkins, 1926), 237.

74. Hamilton, *Recent Changes in the Painters' Trade*, 1.

75. Frederick L. Hoffman, "Lead Poisoning Statistics for 1933," *American Public Health Yearbook*, supplement to the *American Journal of Public Health* (1935), 25: 93, 99.

Chapter 5   **Children and the Lead Industries Association, 1925–1935**

1. Henry M. Thomas and Kenneth D. Blackfan, "Recurrent Meningitis, Due to Lead, in a Child of Five Years," *American Journal of Diseases of Children* (1914), 8: 377–380; Kenneth D. Blackfan, "Lead Poisoning in Children: With Especial Reference to Lead as a Cause of Convulsions," *American Journal of the Medical Sciences* (1917), 153: 877–887; L. Emmett Holt, Jr., "Lead Poisoning in Infancy," *American Journal of Diseases of Children* (1923), 25: 229–233.
2. Robert A. Strong, "Meningitis, Caused by Lead Poisoning, in a Child of Nineteen Months," *Archives of Pediatrics* (1920), 37: 532–537.
3. John C. Ruddock, "Lead Poisoning in Children, with Special Reference to Pica," *Journal of the American Medical Association* (1924), 82: 1682–1683.
4. Isaac A. Abt, ed., *Pediatrics, by Various Authors* (Philadelphia: W. B. Saunders, 1925), 7: 316.
5. Christian Warren argues that some cases of lead poisoning may have been misdiagnosed as tuberculous meningitis. The same might be true of polio. I do not believe that this would have been common after Blackfan, Holt, and others called attention to the diagnosis of lead poisoning. See Christian Warren, *Brush with Death: A Social History of Lead Poisoning* (Baltimore: Johns Hopkins University Press, 2000), 33–38.
6. Samuel H. Preston and Michael R. Haines, *Fatal Years: Child Mortality in Late Nineteenth-Century America* (Princeton, N.J.: Princeton University Press, 1991), table 1.1 ("Leading Causes of Death among Infants and Children: U.S. Death Registration Area, 1899–1900"), 4–5.
7. Peter C. English, "'Not Miniature Men and Women': Abraham Jacobi's Vision of a New Medical Specialty a Century Ago," in *Children and Health Care: Moral and Social Issues*, ed. Loretta M. Kopelman and John C. Moskop (Dordrecht: Kluwer Academic Publishers, 1986), 247–273; and Richard A. Meckel, *Save the Babies: American Public Health Reform and the Prevention of Infant Mortality, 1850–1929* (Baltimore: Johns Hopkins University Press, 1990).
8. Ruddock, "Lead Poisoning in Children, with Special Reference to Pica," 1682.
9. L. Emmett Holt, *The Diseases of Infancy and Childhood, for the Use of Students and Practitioners of Medicine*, 6th ed. (New York: D. Appleton, 1912), 693.
10. J. P. Crozier Griffith, *The Diseases of Infants and Children* (Philadelphia: W. B. Saunders Co., 1920), 287.
11. Abt, *Pediatrics, by Various Authors*, 7: 314–317.
12. S. S. Blackman, Jr., "Intranuclear Inclusion Bodies in the Kidney and Liver Caused by Lead Poisoning," *Bulletin of the Johns Hopkins Hospital* (1936), 58: 397 (autopsy case no. 14307).
13. Charles F. McKhann, "Lead Poisoning in Children, with Notes on Therapy," *American Journal of Diseases of Children* (1926), 32: 386.
14. "Lead Poisoning in Early Childhood," *Monthly Bulletin, Health Department of the City of Boston* (November 1927): 266.
15. L. Emmett Holt and John Howland, *The Diseases of Infancy and Childhood*, 9th ed. (New York: D. Appleton, 1926), 542.
16. L. W. Holloway, "Lead Poisoning in Children," *Journal of the Florida Medical Association* (1926), 13: 95.
17. F. L. Hoffman, *Deaths from Lead Poisoning*, Bulletin of the Bureau of Labor Statistics, no. 426 (Washington, D.C., 1927), 33–34.
18. Louis I. Dublin, "Chronic Lead Poisoning in Infancy and Early Childhood," *Statistical Bulletin*, Metropolitan Life Insurance Company (August 1930), 11: 4–5.
19. Ibid., 5. Dublin gave more details of his survey in a letter, dated September 14, 1933, to Dr. Ella Oppenheimer of the Children's Bureau, National Archives, Washington, D.C. The *American Journal of Public Health* reported on the Metropolitan Life Insurance

Company survey. "Chronic Lead Poisoning in Infancy and Early Childhood," *American Journal of Public Health* (1931), 21: 18.

20. "Lead-free Paint on Furniture and Toys to Protect Children," *United States Daily* (November 20, 1930), 1.
21. Felix Wormser to R. R. Sayers, November 21, 1930, Bureau of Mines, National Archives.
22. Albert E. Russell to R. R. Sayers, November 26, 1930, Bureau of Mines, National Archives.
23. R. R. Sayers to Felix Wormser, November 29, 1930, Bureau of Mines, National Archives.
24. Wormser discussed the survey with the board of the LIA on December 12, 1930, Minutes, Lead Industries Association, December 12, 1930, Lead Industries Association (LIA) Archives, housed in the offices of Sullivan, Sullivan and Nahigian, Boston, Mass.
25. Frederick L. Hoffman, *Lead Poisoning: Legislation and Statistics* (Newark, N.J.: Prudential Press, 1933), 19.
26. Dublin, "Chronic Lead Poisoning in Infancy and Early Childhood," 5; McKhann, "Lead Poisoning in Children, with Notes on Therapy," 391; and Louis I. Dublin to Ella Oppenheimer, September 14, 1935, Children's Bureau, National Archives.
27. *White House Conference on Child Health and Protection. Section IV: The Handicapped* (New York: Century, 1932), 233.
28. Minutes, Lead Industries Association, June 8, 1932, LIA Archives.
29. Minutes, Lead Industries Association, 1937, LIA Archives.
30. Minutes, Lead Industries Association, 1929–1973, LIA Archives.
31. Minutes, Lead Industries Association, September 30, 1931, LIA Archives.
32. Minutes, Lead Industries Association, 1938, LIA Archives.
33. Gerald Markowitz and David Rosner argue that the LIA used the results of the survey to mislead the public health community about the safety of painted toys and furniture; see Markowitz and Rosner, "'Cater to the Children': The Role of the Lead Industry in a Public Health Tragedy, 1900–1955," *American Journal of Public Health* (2000) 90: 38. Christian Warren concludes, "These manufacturers may or may not have known how much lead was in the pigments in their enamels, but their answers probably reflected their faith that their paints were nontoxic, and in any case were not 'white lead,'" Warren, *Brush with Death*, 140.
34. Glidden Company to Ella Oppenheimer, May 13, 1932; Halsam Products to Oppenheimer, May 2, 1935; Sherwin-Williams to Oppenheimer, May 2, 1935; Newark Varnish Works to Oppenheimer, April 25, 1935; Embossing Company to Oppenheimer, April 22, 1935; Toy Tinkers to Oppenheimer, April 29, 1935; and A. Schoenhut Company, April 17, 1935. All letters from U.S. Children's Bureau, National Archives.
35. Editors, "Lead Hazard in Toys," *Consumer Reports* (May 1936): 11.
36. H. B. Cushing, "Lead Poisoning in Children: Introductory Remarks," *International Clinics* (1934), 1: 190–191.
37. Charles F. McKhann and Edward C. Vogt, "Lead Poisoning in Children," *Journal of the American Medical Association* (1933), 101: 1131.
38. In 1933, John S. Crutcher, a physician from Nashville, Tennessee, commented while describing an epidemic of lead poisoning from burning battery casings: "With the reduction in the use of lead-containing paints and with the reduction in the use of lead water pipes, we have begun to think of lead poisoning as only infrequently occurring in those people not engaged in lead industries" (Crutcher, "Lead Poisoning in Children," *Journal of the Tennessee Medical Association* [1933], 26: 20). In 1937, C. M. Jephcott described the situation in Ontario: "At the present time lead-free paints are readily available and, in Ontario, manufacturers of children's cots, play-

pens and toys select their paints with this point in mind" (Jephcott, "Lead in Certain Coloured Chalks and the Danger to Children," *Canadian Public Health Journal* [1937], 20: 392). In 1943, Randolph K. Byers and Elizabeth E. Lord reflected the medical view that new toys and cribs no longer contained lead-based paint: "In many instances the parents stated that they had repainted the crib, a practice which would vitiate the use of lead-free paint by the most conscientious of furniture manufacturers" (Byers and Lord, "Late Effects of Lead Poisoning on Mental Development," *American Journal of Diseases of Children* [1943], 66: 478).

39. John McDonald, M.D., comments in *Symposium on Lead Poisoning* (American Medical Association, 1947), 51. In 1947, Philip Drinker reemphasized the accepted view: "Severe lead poisoning of children who have chewed lead-painted objects has occurred in various parts of the world. In the United States, it is becoming rare because lead-painted toys and furniture are rare—toy manufacturers are advised not to use lead paint for these purposes, and compliance with this advice is good" (Drinker, "Public Exposure to Lead," *Occupational Medicine* [1947], 3: 146). In 1948 Charles McKhann reiterated the consensus opinion: "The manufacturers of cribs and toys, informed of the danger to small children from the ingestion of lead paint, have substituted other types of pigments for some of the lead pigments formerly used. New cribs are seldom painted with lead paint, and the better grades of toys are largely free from lead pigment" (McKhann, "Lead Poisoning," in *Brennemann's Practice of Pediatrics*, ed. Irvine McQuarrie (Hagerstown, Md.: W. F. Prior, 1948), 1). In 1951, in response to a query about the status of childhood lead poisoning from cribs and toys, submitted by Thomas Rumore, a physician from West Brentwood, Long Island, the editors of the *Journal of the American Medical Association* replied: "At present the incidence of lead poisoning among children from their gnawing on baseboards, furniture or toys is low. At present few coating materials for interiors or furniture contain lead, for economic reasons. Lithopone and titanium dioxide have largely replaced lead compounds. Some lead may appear in the pigments, such as the greens and oranges. No substantial toy manufacturer now uses lead paints" ("Lead Poisoning from Biting Furniture," Queries and Minor Notes, *Journal of the American Medical Association* [1951], 145: 531). Reflecting this view was Horst A. Agerty, a physician in Philadelphia, who wrote in 1952: "Although it is now a seemingly universal practice to exclude lead-containing paint from use on children's furniture and toys and all indoor woodwork, in many substandard living situations contact with hand-me-down repainted toys, reused nursery furniture and many-times repainted woodwork such as window sills still poses a great threat. Though indoor paint is free from lead, the content of outdoor paint may vary considerably and in many cases may still be high" (Agerty, "Lead Poisoning in Children," *Medical Clinics of North America* [1952], 36: 1587). In 1957, in the most definitive statement about the absence of lead paint on toys, the American Academy of Pediatrics, after an informal polling of over thirty Poison Control Centers, concluded: "The American Academy of Pediatrics has long been concerned with the problem of lead poisoning in children. . . . Verbal impromptu polling of all these representatives failed to reveal any cases of lead poisoning attributed to the ingestion of paint from children's toys. This included centers from the cities of New York and Cincinnati where careful exploration and epidemiologic studies of lead poisoning over a period of several years (including a series of 600 cases in New York City) had been done" ("Lead Poisoning Hazard from Paint on Children's Toys," *Journal of the American Medical Association* [1957], 165: 1996.)

40. Robert Kehoe to Frederick Hoffman, June 26, 1937, Kehoe Papers, Robert A. Kehoe Archives, Cincinnati Medical Heritage Center, University of Cincinnati Medical Center.

41. Robert Kehoe to A. J. Lanza, March 18, 1938, Kehoe Papers.

42. Henry A. Gardner to John M. McDonald, director, Bureau of Occupational Diseases, Baltimore City Health Department, September 14, 1937, Baltimore Health Department (BHD) Archives.
43. Joseph C. Aub to Felix Wormser, January 22, 1945, LIA Archives.
44. Joseph C. Aub to Felix Wormser, May 17, 1945, LIA Archives.
45. LIA Minutes, 1932; LIA Minutes, December 12, 1930, LIA Archives.
46. LIA Minutes, 1932, LIA Archives.
47. LIA Minutes, 1935, LIA Archives.
48. LIA Minutes, June 5, 1934, 1, LIA Archives.
49. "Revised Rules, Regulations, and Recommendations Pertaining to Structural Painting," Massachusetts Department of Labor and Industries, November 1, 1933, 8.
50. LIA Executive Committee Minutes, November 22, 1935, 3, LIA Archives.

Chapter 6 **Baltimore, Boston, and Robert Kehoe, 1930–1940**

1. Abraham Levinson and Mary Zeldes, "Lead Intoxication in Children, a Study of 26 Cases," *Archives of Pediatrics* (1939), 56: 738–748; Alexander J. Alexander and R. E. Dowling, "Lead Poisoning in Children: Report of an Epidemic Due to the Burning of Storage Battery Casings as Fuel," *International Clinics* (1941), 2: 229–242; and Levinson and Leonard H. Harris, "Lead Encephalopathy in Children," *Journal of Pediatrics* (1936), 8: 315–329.
2. Murray H. Bass and Sidney Blumenthal, "Fatal Lead Poisoning in a Nursing Infant Due to Prolonged Use of Lead Nipple Shields," *Journal of Pediatrics* (1939), 15: 724–732; and Milton Rapoport and Athol S. Kenney, "A Case of Lead Encephalopathy in a Breast-Fed Infant Due to the Use of Lead Nipple Shields by the Mother," *Journal of the American Medical Association* (1939), 112: 2040–2042.
3. John Caffey, "Lead Poisoning Associated with Active Rickets: Report of a Case with Absence of Lead Lines in the Skeleton," *American Journal of Diseases of Children* (1938), 55: 798–806.
4. Andrew J. Akelaitis, "Lead Encephalopathy in Children and Adults: A Clinico-Pathological Study," *Journal of Nervous and Mental Diseases* (1941), 93: 313–332.
5. Milton Rapoport and Mitchell I. Rubin, "Lead Poisoning, A Clinical and Experimental Study of the Factors Influencing the Seasonal Incidence in Children," *American Journal of Diseases of Children* (1941), 61: 245–255.
6. L. Emmett Holt, Jr., and Rustin McIntosh, *Holt's Diseases of Infancy and Childhood: A Textbook for the Use of Students and Practitioners* (New York: Appleton-Century-Crofts, 1940), 1368.
7. Edward C. Vogt, "The Roentgen Sign of Plumbism: The Lead Line Growing Bone," *American Journal of Roentgenology* (1930), 24: 550–553.
8. John Caffey, "Clinical and Experimental Lead Poisoning: Some Roentgenologic and Anatomic Changes in Growing Bones," *Radiology* (1931), 17: 957–983.
9. Edwards A. Park, Deborah Jackson, and Laslo Kajdi, "Shadows Produced by Lead in the X-Ray Pictures of the Growing Skeleton," *American Journal of Diseases of Children* (1931), 41: 485–499. See also Robert Drane, "Lead Poisoning: The Bone Changes Roentgenologically Considered," *Southern Medical Journal* (1932), 25: 907–909.
10. This collaboration appears to have prompted the diagnosis of the first British case. See T. Stanley Rodgers, J.R.S. Peck, and M. H. Jupe, "Lead Poisoning in Children: With a Case Record," *Lancet* (1934), 2: 129–133.
11. Charles F. McKhann, "Lead Poisoning in Children: The Cerebral Manifestations," *Archives of Neurology and Psychiatry* (1932), 27: 294.
12. Edward C. Vogt, "Roentgenologic Diagnosis of Lead Poisoning in Infants and Children," *Journal of the American Medical Association* (1932), 98: 125–129.

13. Charles F. McKhann and Edward C. Vogt, "Lead Poisoning in Children," *Journal of the American Medical Association* (1933), 101: 1134.
14. Edward C. Vogt and Charles F. McKhann, "Lead Poisoning in Infants and Children: Roentgenological Findings," *Radiology* (1934), 22: 87.
15. William F. Ashe, "Robert Arthur Kehoe, MD," *Archives of Environmental Health* (1966), 13: 138–142; and Irene R. Campbell, "The House That Robert A. Kehoe Built," *Archives of Environmental Health* (1966), 13: 143–151.
16. Walter Bauer, William T. Salter, and Joseph C. Aub, "Studies of Calcium and Phosphorus Metabolism: Xa. The Use of Calcium Chloride to Relieve Peristaltic Pain," *Journal of the American Medical Association* (1931), 96: 1216–1217; Aub, George C. Robb, and Elsie Rossmeisl, "Significance of Bone Trabeculae in the Treatment of Lead Poisoning: Lead Studies XVII," *American Journal of Public Health* (1932), 22: 825–830; and Aub, "The Biochemical Behavior of Lead in the Body," *Journal of the American Medical Association* (1935), 104: 87–90.
17. Lawrence T. Fairhall and J. William Heim, "The Problem of the Possible Health Hazard of Lead-Weighted Silk Fabric," *Journal of Industrial Hygiene* (1932), 14: 317–327; Fairhall, "Note on the Accuracy of Lead Analyses," *Journal of Industrial Hygiene* (1933), 15: 289; Fairhall, "The Lead Content of Evaporated Milk," *Journal of Industrial Hygiene and Toxicology* (1937), 19: 491–497; Fairhall, "Precision Methods in the Determination of the Heavy Metals," *American Journal of Public Health* (1938), 28: 825–831; Fairhall and Paul A. Neal, "The Absorption and Excretion of Lead Arsenate in Man," *Public Health Reports* (1938), 53: 1231–1245; Fairhall and R. R. Sayers, "The Significance of the Excretion of Lead in the Urine," *Public Health Reports* (1939), 54: 2016–2019; Fairhall, "The Solubility of Lead Arsenate in Body Fluids," *Public Health Reports* (1939), 54: 1636–1642; Fairhall and John W. Miller, "The Deposition and Removal of Lead in the Soft Tissues (Liver, Kidneys, and Spleen)," *Public Health Reports* (1941), 56: 1641–1650; Fairhall and Miller, "A Study of the Relative Toxicity of the Molecular Components of Lead Arsenate," *Public Health Reports* (1941), 56: 1610–1625; Fairhall and F. Lloyd Weaver, "The Effect of Arsenates on the Storage of Lead," *Public Health Reports* (1943), 58: 955–959; Fairhall, Wendell V. Jenrette, Stuart W. Jones, and E. A. Pritchard, "The Toxicity of Lead Azide," *Public Health Reports* (1943), 58: 607–617; and Fairhall, "The Identification and Localization of Lead in Bone Tissue," *Public Health Reports* (1943), 58: 209–216.
18. In 1942, Kehoe complained to members of the board of the Lead Industries Association that their money would be better spent funding the Kettering Laboratory; see Robert Kehoe to Schaeffer, January 1942, Kehoe Papers, Robert A. Kehoe Archives, Cincinnati Medical Heritage Center, University of Cincinnati Medical Center.
19. Raymond R. Suskind, "Kettering Laboratory: A Pioneer in Lead Research," *American Journal of Public Health* (1990), 80: 1001–1002.
20. William Graebner, "Hegemony through Science: Information Engineering and Lead Toxicology, 1925–1965" (140–159) and David Rosner and Gerald Markowitz, "'A Gift from God'?: The Public Health Controversy over Leaded Gasoline during the 1920s" (121–139), in *Dying for Work: Workers' Safety and Health in Twentieth-Century America*, ed. David Rosner and Gerald Markowitz (Bloomington: Indiana University Press, 1989); and Richard P. Wedeen, "Shaping Environmental Research: The Lead Industries Association, 1928–1946," *Economic Interests and Science* (1995), 62: 386–389.
21. Christopher C. Sellers, *Hazards of the Job: From Industrial Disease to Environmental Health Science* (Chapel Hill: University of North Carolina Press, 1997).
22. Christian Warren, *Brush with Death: A Social History of Lead Poisoning* (Baltimore: Johns Hopkins University Press, 2000), 149–150.
23. Robert A. Kehoe, "On the Diagnosis and Treatment of Lead Poisoning," *Journal of Medicine* (1930), 11: 4.

24. Robert A. Kehoe, "The Diagnosis of Lead Poisoning in the Light of Recent Information," *Journal of Medicine* (1935), 16: 528.
25. Robert A. Kehoe and Frederick Thamann, "The Excretion of Lead," *Journal of the American Medical Association* (1929), 92: 1418–1421; Kehoe, "The Determination of Lead in Excreta and Tissues," *American Journal of Clinical Pathology* (1935), 5: 13–20; and Kehoe and Thamann, "The Behavior of Lead in the Animal Organism-I," *American Journal of Public Health* (1928), 18: 555–564.
26. Peter C. English, *Rheumatic Fever in America and Britain: A Biological, Epidemiological, and Medical History* (New Brunswick, N.J.: Rutgers University Press, 1999).
27. Kehoe, "On the Diagnosis and Treatment of Lead Poisoning"; Kehoe, "The Diagnosis of Lead Poisoning in Light of Recent Information"; and Kehoe, "Recognition and Prevention of Lead Poisoning," *Surgery, Gynecology, and Obstetrics* (1938), 66: 444–447.
28. Robert A. Kehoe, Frederick Thamann, and Jacob Cholak, "On the Normal Absorption and Excretion of Lead. I. Lead Absorption and Excretion in Primitive Life," *Journal of Industrial Hygiene* (1933), 15: 257–272.
29. Robert A. Kehoe, Frederick Thamann, and Jacob Cholak, "On the Normal Absorption and Excretion of Lead. II. Lead Absorption and Lead Excretion in Modern American Life," *Journal of Industrial Hygiene* (1933), 15: 273–288.
30. Robert A. Kehoe, Frederick Thamann, and Jacob Cholak, "Lead Absorption and Excretion in Certain Lead Trades," *Journal of Industrial Hygiene* (1933), 15: 306-319.
31. Robert A. Kehoe, Frederick Thamann, and Jacob Cholak, "On the Normal Absorption and Excretion of Lead. III. The Sources of Normal Lead Absorption," *Journal of Industrial Hygiene* (1933), 15: 290–300.
32. Robert A. Kehoe, Frederick Thamann, and Jacob Cholak, "Lead Absorption and Excretion in Relation to the Diagnosis of Lead Poisoning," *Journal of Industrial Hygiene* (1933), 15: 320–340.
33. Robert Kehoe to Charles McKhann, June 31, 1931, Kehoe Papers.
34. Kehoe, Thamann, and Cholak, "On the Normal Absorption and Excretion of Lead. II. Lead Absorption and Excretion in Modern American Life."
35. Robert A. Kehoe, Jacob Cholak, Donald M. Hubbard, Karl Bambach, Robert R. McNary, and Robert V. Story, "Experimental Studies on the Ingestion of Lead Compounds," *Journal of Industrial Hygiene and Toxicology* (1940), 22: 381–400; Kehoe, Cholak, Hubbard, Bambach, and McNary, "Experimental Studies on Lead Absorption and Excretion and Their Relation to the Diagnosis and Treatment of Lead Poisoning," *Journal of Industrial Hygiene and Toxicology* (1943), 25: 71–79; Kehoe, "Lead Absorption and Lead Poisoning," *Medical Clinics of North America* (1942), 26: 1261–1279; Cholak and Bambach, "Measurement of Industrial Lead Exposure by Analyses of Blood and Excreta of Workmen," *Journal of Industrial Hygiene and Toxicology* (1943), 25: 47–54; and Lester W. Sanders, "Measurement of Industrial Lead Exposure by Determination of Stippling of the Erythrocytes," *Journal of Industrial Hygiene and Toxicology* (1943), 25: 38–46.
36. Robert A. Kehoe, Frederick Thamann, and Jacob Cholak, "An Appraisal of the Lead Hazards Associated with the Distribution and Use of Gasoline Containing Tetraethyl Lead, Part I," *Journal of Industrial Hygiene* (1934), 16: 100–128; and "Part II, The Occupational Lead Exposure of Filling Station Attendants and Garage Mechanics," *Journal of Industrial Hygiene and Toxicology* (1936), 18: 42–68.
37. Robert Kehoe to Kenneth Blackfan, June 7, 1937, Kehoe Papers.
38. Pepsodent/Kehoe correspondence, January 1942, Kehoe Papers.
39. Loew Brothers Company/Robert Kehoe correspondence, February 1942, Kehoe Papers.
40. Univis Lens Company/Robert Kehoe correspondence, September 1942, Kehoe Papers.
41. Robert A. Kehoe, Frederick Thamann, and Jacob Cholak, "On the Normal Absorp-

tion and Excretion of Lead. IV. Lead Absorption and Excretion in Infants and Children," *Journal of Industrial Hygiene* (1933), 15: 301–305.

42. Robert A. Kehoe, "Lead Studies in Children," *American Journal of Diseases of Children* (1932), 43: 779.

43. *Report*, Baltimore Health Department, 1933, 15, Baltimore Health Department (BHD) Archives.

44. Francis F. Schwentker, "Children Who Eat Paint," *Keeping Well; The Second Series of Radio Talks Broadcast by the Baltimore City Health Department and the Medical and Chirurgical Faculty of Maryland, November 21, 1933–April 21, 1936* (Baltimore: Baltimore City Health Department, 1936), 122.

45. *Report*, Baltimore Health Department, 1937, 162, BHD Archives.

46. Elizabeth Fee, "Public Health in Practice: An Early Confrontation with the 'Silent Epidemic' of Childhood Lead Paint Poisoning," *Journal of the History of Medicine and Allied Sciences* (1990), 45: 570–606.

47. "Paint-Eating Children," *Baltimore Health News* (1932), 9: 83.

48. Huntington Williams, Wilmer H. Schulze, H. B. Rothchild, A. S. Brown, and Frank R. Smith, "Lead Poisoning from the Burning of Battery Casings," *Journal of the American Medical Association* (1933), 100: 1485–1489.

49. E. A. Park, D. Jackson, T. C. Goodwin, and L. Kajdi, "X-Ray Shadows in Growing Bones Produced by Lead: Their Characteristics, Cause, Anatomical Counterpart in the Bone and Differentiation," *Journal of Pediatrics* (1933), 3: 265–298.

50. Fee, "Public Health in Practice," 580.

51. P. G. Shipley, T. F. McNair Scott, and H. Blumberg, "The Spectrographic Detection of Lead in the Blood as an Aid to the Clinical Diagnosis of Plumbism," *Bulletin of the Johns Hopkins Hospital* (1932), 51: 327–328; and Blumberg and Scott, "The Plasma-Cell Partition of Blood Lead in Clinical Lead Poisoning," *Bulletin of the Johns Hopkins Hospital* (1935), 56: 311–316.

52. John M. McDonald and Emanuel Kaplan, "Incidence of Lead Poisoning in the City of Baltimore," *Journal of the American Medical Association* (1942), 119: 871.

53. Emanuel Kaplan and John M. McDonald, "Blood Lead Determinations as a Health Department Laboratory Service," *American Journal of Public Health* (1942), 32: 482.

54. Ibid., table 1.

55. Ibid., 482.

56. Robert A. Kehoe, "Exposure to Lead," *Occupational Medicine* (1947), 3: 156–171.

57. Sidney Lionel Tompsett and Alan Bruce Anderson, "Lead-Poisoning: Lead Content of Blood and of Excreta," *Lancet* (1939), 1: 559–562; and Tompsett and J.N.M. Chalmers, "Studies in Lead Mobilization," *British Journal of Experimental Pathology* (1939), 20: 408–417.

58. J. N. Marshall Chalmers, "Lead Content of Human Blood," *Lancet* (1940), 1: 447–450.

59. Carl E. Willoughby and Elwood S. Wilkins, Jr., "The Lead Content of Human Blood," *Journal of Biological Chemistry* (1938), 124: 639–657.

60. Harold Blumberg and T. F. McNair Scott, "The Quantitative Spectrographic Estimation of Blood Lead and Its Value in the Diagnosis of Lead Poisoning," *Bulletin of the Johns Hopkins Hospital* (1935), 56: 291.

61. Huntington Williams, Emanuel Kaplan, Charles E. Couchman, and R. R. Sayers, "Lead Poisoning in Young Children," *Public Health Reports* (1952), 67: 230–236.

62. Fee, "Public Health in Practice," 584n47.

63. "Lead Poisoning in Children," *Baltimore Health News* (April 1937), 14: 109–110, BHD Archives. For postmortem analysis, see S. S. Blackman, "Intranuclear Inclusion Bodies in the Kidney and Liver Caused by Lead Poisoning," *Bulletin of the Johns Hopkins Hospital* (1936), 58: 384–404; and Blackman, "The Lesions of Lead Encephalitis in Children," *Bulletin of the Johns Hopkins Hospital* (1937), 61: 1–61.

64. Schwentker, "Children Who Eat Paint," 199-200.
65. "Lead Poisoning Kills Children," *Baltimore Health News* (1939), 134.
66. *Annual Report*, Baltimore City Central Purchasing Bureau, 1936, 3; and "Baltimore's City Government Specifies White Lead," *Lead* (1941–1942), 10–11.
67. "Lead Poisoning from Toys," *Child Welfare* (1931), 25: 608.
68. "Poisoning from Toys," *What to Tell the Public about Health*, 2d ed. (New York: American Public Health Association, 1936), 20.
69. Ralph Netzley, "Lead Encephalitis Precipitated by Acute Infection," *California and Western Medicine* (1937), 46: 308, discussion.
70. Holt and McIntosh, *Holt's Diseases of Infancy and Childhood*, 1372.
71. F. H. Lewy, "Toys and Lead Poisoning," *Safety Education* (1939), 19: 169.
72. "Lead Toys—Lead Paint—Lead Poisoning," *Safety Education* (1942), 22: 194.
73. H. S. Mitchell, "Lead Poisoning in Children," *Canadian Medical Association Journal* (1932), 26: 546–549.
74. Cushing stated the source of lead: "There was usually a history of chewing paint off their cribs, toys, pencils, etc. The country lately has been flooded with cheap wooden painted toys and this seems to have led to the increase in lead poisoning cases." H. B. Cushing, "Lead Poisoning in Children: Introductory Remarks," *International Clinics* (1934), 1: 190.
75. Ibid., 190–191.
76. Ibid., 191. Additional papers presented at the symposium include "Roentgenray Observations," "Chemistry of Lead," "Pathology," "Observations of Cases," and "Treatment." A. E. Childe, "The Roentgen Ray Diagnosis of Lead Poisoning in Children," *International Clinics* (1934), 1: 192–195; I. M. Rabinowitch, "Some of the Biochemical Aspects of Lead Poisoning," *International Clinics* (1934), 1: 196–201; Lawrence J. Rhea, "Pathology of Lead Poisoning: With Special Reference to the Lesions of Bones and Brain in Children," *International Clinics* (1934), 1: 202–206; H. S. Mitchell, "Lead Poisoning in Children," *International Clinics* (1934), 1: 207–216; and S. G. Ross, "The Treatment of Lead Poisoning," *International Clinics* (1934), 1: 217–220.
77. John R. Ross and Alan Brown, "Poisonings Common to Children," *Canadian Public Health Journal* (1935), 26: 241.
78. Ibid., 242.
79. Ibid., 243.
80. Williams, Kaplan, Couchman, and Sayers, "Lead Poisoning in Young Children," note 17.
81. C. M. Jephcott, "Lead in Certain Coloured Chalks and the Danger to Children," *Canadian Public Health Journal* (1937), 28: 391.

Chapter 7   A 1950s Transformation

1. Huntington Williams, Emanuel Kaplan, Charles E. Couchman, and R. R. Sayers, "Lead Poisoning in Young Children," *Public Health Reports* (1952), 67: 230–236.
2. Ibid., 233.
3. "Lead Poisoning Killed 83 Children: Occurrence by Months of 293 Cases, 1931–1951," *Baltimore Health News* (1951), 28: 114.
4. Ibid.
5. Baltimore City Health Department, Ordinance on the Hygiene of Housing, No. 384 (approved March 6, 1941), Baltimore Health Department (BHD) Archives.
6. Huntington Williams, "Housing as a Health Officer's Opportunity," *American Journal of Public Health* (1942), 32: 1001.
7. "St. John's Court Is No More," *Baltimore Health News* (March 1940), 17: 17–19; "Winter Street—Before and After," *Baltimore Health News* (April 1941), 18: 129–130; Huntington Williams, "City Health Department Aids Slum Clearance, Four Years'

Progress, Capped by an Important Court Decision," *The American City* (September 1943), 58: 59–60; Huntington Williams, "Studies of the Effect of the Provision of Good Housing on Health" (tentative proposal by the Joint Committee on Housing and Health of the American Public Health Association and the National Association of Housing Officials), Huntington Williams Papers, July 24, 1945, George Huntington Williams Collection, Alan Mason Chesney Medical Archives, Johns Hopkins Medical Institutions, Baltimore, Md.; Huntington Williams, "Coordinated Effort in Housing Law Enforcement," *Journal of Housing* (September 1946), 193; and Huntington Williams and Wilmer H. Schultze, "Housing Law Enforcement and the City Health Department's Attack on Slums," *Baltimore Health News* (December 1948), 25: 81–87.

8. Presentation, Citizen's Planning and Housing Association of Baltimore, 1947, Huntington Williams Papers.

9. "Lead Poisoning in Children," *Baltimore Health News* (April 1937), 14: 109–110.

10. Williams, Kaplan, Couchman, and Sayers, "Lead Poisoning in Young Children," 230.

11. Ibid., 233.

12. Ibid., 232-233.

13. Charles F. McKhann, "Lead Poisoning in Children: The Cerebral Manifestation," *Archives of Neurology and Psychiatry* (1932), 27: 294.

14. "Paint Eaters," *Time* (December 20, 1943), 49.

15. Felix Wormser to Robert Kehoe, January 19, 1944, Kehoe Papers, Robert A. Kehoe Archives, Cincinnati Medical Heritage Center, University of Cincinnati Medical Center.

16. For a discussion, see Anthony J. Leone, Jr., "On Lead Lines," *American Journal of Roentgenology, Radium Therapy, and Nuclear Medicine* (1968), 103: 165–168; and Reuben Eisenstein and Setsuo Kawanoue, "The Lead Line in Bone—A Lesion Apparently Due to Chondroclastic Indigestion," *American Journal of Pathology* (1975), 80: 309–316.

17. Robert Kehoe to Felix Wormser, February 7, 1944, Kehoe Papers.

18. Bibliography attached to Robert Kehoe to Felix Wormser, May 23, 1944, Kehoe Papers.

19. Felix Wormser to Robert Kehoe, May 4, 1944; Felix Wormser to Robert Kehoe, May 17, 1944; and Felix Wormser to Robert Kehoe, November 27, 1945, Kehoe Papers.

20. J. H. Schaefer to Felix Wormser, June 27, 1944, Kehoe Papers.

21. Confidential letter, Felix Wormser to Members of the Lead Industries Association, December 8, 1944, Lead Industries Association (LIA) Archives, Housed in the offices of Sullivan, Sullivan and Nahigian, Boston, Mass.

22. "Lead Hygiene and Safety Bulletin" no. 40, December 1944; and LIA Minutes, May 29, 1945, 4, LIA Archives.

23. LIA Minutes, April 2, 1948, LIA Archives.

24. "In the diagnostic files of this hospital I found 65 cases labeled as lead poisoning, of whom 20 were obviously spurious. They had just one X-ray or a stipple cell or a coproporphyrin reaction. One youngster came down with polio the next day." Randolph Byers, "Clinical Pathological Conference, The Children's Medical Center Boston, Massachusetts," *Journal of Pediatrics* (1959), 55: 108.

25. Randolph K. Byers, unpublished memoirs, June 1986, 83–84.

26. "A Safety and Hygiene Program for the Lead Industries Association," December 28, 1945, LIA Archives.

27. Felix Wormser to Joseph Aub, January 24, 1946; and memorandum on agenda for symposium, February 7, 1946, LIA Archives.

28. LIA Minutes, May 8, 1947, LIA Archives.

29. "The Use of CaEDTA in Cases of Lead Intoxication," July 1952, LIA Archives.

30. Charles E. Couchman to Thurber Fales, January 3, 1949, BHD Archives.

31. Manfred Bowditch to W. H. Schultze, February 18, 1949, BHD Archives.
32. Unknown to Manfred Bowditch, March 30, 1949, BHD Archives.
33. "Lead Poisoning in Children Is Preventable and Can Be Fatal," *Baltimore Health News* (May 1949), 26: 122.
34. T. Campbell Goodwin, "Lead Poisoning Kills Children," *Baltimore Health News* (1939): 132–134.
35. Memo, Dr. M. Alexander Novey to Charles Couchman, July 1, 1949, BHD Archives.
36. Huntington Williams to Manfred Bowditch, July 1, 1949; and Huntington Williams to Manfred Bowditch, July 5, 1949, BHD Archives.
37. Anna Baetjer and Mary Watt, "Report on Child Lead Cases Occurring in Baltimore, from January 1948 to August 1949," BHD Archives.
38. Anna Baetjer to Huntington Williams, October 3, 1949, BHD Archives.
39. Manfred Bowditch to Randolph K. Byers, December 21, 1949, BHD Archives.
40. "Toxic Finishes Law," Chapter 517 of the Acts of 1949, Article 27: Crimes and Punishment, paragraph 323, BHD Archives.
41. J. Davis Donovan (Chief, Division of Legal Services, Maryland Department of Health), memo, July 1, 1949; Emanuel Kaplan to Charles Couchman, August 8, 1949; and Wilmer H. Schultz to Charles Couchman, "Conference to Repeal Chapter 517 of the Acts of 1949 of the Maryland State Law," February 6, 1950, BHD Archives.
42. *Baltimore Sun*, February 24, 1950.
43. LIA Minutes, March 10, 1950, 4, LIA Archives.
44. The study did not begin until 1951. Manfred Bowditch to R. R. Sayers, January 16, 1951, BHD Archives.
45. For example, in a letter to Charles Couchman, director of Baltimore's Bureau of Industrial Hygiene, on October 9, 1950, Bowditch wrote: "I should have acknowledged before this your good letter of September 26. I was particularly glad to receive it as it enabled me to discuss with Doctor Sayers some aspects of the childhood plumbism headache with which all of us are trying to cope. . . . Your figures on this year's cases add stimulus to our determination to get the Johns Hopkins study under way. I have had several recent telephone talks with Doctor Baetjer, and Dr. Sayers has promised to confer with her as to ways and means. I had heard something of Doctor Goldman's [Bureau of Public Health Engineering, Washington, D.C.] plans and only hope that his approach will be adequate in all respects. The more investigations the better, provided that the work is well and thoroughly done." Manfred Bowditch to Charles E. Couchman, October 9, 1950, BHD Archives.
46. May R. Mayers to Manfred Bowditch, January 12, 1950, attached, "Report on Lead Poisoning in Infants in Baltimore," 1, LIA Archives.
47. Charles E. Couchman to Joseph C. Willett, April 12, 1950, BHD Archives.
48. Charles E. Couchman to E. G. Frederick, April 28, 1950, BHD Archives.
49. Charles E. Couchman to Harry E. Seifert, May 16, 1950, BHD Archives.
50. Charles E. Couchman to Frederick E. Goldman, July 21, 1950, BHD Archives.
51. H. Breiger to Charles E. Couchman, August 8, 1950, BHD Archives.
52. J. S. Felton to Charles E. Couchman, August 31, 1950, BHD Archives.
53. New York City Bureau of Preventable Diseases, "Report of Activities, May 1950. Epidemiological Notes: Lead Poisoning," June 7, 1950, 2.
54. Manfred Bowditch to R. R. Sayers, December 4, 1950, BHD Archives. For example, Bowditch passed the Cincinnati cases to Baltimore, Manfred Bowditch to R. R. Sayers, April 11, 1951, BHD Archives; Bowditch passed along Boston cases to Cincinnati, Manfred Bowditch to Robert Kehoe, August 14, 1951, BHD Archives; Bowditch sent Cincinnati findings to Baltimore, Manfred Bowditch to Francis F. Schwentker, August 15, 1951, BHD Archives; Robert Kotte sent a detailed analysis of Cincinnati's cases to Bowditch and George Wheatley, Robert Kotte to Manfred Bowditch, August 22, 1951, Kehoe Papers. Bowditch, in turn, sent all the correspondence and case

reports from Cincinnati and Boston to Baltimore, R. R. Sayers to Manfred Bowditch, August 23, 1951, BHD Archives; and more Cincinnati cases to Bowditch and George Wheatley, Robert Kotte to Manfred Bowditch, September 10, 1951, BHD Archives.

Chapter 8   The Urban Ecology

1. (Boston) Randolph K. Byers, Clarence A. Maloof, and Margaret Cushman, "Urinary Excretion of Lead in Children: Diagnostic Application," *American Journal of Diseases of Children* (1954), 87: 548–558; Byers and Maloof, "Edathamil Calcium-Disodium (Versenate) in Treatment of Lead Poisoning in Children," *American Journal of Diseases of Children* (1954), 87: 559–569; (Baltimore) J. Julian Chisholm, Jr., and Harold E. Harrison, "The Exposure of Children to Lead," *Pediatrics* (1956), 18: 943–958; (Cincinnati) Hugo Dunlap Smith, "Lead Poisoning in Children and Its Therapy with EDTA," *Industrial Medicine and Surgery* (1959), 28: 148–155; Smith, "Pediatric Lead Poisoning," *Archives of Environmental Health* (1964), 8: 256–261; (New York City) Harold Jacobziner and Harry W. Raybin, "Lead Poisoning in Young Children—Fatal and Nonfatal," *New York State Journal of Medicine* (1960), 60: 273–277; (Minneapolis) Evelyn E. Hartman, Wilford E. Park, and H. Godfrey Nelson, "The Peeling House Paint Hazard to Children," *Public Health Reports* (1960), 75: 623–629; (Philadelphia) Emil A. Tiboni and Raymond L. Tyler, "Childhood Lead Poisoning in Philadelphia," *Philadelphia Medicine* (1960), 56: 668–669; (Chicago) Joseph R. Christian, "Lead Poisoning in Children," *Chicago Medicine* (June 24, 1961), 15–18; (Cleveland) Robert C. Griggs, Irving Sunshine, Vaun A. Newill, Burritt W. Newton, Stuart Buchanan, and Cleo A. Rasch, "Environmental Factors in Childhood Lead Poisoning," *Journal of the American Medical Association* (1964), 187: 703–707.
2. "Lead Poisoning in Children," *Baltimore Health News* (April 1937), 14: 109–110.
3. Huntington Williams, Emanuel Kaplan, Charles E. Couchman, and R. R. Sayers, "Lead Poisoning in Young Children," *Public Health Reports* (1952), 67: 233.
4. "Lead Poisoning Killed 83 Children; Occurrence by Months of 293 Cases, 1931–1951," *Baltimore Health News* (1951), 28: 114.
5. Robert B. Mellins and C. David Jenkins, "Epidemiological and Psychological Study of Lead Poisoning in Children," *Journal of the American Medical Association* (1955), 158: 16.
6. Mary Culhane McLaughlin, "Lead Poisoning in Children in New York City, 1950–1954: An Epidemiologic Study," *New York State Journal of Medicine* (1956), 56: 3713.
7. Hugo Dunlap Smith, "Lead Poisoning in Children and Its Therapy with EDTA," *Proceedings of the Lead Hygiene Conference*, sponsored by the Lead Industries Association (November 6–7, 1958), *Industrial Medicine and Surgery* (1959), 28: 149.
8. Ian C. Bristow, *Interior House-Painting Colours and Technology, 1615–1840* (New Haven: Yale University Press, 1996); Michael Jacobs and Gelvin Stevenson, "Health and Housing: A Historical Examination of Alternative Perspectives," *International Journal of Health Services* (1981), 11: 105–122.
9. George B. Heckel, *The Paint Industry: Reminiscences and Comments* (St. Louis: American Paint Journal Company, 1931).
10. Paul M. Tyler, *Trends in White-Pigment Consumption*, U.S. Bureau of Mines, Information Circular 6881, April 1936, 2.
11. Nancy Tomes, *The Gospel of Germs: Men, Women, and the Microbe in American Life* (Cambridge, Mass.: Harvard University Press, 1998), 167.
12. Sophronia Maria Elliott, *Household Hygiene* (Chicago: American School of Home Economics, 1907), 154.
13. Henry A. Gardner, *Papers on Paint and Varnish, and the Material Used in Their Manufacture* (Washington, D.C.: Paint and Varnish Manufacturers Association, 1920), 401–402.

14. Robert W. DeForest and Lawrence Veiller, *The Tenement House Problem, Including the Report of the New York State Tenement House Commission of 1900; by Various Writers* (New York: Macmillan Co., 1903), 1: 25, 106, 454, ("All walls in lodging houses and tenement houses should be painted; the use of wall paper should be prohibited, as should also the use of carpets, mattings, or any textile fabrics on the walls and stairways"), 2: 137, 138, 305; Lawrence Veiller, *Housing Reform: A Hand-Book for Practical Use in American Cities* (New York: Russell Sage Foundation, 1910), 3, 5, 8, 10, 113; Lawrence Veiller, *A Model Housing Law*, rev. ed. (New York: Russell Sage Foundation, 1920), 215, 216, 221, 222, 245, 246; Jacob A. Riis, *The Battle with the Slum* (New York: Macmillan Co., 1902), 1, 90, 94, 264–309; Jacob A. Riis, *The Peril and the Preservation of the Home, Being the William L. Bull Lectures for the Year 1903* (Philadelphia: George W. Jacobs & Co., 1903), 79. See also Jacob A. Riis, *Children of the Tenements* (New York: Macmillan Co., 1903); Riis, *How the Other Half Lives: Studies Among the Tenements of New York, with 100 Photographs from the Jacob A. Riis Collection, the Museum of the City of New York* (New York: Dover Publications, 1971); Riis, *The Children of the Poor* (New York: Charles Scribner's Sons, 1892); Keith Gandal, *The Virtues of the Vicious: Jacob Riis, Stephen Crane, and the Spectacle of the Slum* (New York: Oxford University Press, 1997), 115–121; and Roy Lubove, *The Progressives and the Slums: Tenement House Reform in New York City, 1890–1917* (Pittsburgh: University of Pittsburgh Press, 1962).
15. Percy Hargraves Walker and Eugene F. Hickson, *Use of United States Government Specification Paint and Paint Materials*, Technologic Papers of the Bureau of Standards, paper no. 274 (Washington, D.C.: Government Printing Office, 1924), 32; "Paint Pigments–White," Technical Information on Building Material for Use in the Design of Low-Cost Housing, National Bureau of Standards (TIBM-30), August 15, 1936; "Federal Specification Paint Pigments and Mixing Formulas," Technical Information on Building Materials for Use in the Design of Low-Cost Housing, National Bureau of Standards (TIBM-33), September 15, 1936; "Federal Specification Ready-Mixed Paints, Semipaste Paints, and Mixing Formulas," Technical Information on Building Material for Use in the Design of Low-Cost Housing, National Bureau of Standards (TIBM-34), September 18, 1936; "Preparation of Paints from Paste and Dry Pigments," Technical Information on Building Materials for Use in the Design of Low-Cost Housing, National Bureau of Standards (TIBM-35), September 23, 1936; "Outside House Painting," National Bureau of Standards (LC-603), July 5, 1940; and Percy Hargraves Walker and Eugene F. Hickson, *Paint Manual, with Particular Reference to Federal Specifications*, Building Materials and Structures Report BMS105 (Washington, D.C.: Government Printing Office, 1945).
16. Alice Hamilton, *Hygiene of the Painters' Trade*, Bulletin of the United States Bureau of Labor Statistics, no. 120 (Washington, D.C.: Government Printing Office, 1913), 8.
17. Henry A. Gardner, *Paint Researches and Their Practical Application* (Washington, D.C.: Judd and Detweiler, 1917), 242; and National Lead Company, *Handy Book on Painting* (Cleveland: National Lead Company, 1920).
18. Paul M. Tyler, *Trends in White-Pigment Consumption*. Information Circular (I.C. 6881), Bureau of Mines, April 1936, 8.
19. Alice Hamilton, *Recent Changes in the Painters' Trade*, United States Division of Labor Standards, Bulletin no. 7 (Washington, D.C.: Government Printing Office, 1936), 1, 6, 15, 23, 28, 29, 41.
20. Walker and Hickson, *Paint Manual, with Particular Reference to Federal Specifications*, 73-78. In 1945, for example, the U.S. Department of Commerce's National Bureau of Standards recommended lead pigment for exteriors. The War Production Board's Office of Price Administration (OPA) kept track of many commodities during World War II as part of its program of price controls. In a discussion of household paints, one administrator concluded: "The use of Basic Carbonate of White Lead in the paint,

varnish and lacquer industry for interior paints is negligible. For all practical purposes we can say that the entire consumption of B.C.W.L. is in exterior paints required for the maintenance of property." W. F. Twombley, Assistant Director, Chemical Division (War Production Board, Office of Price Administration) to Erwin Vegelsang, Director Tin, Lead and Zinc Division, "Lead Requirements for the Paint, Varnish, and Lacquer Industry," December 11, 1946, 1. In 1955, the U.S. Department of Agriculture concluded: "The outstanding merits of pure white lead paint are its exceptionally great resistance to adverse conditions of service and its wide tolerance for differing programs of maintenance." *Wood Handbook, Basic Information on Wood as a Material of Construction with Data for Its Use in Design and Specification, Prepared by the Forest Products Laboratory, Forest Service, U.S. Department of Agriculture* (Washington, D.C.: Government Printing Office, 1955), 363. These sentiments were echoed in other Department of Agriculture consumer publications a year later. See Forest Products Laboratory, *Wood Siding, How to Install It, Paint It, Care for It*, Home and Garden Bulletin no. 52 (Washington, D.C.: U.S. Department of Agriculture, Government Printing Office, 1956), 6.

21. Donald Barltrop and N.J.P. Killala, "Factors Influencing Exposure of Children to Lead," *Archives of Diseases in Childhood* (1969), 44: 477.

22. J. Julian Chisholm, Jr., "Treatment of Lead Poisoning," *Modern Treatment* (1967), 4: 712.

23. Robert Halpern, *Rebuilding the Inner City: A History of Neighborhood Initiatives to Address Poverty in the United States* (New York: Columbia University Press, 1995), 57–82; David M. Cutler, Edward L. Glaeser, and Jacob L. Vigdor, *The Rise and Decline of the American Ghetto*, Working Paper 5881 (Cambridge, Mass.: National Bureau of Economic Research, 1997), 1–37; Jon C. Teaford, *The Rough Road to Renaissance: Urban Revitalization in America, 1940–1985* (Baltimore: Johns Hopkins University Press, 1990), 10–43.

24. *Housing for Health: Papers Presented under the Auspices of the Committee on the Hygiene of Housing of the American Public Health Association* (Lancaster, Pa.: Science Press Printing Co., 1941), app. A, 184–216; Committee on the Hygiene of Housing, American Public Health Association, "An Appraisal Method for Measuring the Quality of Housing: A Yardstick for Health Officers, Housing Officials and Planners, Part II. Appraisal of Dwelling Conditions, Volume B. Field Procedures," 1946.

25. Margaret Galbreath, "Lead Poisoning in Young Children," *Safety Education* (1952), 32: 16.

26. J. Julian Chisholm, Jr., and Harold E. Harrison, "The Exposure of Children to Lead," *Pediatrics* (1956), 18: 943.

27. Arnold L. Tanis, "Lead Poisoning in Children: Including Nine Cases Treated with Edathamil Calcium-Disodium," *American Journal of Diseases of Children* (1955), 89: 325.

28. C. David Jenkins and Robert B. Mellins, "Lead Poisoning in Children: A Study of 46 Cases," *Archives of Neurology and Psychiatry* (1957), 77: 70.

29. Joseph Greengard, Lowell Zollar, and Manoucher Sharifi, "Medical Progress in the Prevention of Childhood Lead Intoxication," *Illinois Medical Journal* (1968), 133: 615.

30. Jacobziner and Raybin, "Lead Poisoning in Young Children—Fatal and Nonfatal," 277.

31. Hugo Dunlap Smith, "Pediatric Lead Poisoning," *Archives of Environmental Health* (1964), 4: 259.

32. Jerome Trichter, "Report on Housing in New York City," presented to the Board of Health, January 5, 1959, 18, 21.

33. Roger Starr, *The Rise and Fall of New York City* (New York: Basic Books, 1985), 84–104; Peter D. Salins, *The Ecology of Housing Destruction: Economic Effects of Public Intervention in the Housing Market* (New York: New York University Press, 1980); and

Peter D. Salins and Gerard C. S. Mildner, *Scarcity by Design: The Legacy of New York City's Housing Policies* (Cambridge, Mass.: Harvard University Press, 1992).

34. Trichter, "Report on Housing in New York City," 22.

35. (Baltimore) "Lead Poisoning Killed 83 Children; Occurrence by Months of 293 Cases, 1931–1951," 115; (Cincinnati) Hugo D. Smith, "Lead Poisoning in Children and Its Therapy with EDTA," *Proceedings of the Lead Hygiene Conference,* sponsored by the Lead Industries Association, November 6–7, *Industrial Medicine and Surgery* (1959), 28: 150; (Philadelphia) Theodore H. Ingalls, Emil A. Tiboni, and Milton Werrin, "Lead Poisoning in Philadelphia, 1955–1960," *Archives of Environmental Health* (1961), 3: 577; (Chicago) Joseph R. Christian, Bohdan S. Celewycz, and Samuel L. Andelman, "A Three-Year Study of Lead Poisoning in Chicago: Part 1. Epidemiology," *American Journal of Public Health* (1964), 54: 1244; (New York City) Harold Jacobziner and Harry W. Raybin, "The Epidemiology of Lead Poisoning in Children," *Archives of Pediatrics* (1962), 79: 73.

36. Jacobziner and Raybin, "The Epidemiology of Lead Poisoning in Children," 72; and Griggs et al., "Environmental Factors in Childhood Lead Poisoning," 703.

37. Robert Halpern, *Rebuilding the Inner City: A History of Neighborhood Initiatives to Address Poverty in the United States* (New York: Columbia University Press, 1995), 57–82; Cutler, Glaeser, and Vigdor, *The Rise and Decline of the American Ghetto,* 1-37; and Jon C. Teaford, *The Rough Road to Renaissance: Urban Revitalization in America, 1940–1985* (Baltimore: Johns Hopkins University Press, 1990), 10–43.

38. Huntington Williams, Emanuel Kaplan, Charles E. Couchman, and R. R. Sayers, "Lead Poisoning in Young Children," *Public Health Reports* (1952), 67: 233.

39. McLaughlin, "Lead Poisoning in Children in New York City, 1950–1954."

40. Jacobziner and Raybin, "Lead Poisoning in Young Children—Fatal and Nonfatal," 277.

41. (Cincinnati) Smith, "Pediatric Lead Poisoning"; (Philadelphia) Theodore H. Ingalls, Emil A. Tiboni, and Milton Werrin, "Lead Poisoning in Philadelphia, 1955–1960," *Archives of Environmental Health* (1961), 3: 575–579; (Chicago) Greengard, Zollar, and Sharifi, "Medical Progress in the Prevention of Childhood Lead Intoxication."

42. Mellins and Jenkins, "Epidemiological and Psychological Study of Lead Poisoning in Children," 16.

43. J. Edmund Bradley and Samuel P. Bessman, "Poverty, Pica, and Poisoning," *Public Health Reports* (1958), 73: 467.

44. Jacobziner and Raybin, "Lead Poisoning in Young Children—Fatal and Nonfatal," 277.

45. Marcia Mann Cooper, *Pica: A Survey of the Historical Literature as well as Reports from the Fields of Veterinary Medicine and Anthropology, the Present Study of Pica in Young Children, and a Discussion of Its Pediatric and Psychological Implications* (Springfield, Ill.: Charles C. Thomas, 1957), 57–69.

46. Frances K. Millican, Emma M. Layman, Reginald D. Lourie, Lily Y. Takahashi, and Christina C. Dublin, "The Prevalence of Ingestion and Mouthing of Non-edible Substances by Children," *Clinical Proceedings of the Children's Hospital of Washington, D.C.* (1962), 18: 213.

47. J. Julian Chisholm, Jr., and Eugene Kaplan, "Lead Poisoning in Childhood—Comprehensive Management and Prevention," *Journal of Pediatrics* (1968), 73: 942.

48. Ibid., 943.

49. *Annual Report,* Baltimore Health Department, 1957, BHD Archives. In Boston, African American children with pica greatly out-numbered white children with pica; see Donald Barltrop, "The Prevalence of Pica," *American Journal of Diseases of Children* (1966), 112: 116–123.

50. Smith, "Lead Poisoning in Children and Its Therapy with EDTA," 57.

51. J. Edmund Bradley and Samuel P. Bessman, "Poverty, Pica, and Poisoning," *Public Health Reports* (1958), 73: 467.

52. George J. Cohen and Walter E. Ahrens, "Chronic Lead Poisoning; A Review of Seven Years' Experience at the Children's Hospital, District of Columbia," *Journal of Pediatrics* (1959), 54: 271.
53. Emil A. Tiboni and Raymond L. Tyler, "Childhood Lead Poisoning in Philadelphia," 668.
54. Chisholm and Kaplan, "Lead Poisoning in Childhood—Comprehensive Management and Prevention," 942.
55. Emanuel Kaplan to Charles Couchman, November 23, 1948, BHD Archives.

Chapter 9 New Therapies

1. For a summary of animal experiments, see Frederick G. Germuth, Jr., and Harry Eagle, "The Efficacy of BAL (2,3-Dimercaptopropanol) in the Treatment of Experimental Lead Poisoning in Rabbits," *Journal of Pharmacology and Experimental Therapeutics* (1948), 92: 397–410; M. Weatherall, "Effects of BAL and BAL Glucoside in Acute Lead Acetate Poisoning," *British Journal of Pharmacology* (1948), 3: 137–145; Michael Ginsburg and Miles Weatherall, "Dimercaprol and the Biliary Excretion of Lead in Rabbits," *British Journal of Pharmacology* (1949), 4: 274–276; A. B. Anderson, "The Effect of Dimercaprol on Lead Poisoning in Mice," *British Journal of Pharmacology* (1949), 4: 348–350; K. R. Adam, M. Ginsburg, and M. Weatherall, "The Effects of Dimercaprol and Parathyroid Extract on the Subacute Distribution of Lead (Acetate) in Rabbits," *British Journal of Pharmacology* (1949), 4: 351–358.
2. Henry W. Ryder, Jacob Cholak, and Robert A. Kehoe, "Influence of Dithiopropanol (BAL) on Human Lead Metabolism," *Science* (1947), 106: 63–64.
3. Kehoe concluded that "the effects of the administration of dithiopropanol are unique in our experience and are of potentially great physiological importance. . . . We also wish to emphasize that dithiopropanol is potentially a dangerous drug, and that lead intoxication is largely a self-limited disease for which the only primary treatment of proved value is the removal of affected men from further exposure to lead." Ibid., 64.
4. Julius M. Ennis and Harold E. Harrison, "Treatment of Lead Encephalopathy with BAL (2,3-Dimercaptopropanol)," *Pediatrics* (1950), 5: 853–868.
5. Garrett E. Dean, Frederick J. Heldrich, Jr., and J. Edmund Bradley, "The Use of BAL in the Treatment of Acute Lead Encephalopathy," *Journal of Pediatrics* (1953), 42: 409–413.
6. Rudolph C. Giannattasio, Michael J. Pirozzi, Andrew V. Bedo, and Kenneth G. Jennings, "BAL Therapy in Chronic Lead Poisoning," *Pediatrics* (1952), 10: 603–611.
7. Rudolph C. Giannattasio and Michael J. Pirozzi, "BAL Therapy in Acute Lead Encephalopathy," *New York State Journal of Medicine* (1953), 53: 3017–3018.
8. "The tremors and twitching subsided on the first and second day of therapy, and the lethargy had completely disappeared by the third day. There was no recurrence of these symptoms." Samuel P. Bessman, Hugh Reid, and Martin Rubin, "Treatment of Lead Encephalopathy with Calcium Disodium Versenate," *Medical Annals of the District of Columbia* (1952), 21: 312–315; for animal studies, see Norman S. MacDonald, Florita Ezmirlian, Patricia Spain, and Donald E. Rounds, "Agents Diminishing Skeletal Accumulation of Lead," *Archives of Industrial Hygiene and Occupational Medicine* (1953), 7: 217–220.
9. Martin Rubin, Solange Gignac, Samuel P. Bessman, and Elston L. Belknap, "Enhancement of Lead Excretion in Humans by Disodium Calcium Ethylenediamine Tetra Acetate," *Science* (1953), 117: 659–660.
10. H. Foreman, H. L. Hardy, T. L. Shipman, and E. L. Belknap, "Use of Calcium Ethylenediaminetetraacetate in Cases of Lead Intoxication," *Archives of Industrial Hygiene and Occupational Medicine* (1953), 7: 148–151; J. B. Sidbury, Jr., J. C. Bynum,

and L. L. Fetz, "Effect of Chelating Agent on Urinary Lead Excretion. Comparison of Oral and Intravenous Administration," *Proceedings of the Society of Experimental Biology and Medicine* (1953), 82: 226–228.

11. Samuel P. Bessman and Ennis C. Layne, Jr., "Distribution of Lead in Blood as Affected by Edathmil Calcium-Disodium," *American Journal of Diseases of Children* (1955), 89: 292–294; Felix E. Karpinski, Jr., Frederic Rieders, and Leonard S. Girsh, "Calcium Disodium Versenate in the Therapy of Lead Encephalopathy," *Journal of Pediatrics* (1953), 42: 687–699; Samuel P. Bessman, Martin Rubin, and Sanford Leikin, "The Treatment of Lead Encephalopathy—A Method for the Removal of Lead during the Acute Stage," *Pediatrics* (1954), 14: 201–208; and James B. Sidbury, Jr., "Lead Poisoning: Treatment with Disodium Calcium Ethylenediamine-tetra-acetate," *American Journal of Medicine* (1955), 18: 932–946.

12. J. Edmund Bradley and Albert M. Powell, Jr., "Oral Calcium EDTA in Lead Intoxication of Children," *Journal of Pediatrics* (1954), 45: 297–301; N. V. O'Donohoe, "Lead Poisoning in Childhood Treated by the Subcutaneous Administration of a Chelating Agent," *Archives of Disease in Childhood* (1956), 31: 321–323.

13. Randolph K. Byers and Clarence Maloof, "Edathamil Calcium-Disodium (Versenate) in Treatment of Lead Poisoning in Children," *American Journal of Diseases of Children* (1954), 87: 559–569.

14. J. Julian Chisholm, Jr., and Harold E. Harrison, "The Exposure of Children to Lead," *Pediatrics* (1956), 18: 943.

15. Rudolph C. Giannattasio, "BAL Therapy in Lead Poisoning," *New York State Journal of Medicine* (1956), 56: 3510–3511; and Giannattasio, "The Management of Lead Intoxication," *New York State Journal of Medicine* (1957), 57: 2394–2396.

16. J. Julian Chisholm, Jr., and Harold E. Harrison, "The Treatment of Acute Lead Encephalopathy in Children," *Pediatrics* (1957), 19: 2–20; J. M. Arena, "Report from the Duke University Poison Control Center: Lead Poisoning, Part Two," *North Carolina Medical Journal* (1961), 22: 73–74; As an editorialist for the *Journal of the American Medical Association* concluded in 1955, "Edathamil calcium-disodium . . . has given the physician his first opportunity to remove lead from the patient's system even during the severe phase of lead encephalopathy without causing an exacerbation of symptoms." "Lead Poisoning" (editorial), *Journal of the American Medical Association* (1955), 158: 47.

17. Cecil E. C. Harris, "A Comparison of Intravenous Calcium Disodium Versenate and Oral Penicillamine in Promoting Elimination of Lead," *Canadian Medical Association Journal* (1958), 79: 664–666; and A. Goldberg, Jacqueline A. Smith, and Ann C. Lochhead, "Treatment of Lead-Poisoning with Oral Penicillamine," *British Medical Journal* (1963), 1: 1270–1275. Both of these studies treated adults only.

18. Robert A. Kehoe, "A Critical Appraisal of Current Practices in the Clinical Diagnosis of Lead Intoxication," *Industrial Medicine and Surgery* (1951), 20: 253–259.

19. Paul V. Woolley, Jr., "Lead Poisoning during Infancy and Early Childhood," *American Journal of Roentgenology, Radium Therapy, and Nuclear Medicine* (1957), 78: 547–549; Peggy Sartain, Jo Anne Whitaker, and Janet Martin, "The Absence of Lead Lines in Bones of Children with Early Lead Poisoning," *American Journal of Roentgenology, Radium Therapy, and Nuclear Medicine* (1964), 91: 597–601.

20. A.J.S. McFadzean and L. J. Davis, "On the Nature and Significance of Stippling in Lead Poisoning, with Reference to the Effect of Splenectomy," *Quarterly Journal of Medicine* (1949), 18: 57–72; Irving J. Wolman and Alfred M. Bongiovanni, "Hematology of Lead Poisoning in Childhood," *American Journal of the Medical Sciences* (1956), 232: 688–694; George Meachim, "The Interpretation of Erythrocyte Stippling in Lead Workers," *American Industrial Hygiene Association Journal* (1962), 23: 245–248.

21. L. T. Fairhall, "Analytic Methods in Diagnosis," *Occupational Medicine* (1947), 3: 13–

19; Elston L. Belknap, "Differential Diagnosis of Lead Poisoning: Accepted Laboratory Criteria," *Journal of the American Medical Association* (1949), 139: 818–823; and Rosedith Sitgreaves and Irving May, "Potential Sources of Error in Blood Lead Determinations Due to Different Methods of Blood Sampling," *Archives of Industrial Hygiene and Occupational Medicine* (1950), 1: 467–470.

22. Rudolph K. Waldman and Roy M. Seideman, "Reliability of the Urinary Porphyrin Test for Lead Absorption," *Archives of Industrial Hygiene and Occupational Medicine* (1950), 1: 290–295; William S. Johnson and Newton E. Whitman, "Coproporphyrinuria as an Index of Lead Absorption," *Archives of Industrial Hygiene and Occupational Medicine* (1950), 2: 170–174; Carey P. McCord, "The Porphyrins: The Significance of Porphyrins in Occupational Diseases," *Industrial Medicine and Surgery* (1951), 20: 185–190; Sherman S. Pinto, Christine Einert, Wesley J. Roberts, Grant S. Winn, and K. W. Nelson, "Coproporphyrinuria: Study of Its Usefulness in Evaluating Lead Exposure," *Archives of Industrial Hygiene and Occupational Medicine* (1952), 6: 496–507; E. S. Parkinson and J. Cholak, "Problems in the Analysis of Urinary Coproporphyrin III," *American Industrial Hygiene Association Quarterly* (1952), 13: 158–162; J. Wyllie, "Urinary Porphyrins in Lead Absorption," *Archives of Industrial Health* (1955), 12: 396–405.

23. Garson H. Tishkoff, Norma B. Granville, Robert Rosen, and William Dameshek, "Excretion of δ-Aminolevulinic Acid in Lead Intoxication," *Acta Haematologica* (1958), 19: 321–326; J. Julian Chisholm, Jr., "Disturbances in the Biosynthesis of Heme in Lead Intoxication," *Journal of Pediatrics* (1964), 64: 174–186; and Kim Cramer and Stig Selander, "Studies in Lead Poisoning: Comparison between Different Laboratory Tests," *British Journal of Industrial Medicine* (1965), 22: 311–314.

24. J. Edmund Bradley, Albert E. Powell, William Niermann, Kathleen R. McGrady, and Emanuel Kaplan, "The Incidence of Abnormal Blood Levels of Lead in a Metropolitan Pediatric Clinic; with Observation on the Value of Coproporphyrinuria as a Screening Test," *Journal of Pediatrics* (1956), 49: 1–6; and Philip F. Benson and J. Julian Chisholm, Jr., "A Reliable Qualitative Urine Coproporphyrin Test for Lead Intoxication in Young Children," *Journal of Pediatrics* (1960), 56: 759–767.

25. Maxwell P. Westerman, Emil Pfitzer, Lawrence D. Ellis, and Wallace N. Jensen, "Concentrations of Lead in Bone in Plumbism," *New England Journal of Medicine* (1965), 273: 1246–1250.

26. Morton J. Robinson, Felix E. Karpinski, Jr., and Heinrich Brieger, "The Concentration of Lead in Plasma, Whole Blood, and Erythrocytes of Infants and Children," *Pediatrics* (1958), 21: 793–797; Otto P. Preuss, "Childhood Plumbism: Doctor, Would You Think of Lead Poisoning?" *Ohio State Medical Journal* (1962), 58: 665–667; and "Lead Poisoning in Children" (editorial), *British Medical Journal* (1964), 1: 1200–1201.

27. Lillis F. Altshuller, Delmar B. Halak, Benjamin H. Landing, and Robert A. Kehoe, "Deciduous Teeth as an Index of Body Burden of Lead," *Journal of Pediatrics* (1962), 60: 224–229.

28. Robert B. Mellins and C. David Jenkins, "Epidemiological and Psychological Study of Lead Poisoning in Children," *Journal of the American Medical Association* (1955), 158: 15–20.

29. Julius B. Richmond, Discussion of J. Julian Chisholm, Jr., "Environmental Factors in Childhood Lead Poisoning," *American Journal of Diseases of Children* (1955), 90: 517.

30. C. David Jenkins and Robert B. Mellins, "Lead Poisoning in Children: A Study of Forty-six Cases," *Archives of Neurology and Psychiatry* (1957), 77: 70–78.

31. "This abnormal eating is a motivated behavior not cured by distracting the child with other activities. Where used, alternative chewing objects did not curtail this dangerous activity. Sometimes not even spanking kept the child from nibbling at the sites of peeling paint. The parents of a girl who loved to eat cigarette ashes place[d] candy on the table near the ash tray. She ignored the candy and scooped up the ashes. Children addicted to pica thus discriminate their favorite substances from food

substance. The latter awareness is shown by their furtive eating of this substance. . . . It is felt that pica is an emotionally caused behavior, perhaps related to feelings of aggression" (ibid., 72).

32. For example, Frances K. Millican, Reginald Lourie, and Emma Layman at the George Washington School of Medicine observed: "Until about the end of the first year of life, lead poisoning must be regarded as accidental. It is one of the many accidental hazards which parents need to be informed of by their physicians in terms of the sources of lead and its dangers. The ages of the children in this study at the time of diagnosis of lead poisoning ranged from 18 to 38 months. The purpose of this study was to learn something of the factors which lead to the persistence of oral activities beyond the normal developmental period." Frances K. Millican, Reginald S. Lourie, and Emma M. Layman, "Emotional Factors in the Etiology and Treatment of Lead Poisoning," *American Journal of Diseases of Children* (1956), 91: 144.

33. Hugo Dunlap Smith, Robert L. Baehner, Thomas Carney, and William Joseph Majors, "The Sequelae of Pica with and without Lead Poisoning: A Comparison of the Sequelae Five or More Years Later: 1. Clinical and Laboratory Observations," *American Journal of Diseases of Children* (1963), 105: 609–616; Hugo Dunlap Smith, "Pediatric Lead Poisoning," *Archives of Environmental Health* (1964), 8: 256–261.

34. J. Edmund Bradley and Ruth J. Baumgartner, "Subsequent Mental Development of Children with Lead Encephalopathy, as Related to Type of Treatment," *Journal of Pediatrics* (1958), 53: 311–315.

Chapter 10   *One Percent Lead Content for Paint*

1. Manfred Bowditch to A. Ashley Weech, November 8, 1950, Baltimore Health Department (BHD) Archives.

2. J. M. Arena, "The Pediatrician's Role in the Poison Control Movement and Poison Prevention," *American Journal of Diseases of Children* (1983), 137: 870–873; John C. Burnham, "How the Discovery of Accidental Childhood Poisoning Contributed to the Development of Environmentalism in the United States," *Environmental History Review* (1995), 19: 57–81; Burnham, "Why Did the Infants and Toddlers Die? Shifts in Americans' Ideas of Responsibility for Accidents—From Blaming Mom to Engineering," *Journal of Social History* (1996), 29: 817–837.

3. "Lead Hygiene and Safety Bulletin," no. 79, December 1, 1950, 1, Lead Industries Association (LIA) Archives, housed in the office of Sullivan, Sullivan, and Nahigian, Boston, Mass.

4. Manfred Bowditch to Robert Kehoe, March 17, 1951, Kehoe Papers, Robert A. Kehoe Archives, Cincinnati Medical Heritage Center, University of Cincinnati Medical Center.

5. Manfred Bowditch to Robert Kehoe, March 30, 1951, Kehoe Papers.

6. Manfred Bowditch to R. R. Sayers, May 2, 1951, BHD Archives.

7. George M. Wheatley, "Can Accidental Trauma Be Prevented?" presented at the meeting of the Massachusetts Medical Society, May 23, 1951, 5, New York City (NYC) Health Department Archives.

8. Manfred Bowditch to R. R. Sayers, September 18, 1951, BHD Archives.

9. Committee on Accident Prevention of the American Academy of Pediatrics, June 1953, American Academy of Pediatrics, pers. comm.

10. Huntington Williams to Mayor Thomas D'Alesandro, July 3, 1951, BHD Archives, and "New Regulation Prohibits Indoor Lead Paint," *Baltimore Health News* (August–September, 1951), 28: 114, BHD Archives.

11. Anon., "Dietary Habits of Baltimore Babies," *American Journal of Public Health* (1951), 1528.

12. J. O. Dean to Katherine Bain, September 17, 1951; National Archives.

13. Morris Greenberg, *Annual Report*, Bureau of Preventable Diseases, 1951, 21, New York City (NYC) Municipal Archives.
14. "Report of the Subcommittee on Laboratory Facilities for the Diagnosis of Poisonings," 1952[?], 1, NYC Health Department Archives.
15. Jerome Trichter to Emanuel Kaplan, December 12, 1952; and Emanuel Kaplan to Jerome Trichter, January 6, 1953, BHD Archives.
16. Manfred Bowditch to Reginald Atwater, December 19, 1951, BHD Archives.
17. LIA Minutes, April 18–19, 1952, 4, LIA Archives; and American Academy of Pediatrics, *Newsletter* (October 1952), 3.
18. Manfred Bowditch, "Lead Poisoning in Infants and Children," *Proceedings of the First Conference on Home Accident Prevention*, January 20, 21, and 22, 1953 (Ann Arbor: University of the Michigan School of Public Health, 1953), 75–77.
19. George Wheatley, "To Curb Lead Poisoning; Health Department Decision Relative to Label on Paint Commended" (letter to the editor), *New York Times* (November 9, 1954), 26: 7.
20. George M. Wheatley, "The Lead Poisoning Problem in Children," presented at the 26th Annual Meeting of the Lead Industries Association, April 22–23, 1954, Chicago, Ill.; see also Wheatley, "Accidental Poisoning in the Home," presented at the American Public Health Association meeting, Kansas City, Mo., November 18, 1955; and Minutes, November 15, 1954, Sectional Committee on Hazards to Children, American Standards Association, 3.
21. See Minutes of the Special Committee to Study Lead Poisoning, National Paint, Varnish, and Lacquer Association, March 24, 1954, LIA Archives; A. J. Lanza, Institute of Industrial Medicine, to Leona Baumgartner, Commissioner, New York City Department of Health, April 12, 1954, NYC Municipal Archives; and Minutes, Subcommittee on Model Labeling, National Paint, Lacquer, and Varnish Association, June 15, 1954, LIA Archives.
22. Minutes, Subcommittee on Model Labeling, National Paint, Varnish, and Lacquer Association, July 15, 1954, LIA Archives. Arnold J. Lehman, chief pharmacologist of the U.S. Food and Drug Administration, made a slightly different calculation based on the possibility of children's chewing up to 12 square inches a day. At this level of consumption, he calculated that 0.3 percent paint would be safe. "Quarterly Report to the Editor on Topics of Current Interest, Lead in Decorative Paint for Children's Toys and Furniture," *Quarterly Bulletin of the Association of Food and Drug Officials* (1956), 20: 36–37; and John H. Foulger, "Precautionary Labeling of Lead Products," *Industrial Medicine and Surgery* (1959), 28: 122–125.
23. Reported in Jerome Trichter to Leona Baumgartner, "Proposed Sanitary Code Amendment to Require a Warning on the Label of Lead-Containing Paints," October 15, 1954, NYC Municipal Archives; and Minutes, American Standards Association, November 15, 1954.
24. Jerome Trichter to Leona Baumgartner, "Proposed Sanitary Code Amendment to Include a Warning on Label of Lead-Containing Paints," May 3, 1954, NYC Municipal Archives.
25. Harold T. Fuerst (epidemiologist) to Morris Greenberg (director), January 26, 1953, NYC Municipal Archives.
26. "Lead Poisoning in Children," report by Morris Greenberg January 28, 1953, NYC Municipal Archives; Jerome Trichter, Summary, March 5, 1953, NYC Municipal Archives; Jerome Trichter to Morris Greenberg, March 19, 1953, NYC Health Department Archives.
27. "City Unit to Seek Lead Poison Curb: Warning on Paint Containers to Be Asked— 15 Deaths in 2 Years Are Cited," *New York Times* (March 29, 1953), 66; see also "Health Board Warns on Lead Paint Poison as 2 More Children in City Are Killed by It," *New York Times* (June 30, 1953).

28. Jerome Trichter to Commissioner of Health, July 1, 1953, NYC Municipal Archives; Minutes, Board of Health, July 14–15, 1953, NYC Health Department Archives.
29. William Sauer, Director, Bureau of Sanitary Inspections, July 1953, NYC Municipal Archives.
30. George Wheatley to William Sauer, September 24, 1953, NYC Municipal Archives.
31. A. J. Lanza to Leona Baumgartner, April 12, 1954; Memo, Manfred Bowditch, April 19, 1954. Lanza and Bowditch asked to present their views in person, Minutes, Commissioner's Staff Meeting, May 3, 1954, NYC Municipal Archives.
32. "A Guide for the Preparation of Warning Labels for Hazardous Chemicals," *Chemical and Engineering News* (1945), 23: 992.
33. Robert E. Mellins to Jerome Trichter, September 3, 1954, NYC Municipal Archives.
34. Jerome Trichter, presentations to the Commissioner's Staff Meeting, August 10, 1954, NYC Health Department Archives.
35. Revised Draft, Proposed American Standard for Safe Labeling of Coatings for Children's Toys and Furniture, August 17, 1954, Eagle Picher Company.
36. Minutes of Meeting of Subcommittee on Model Labeling, National Paint, Varnish, and Lacquer Association, August 12, 1954.
37. *Sanitary Code of the City of New York Including Regulations*, 1954, 274, NYC Charter and Administrative Code of the City of New York, Chapter 22, NYC Municipal Archives.
38. New York City Health Code, enacted by the Board of Health of the City of New York on March 23, 1959. Updated to June 1973, section 211.13, 18–19.
39. Robert C. Griggs, Irving Sunshine, Vaun A. Newill, Burritt W. Newton, Stuart Buchanan, and Cleo A. Rasch, "Environmental Factors in Childhood Lead Poisoning," *Journal of the American Medical Association* (1964), 187: 704.
40. Harold Jacobziner, "Lead Poisoning in Childhood: Epidemiology, Manifestations, and Prevention," *Clinical Pediatrics* (1966), 5: 281.
41. J. Edmund Bradley, "Don't Let Your Child Get Lead Poisoning," *Parade* (July 6, 1956).

Chapter 11   Urban Lead Programs of the 1950s and 1960s

1. For a chronology of Baltimore's struggle with childhood lead poisoning, see "Chronology of Lead Poisoning Control, Baltimore 1931–1971," *Baltimore Health News* (1972), 49: 34–39; and Robert E. Farber, "Child Lead Paint Poisoning Still Prevalent," *Maryland State Medical Journal* (1968), 17: 137–138.
2. Matthew Taback to Charles Couchman, March 19, 1952, Baltimore Health Department (BHD) Archives.
3. *Annual Report*, Baltimore Health Department, 1951.
4. *Annual Report*, Baltimore Health Department, 1950.
5. Bureau of Health Information, Baltimore City Health Department, "Lead Poisoning," episode of weekly, "Your Family Doctor," initially aired May 21, 1953. Script in BHD Archives.
6. Bureau of Health Information, Baltimore City Health Department, "Death at the Window Sill," initially broadcast March 2, 1953. Script located in BHD Archives.
7. "Lead Poisoning in Children," pamphlet passed out at well-child visits beginning in 1949, BHD Archives.
8. *Annual Report*, Baltimore Health Department, 1952.
9. Baltimore City Health Department, *City Housing Code*, Regulation 17, "Interior Painting: No paint shall be used for interior painting of any dwelling or dwelling unit or any part thereof unless the paint is free from any lead pigment" (June 19, 1951), 11.
10. Housing Bureau, Baltimore City Health Department, "The Baltimore Plan of Housing Law Enforcement," May 1952, 29 pages, Huntington Williams Papers; see also "Housing Code Enforcement: A Report to Mayor J. Harold Grady, Technical Re-

port on the Baltimore Experience and Possibilities for Reorganization," February 1961, Huntington Williams Papers, George Huntington Williams Collection, Alan Mason Chesney Medical Archives, Johns Hopkins Medical Institutions, Baltimore, Md.

11. *Annual Report*, Baltimore Health Department, 1953, 1954, 1955.

12. J. Julian Chisholm, Jr., and Harold E. Harrison, "The Exposure of Children to Lead," *Pediatrics* (1956), 18: 955.

13. Huntington Williams to Mayor Thomas D'Alesandro, August 17, 1956; "Poisoning Study Unit Formed," *Evening Sun* (Baltimore), August 18, 1956.

14. Minutes, Baltimore Lead Paint Poisoning Prevention Committee, August 14, 1956, BHD Archives and Huntington Williams Archives, Membership included: William Sallow, assistant director, Housing Bureau; Charles Couchman, director of Industrial Hygiene; Clinton Ewing, Bureau of Laboratories; Robert Farber, Bureau of Communicable Diseases; Joseph Gordon, Bureau of Health Information; Emanuel Kaplan, assistant director, Bureau of Laboratories; R. R. Sayers, Occupational Diseases; George Schucker, Bureau of Environmental Diseases; Wilner Schulze, Sanitation Section; Matthew Tayback, Statistical Section; and Bertram Haines, Medical Care Research.

15. Charles E. Couchman to Huntington Williams, "Child Lead Poisoning among Migrants," BHD Archives.

16. After World War II, many Jews and middle-class African Americans moved away from Baltimore's urban center. In their place came African Americans from the South. For a discussion, see Marcia Mann Cooper, *Pica: A Survey of the Historical Literature as well as Reports from the Fields of Veterinary Medicine and Anthropology, the Present Study of Pica in Young Children, and a Discussion of Its Pediatric and Psychological Implications* (Springfield, Ill.: Charles C. Thomas, 1957), 62–69.

17. *Annual Report*, Baltimore Health Department, 1957.

18. Letter to parents, "Don't Let Your Child Get Sick by Nibbling Paint in Your Home," Huntington Williams Papers, 1958.

19. Baltimore City Health Department and Baltimore Urban Renewal and Housing Agency, "Progress Report on Leaded Paint Inspection Program," 1957. This survey indicated that 70 percent of inspected housing units contained lead paint. Huntington Williams Papers.

20. Huntington Williams to Mayor Thomas D'Alesandro, August 2, 1957. "By August 1 a total of 611 notices to remove lead paint from dwelling unit interiors had been issued and 391 corrections had been made. Landlords and home owners have been very cooperative in this program and so far it has been necessary in only 5 instances to take recalcitrant property owners to Housing Court," Huntington Williams Papers.

21. Baltimore City Health Department and Baltimore Urban Renewal and Housing Agency, "Progress Report on Leaded Paint Inspection Program," 1957, Huntington Williams Papers; see also George O. Motry to Huntington Williams, "Lead Paint Survey—1957," March 22, 1961, BHD Archives.

22. Bureau of Laboratories, Baltimore City Health Department, "Rapid Screening Method for Lead in Paint at the One Percent Level," 1961.

23. George O. Motry to George W. Schucker, "Proposed Statement of Policy on Lead Paint Removal," February 5, 1960, BHD Archives; and Baltimore City Health Department, "Questions and Answers Concerning Lead Paint Removal," 1960, BHD Archives.

24. George Schucker to Huntington Williams, Conference at City Hospitals Concerning Lead Paint Poisoning, November 7, 1960, BHD Archives.

25. Huntington Williams to Leona F. Baumgartner (commissioner of health, New York City Department of Health), June 5, 1958, Huntington Williams Archives.

26. *Baltimore Health News* (August 1958), 35: 58.

27. *Annual Report*, Baltimore Health Department, 1958, 44.

28. *Baltimore Health News* (December 1958), 35: 89.

29. Huntington Williams to Paint Dealers, May 12, 1958, BHD Archives.
30. G. M. Hammond (manager, Trade Sales, National Lead Company) to Huntington Williams, September 17, 1958, with copy of proposed Dutch Boy label, BHD Archives.
31. Melvin Sklar, Chairman of Legislative Committee, Baltimore Paint, Varnish, and Lacquer Association, to Hon. Walter Dixon, Chairman, Committee on Health, Baltimore City Council, April 24, 1958, Huntington Williams Papers; and Huntington Williams to G. M. Hammond, September 18, 1958, BHD Archives.
32. G. M. Hammond to Huntington Williams, September 22, 1958, BHD Archives.
33. See label of the Baltimore Copper Paint Company, BHD Archives.
34. Minutes, Lead Paint Labeling Meeting, March 26, 1959, held in Huntington Williams's office. Attending were representatives of the National Paint, Varnish, and Lacquer Association, Sapolin Paints, the Sherwin-Williams Company, Inter-Coastal Paint Corporation, the O'Brien Corporation, and the New York City Department of Health, BHD Archives.
35. Rules and Regulations Governing Lead Paint Labeling, April 27, 1959, BHD Archives.
36. *Annual Report*, Baltimore Health Department, 1958.
37. *Annual Report*, Baltimore Health Department, 1959.
38. BHD Archives.
39. *Annual Report*, Baltimore Health Department, 1960.
40. Minutes, Baltimore Lead Paint Poisoning Prevention Committee, January 11, 1962, February 8, 1962, BHD Archives.
41. Minutes, Baltimore Lead Paint Poisoning Prevention Committee, July 16, 1964, BHD Archives.
42. Alice Sundberg and Charles Couchman to Huntington Williams, "Child Lead Poisoning—Cooperation with Dr. Chisholm," April 17, 1957. Papers of the Baltimore City Department of Health, BHD Archives.
43. Huntington Williams to William A. Kressler, State of New Jersey Department of Health, June 22, 1959, BHD Archives.
44. Robert E. Farber to Forbes Shepherd, Executive Director, Independent Voters of Illinois, August 13, 1963, BHD Archives.
45. C. E. Couchman, "Non-Fatal vs. Fatal Cases of Lead Poisoning for Various Blood Lead Values, Diagnosed Cases in Children January 1, 1936–October 1, 1953," BHD Archives.
46. George J. Cohen and Walter E. Ahrens, "Chronic Lead Poisoning: A Review of Seven Years' Experience at the Children's Hospital, District of Columbia," *Journal of Pediatrics* (1959), 54: 279.
47. *Annual Reports*, Baltimore Health Department, 1961–1965.
48. *Annual Report*, Baltimore Health Department, 1966.
49. *Annual Reports*, Baltimore Health Department, 1967–1971.
50. George Schucker, Edward H. Vail, Elizabeth B. Kelley, and Emanuel Kaplan, "Prevention of Lead Paint Poisoning among Baltimore Children: A Hard-Sell Program," *Public Health Reports* (1965), 80: 969–974.
51. Robert E. Farber, "Lead Paint Poisoning Still with Us," *Maryland State Medical Journal* (1963), 12: 296.
52. Randolph K. Byers, Clarence A. Maloof, and Margaret Cushman, "Urinary Excretion of Lead in Children: Diagnostic Application," *American Journal of Diseases of Children* (1954), 87: 548–558; and R. K. Byers, "Lead Poisoning: Review of the Literature and Report on 45 Cases," *Pediatrics* (1959), 23: 585–603.
53. Nicholas Freudenberg and Maxine Golub, "Health Education, Public Policy, and Disease Prevention: A Case History of the New York City Coalition to End Lead Poisoning," *Health Education Quarterly* (1987), 14: 387–401; and Diana R. Gordon, *City*

Limits: Barriers to Change in Urban Government (New York: Charterhouse, 1973), 17–62.

54. *Annual Report*, Bureau of Preventable Diseases, New York City Health Department, 1950.
55. *Annual Report*, Bureau of Preventable Diseases, New York City Health Department, 1951.
56. *Annual Report*, Bureau of Preventable Diseases, New York City Health Department, 1952.
57. *Annual Report*, Bureau of Preventable Diseases, New York City Health Department, 1954; see also Mary Culhane McLaughlin, "Lead Poisoning in Children in New York City, 1950–1954: An Epidemiologic Study," *New York State Journal of Medicine* (1956), 56: 3711–3714.
58. Morris Greenberg, Harold Jacobziner, Mary C. McLaughlin, Harold T. Fuerst, and Ottavio Pellitteri, "A Study of Pica in Relation to Lead Poisoning," *Pediatrics* (1958), 22: 756–760; Harold Jacobziner and Harry W. Raybin, "Public Health Aspects of Lead Poisoning in Infancy and Young Children," *New York State Journal of Medicine* (1958), 58: 730–734; Jacobziner and Raybin, "Lead Poisoning and Pica in Children," *New York State Journal of Medicine* (1959), 59: 1606–1610; and Jacobziner and Raybin, "Lead Poisoning in Young Children—Fatal and Nonfatal," *New York State Journal of Medicine* (1960), 60: 273–277.
59. Harold Jacobziner and Harry Raybin, "The Epidemiology of Lead Poisoning in Children," *Archives of Pediatrics* (1962), 79: 72–76; and Harold Jacobziner, "Lead Poisoning in Childhood: Epidemiology, Manifestations, and Prevention," *Clinical Pediatrics* (1966), 5: 279.
60. Vincent F. Guinee, "Pica and Lead Poisoning," *Nutrition Reviews* (1971), 29: 267–268.
61. Ibid., 268.
62. Gordon, *City Limits*, 17–62.
63. Mark W. Oberle, "Lead Poisoning: A Preventable Childhood Disease of the Slums," *Science* (1969), 165: 991–992.
64. As she phrased it: "By pinching here and begging there, I was able to get together $150,000 for a crash program. Everyone said 'That's great!' But it was not great; it was just a stop gap. It was not getting at the root of the problem." Mary C. McLaughlin, "Two Health Problems: One Solution," *Bulletin of the New York Academy of Medicine* (1970), 46: 454–455.
65. Lloyd A. Thomas, Rita G. Harper, and Dorothy L. Trice, "A Community Centered Approach to the Problem of Lead Poisoning," *Journal of the National Medical Association* (1970), 62: 106–108.
66. Michael A. Pawel, Christopher N. Frantz, and Ingrid B. Pisetsky, "Screening for Lead Poisoning with the Urinary ALA Test," *HSMHA Health Reports* (1971), 86: 1030–1036.
67. Jack Newfield, "Lead Poisoning: Silent Epidemic in the Slums," *Village Voice* (September 18, 1969), 1.
68. Vincent F. Guinee, "Lead Poisoning in New York City," *Transactions of the New York Academy of Sciences* (1971), 33: 539–551; Guinee, "Lead Poisoning" (editorial), *American Journal of Medicine* (1972), 52: 283–288; Gary Eidsvold, Anthony Mustalish, and Lloyd F. Novik, "The New York City Department of Health: Lessons in a Lead Poisoning Control Program," *American Journal of Public Health* (1974), 64: 956–962; and Freudenberg and Golub, "Health Education, Public Policy and Disease Prevention."
69. J. Earle Smith, B. W. Lewis, and Herbert S. Wilson, "Lead Poisoning: A Case Finding Program," *American Journal of Public Health* (1952), 42: 417–421.
70. *Cincinnati's Health: Annual Report [of the] Cincinnati Health Department* (Cincinnati: Cincinnati Board of Health, 1944).

71. *Cincinnati's Health* (1948), 5. See also Robert B. Fairbanks, *Making Better Citizens: Housing Reform and the Community Development Strategy in Cincinnati, 1890–1960* (Urbana: University of Illinois Press, 1988).
72. *Cincinnati's Health* (1949).
73. *Cincinnati's Health* (1950).
74. *Cincinnati's Health* (1951), 20.
75. *Cincinnati's Health* (1953), 21.
76. *Cincinnati's Health* (1958).
77. *Cincinnati's Health* (1959). See also Hugo Dunlap Smith, "Pediatric Lead Poisoning," *Archives of Environmental Health* (1964), 8: 256–261.
78. Emil A. Tiboni and Raymond L. Tyler, "Childhood Lead Poisoning in Philadelphia," *Philadelphia Medicine* (1960), 56: 668–669.
79. Theodore H. Ingalls, Emil A. Tiboni, and Milton Werrin, "Lead Poisoning in Philadelphia, 1955–1960," *Archives of Environmental Health* (1961), 3: 575–579.
80. Emil A. Tiboni, "Control of Childhood Lead Poisoning," *Public Health Reports* (1964), 79: 167–174.
81. Arnold L. Tanis, "Lead Poisoning in Children: Including Nine Cases Treated With Edathamil Calcium-Disodium," *American Journal of Diseases of Children* (1955), 89: 325–331.
82. Joseph Greengard, William Rowley, Harry Elam, and Meyer Perlstein, "Lead Encephalopathy in Children: Intravenous Use of Urea in Its Management," *New England Journal of Medicine* (1961), 264: 1027–1030; and Joseph R. Christian, "Lead Poisoning in Children," *Chicago Medicine* (June 24, 1961), 15–18.
83. "Lead Paint in Chicago," *Time* (August 9, 1963), 36.
84. Joseph R. Christian, Bohdan S. Celewycz, and Samuel L. Andelman, "A Three-Year Study of Lead Poisoning in Chicago, Part I: Epidemiology," *American Journal of Public Health* (1964), 54: 1241–1245.
85. Joseph R. Christian, Bohdan S. Celewycz, and Samuel L. Andelman, "A Three-Year Study of Lead Poisoning in Chicago, Part II: Case Finding in Asymptomatic Children Using Urinary Coproporphyrin as a Screening Test," *American Journal of Public Health* (1964), 54: 1245–1251.
86. Philip F. Benson, "Influence of Climatic Factors on Blood Lead Levels in Children with Pica," *Guy's Hospital Reports* (1962), 111: 306–312.
87. Anna M. Baetjer, "Effects of Season and Temperature on Childhood Plumbism," *Industrial Medicine* (1959), 28: 137–143; A. M. Baetjer, S.N.D. Joardar, and W. A. McQuary, "Effect of Environmental Temperature and Humidity on Lead Poisoning in Animals," *Archives of Environmental Health* (1960), 1: 463–477.
88. United States Public Health Service, Advisory Committee on Tetraethyl Lead, *Public Health Aspects of Increasing Tetraethyl Lead Content in Motor Fuel* (Washington, D.C.: U.S. Public Health Service, Division of Special Services, Occupational Health Program, 1959); Richard S. Brief, Allen R. Jones, and John D. Yoder, "Lead, Carbon Monoxide, and Traffic: A Correlation Study," *Journal of the Air Pollution Control Association* (1960), 10: 384–388.
89. J. Cholak, L. J. Schafer, and T. D. Sterling, "The Lead Content of the Atmosphere," *Journal of the Air Pollution Control Association* (1961), 11: 281–288. Jacob Cholak questioned the findings of the three-city study; see Cholak, "Further Investigations of Atmospheric Concentration of Lead," *Archives of Environmental Health* (1964), 8: 314–324. See also D. H. Hofreuter, E. J. Catcott, R. G. Keenan, and C. Xintaras, "The Public Health Significance of Atmospheric Lead," *Archives of Environmental Health* (1961), 3: 570, table 3.
90. Theodore D. Sterling, "Epidemiology of Disease Associated with Lead," *Archives of Environmental Health* (1964), 8: 333–348.
91. Katherine Bain, "Death Due to Accidental Poisoning in Young Children," *Journal of Pediatrics* (1954), 44: 616–623.

92. Ibid., 620. See also John Aikman, "The Problem of Accidental Poisoning in Child-hood," *Journal of the American Medical Association* (1934), 103: 640–643; and Alexander King, "Ingestion by Children of Various Substances, Including Poisons," *Permanente Foundation Medical Bulletin* (1947), 5: 20–28.
93. Robert W. Harris and William R. Elsea, "Ceramic Glaze as a Source of Lead Poison-ing," *Journal of the American Medical Association* (1967), 202: 544–546; J. R. McNiel and M. C. Reinhard, "Lead Poisoning from Home Remedies," *Clinical Pediatrics* (1967), 6: 150–156; William R. Law and Erland R. Nelson, "Gasoline-Sniffing by an Adult: Report of a Case with Unusual Complication of Lead Encephalopathy," *Journal of the American Medical Association* (1968), 204: 1002–1004; Paul A. Palmisano, Raphael C. Sneed, and George Cassady, "Untaxed Whiskey and Fetal Lead Exposure," *Journal of Pediatrics* (1969), 75: 869–872.
94. Report of Subcommittee on Accidental Poisoning, "Statement on Diagnosis and Treatment of Lead Poisoning in Childhood," *Pediatrics* (1961), 27: 676.
95. Ibid.
96. Ibid., 679.
97. Ibid., 679–680.

Chapter 12 **Children and Lead, 1960–1965**

1. Robert A. Kehoe, "The Harben Lectures, 1960: The Metabolism of Lead in Man in Health and Disease; Lecture I: The Normal Metabolism of Lead," *Journal of the Royal Institute of Public Health and Hygiene* (1961), 24: 96. For a brief summary of his Harben Lectures, see Robert A. Kehoe, "The Metabolism of Lead in Man in Health and Dis-ease," *Archives of Environmental Health* (1961), 2: 418–422; and for another assess-ment of lead in daily life, see Robert T. P. Treville, "Natural Occurrence of Lead," *Archives of Environmental Health* (1964), 8: 212–221.
2. Morton J. Robinson, Felix Karpinski, Jr., and Heinrich Brieger, "The Concentration of Lead in Plasma, Whole Blood, and Erythrocytes of Infants and Children," *Pediat-rics* (1958), 21: 794, table 1.
3. Otto P. Preuss, "Childhood Plumbism: Doctor, Would You Think of Lead Poison-ing?" *Ohio State Medical Journal* (1962), 58: 667; and "Lead Poisoning in Children" (editorial), *British Medical Journal* (1964), 1: 1200–1201.
4. Robert A. Kehoe, "The Harben Lectures, 1960: The Metabolism of Lead in Man in Health and Disease; Lecture III: "Present Hygienic Problems Relating to the Absorp-tion of Lead," *Journal of the Royal Institute of Public Health and Hygiene* (1961), 24: 177–261.
5. Clair C. Patterson, "Contaminated and Natural Lead Environments of Man," *Ar-chives of Environmental Health* (1965), 11: 344–360.
6. Herbert L. Needleman, "Clair Patterson and Robert Kehoe: Two Views of Lead Tox-icity," *Environmental Research* (1998), 78: 79–85; and Jerome O. Nriagu, "Clair Patterson and Robert Kehoe's Paradigm of 'Show Me the Data' on Environmental Lead Poisoning," *Environmental Research* (1998), 78: 71–78.
7. See also A. C. Aufderheide, F. D. Neiman, L. E. Wittmers, Jr., and G. Rapp, "Lead in Bone. II: Skeletal-Lead Content as an Indicator of Lifetime Ingestion and the So-cial Correlates in an Archeological Population," *American Journal of Anthropology* (1981), 55: 285–291; H. A. Waldron, "Lead in Bones: A Cautionary Tale," *Ecology of Disease* (1982), 1: 191–196; C. C. Patterson, H. Shirahata, and J. E. Ericson, "Lead in Ancient Human Bones and Its Relevance to Historical Developments of Social Problems with Lead," *Science of the Total Environment* (1987), 61: 167–200; P. Grandjean, "International Perspectives of Lead Exposure and Lead Toxicity," *Neurotoxicology* (1993), 14: 9–14.
8. A. S. Minot, "The Physiological Effects of Small Amounts of Lead: An Evaluation of the Lead Hazard of the Average Individual," *Physiological Review* (1938), 18: 562–563.

9. Ibid., 573.
10. Robert Kehoe to Anne Minot, December 13, 1938, Kehoe Papers, Robert A. Kehoe Archives, Cincinnati Medical Heritage Center, University of Cincinnati Medical Center.
11. U.S. Department of Health, Education, and Welfare (Public Health Service), *Symposium on Environmental Lead Contamination, Sponsored by the Public Health Service, December 13–15, 1965,* Public Health Service Publication no. 1440 (Washington, D.C.: Government Printing Office, 1966).
12. Robert A. Kehoe, "Under What Circumstances Is Ingestion of Lead Dangerous?" in ibid., 54.
13. Ibid., 55.
14. Ibid., 57.
15. Harriet L. Hardy, "Lead," in U.S. Department of Health, Education, and Welfare (Public Health Service), *Symposium on Environmental Lead Contamination, December 13–15, 1965,* 81.
16. Discussion, in U.S. Department of Health, Education, and Welfare (Public Health Service), *Symposium on Environmental Lead Contamination, December 13–15, 1965,* 149.
17. Ibid., 150–151.
18. Robert A. Kehoe, "Summary: Risk of Exposure and Absorption to Lead," in U.S. Department of Health, Education, and Welfare (Public Health Service), *Symposium on Environmental Lead Contamination, December 13–15, 1965,* 154-157.
19. Discussion, in U.S. Department of Health, Education, and Welfare (Public Health Service), *Symposium on Environmental Lead Contamination, December 13-15, 1965,* 164.
20. Robert Kehoe to Harriet Hardy, April 1965; and Kehoe to Hardy, December 1965, Kehoe Papers.
21. Edward Press, "Poisoning Hazards in the Home Environment," *Archives of Environmental Health* (1966), 13: 525.
22. J. Julian Chisholm, Jr., "Chronic Lead Intoxication in Children," *Developmental Medicine and Child Neurology* (1965), 7: 529–536.
23. Harriet L. Hardy, "What Is the Status of Knowledge of the Toxic Effect of Lead on Indentifiable Groups in the Population?" *Clinical Pharmacology and Therapeutics* (1966), 7: 713–722; Henry A. Schroeder and Isabel H. Tipton, "The Human Body Burden of Lead," *Archives of Environmental Health* (1968), 17: 965–978.
24. Harriet L. Hardy, Richard I. Chamberlin, Clarence C. Maloof, George W. Boylen, Jr., and Mary C. Howell, "Lead as an Environmental Poison" (review article), *Clinical Pharmacology and Therapeutics* (1971), 12: 982–1002.
25. Chisholm, "Chronic Lead Intoxication in Children," 532–533.
26. J. Julian Chisholm, Jr., "Increased Lead Absorption: Toxicological Considerations," *Pediatrics* (1971), 48: 349–352.

Chapter 13   A "Submerged" National Epidemic

1. Lorry A. Blanksma, Henrietta K. Sachs, Edward F. Murray, and Morgan J. O'Connell, "Incidence of High Blood Lead Levels in Chicago Children," *Pediatrics* (1969), 44: 661.
2. Ibid., 661-667.
3. Henrietta Sachs, Lorry A. Blanksma, Edward F. Murray, and Morgan J. O'Connell, "Ambulatory Treatment of Lead Poisoning: Report of 1,155 Cases," *Pediatrics* (1970), 46: 389–396. For additional descriptions of the Chicago program, see Joseph Greengard, Lowell Zollar, and Manoucher Sharifi, "Medical Progress in the Prevention of Childhood Lead Intoxication," *Illinois Medical Journal* (1968), 133: 615–618;

Joseph R. Christian, "Childhood Lead Poisoning: A Major Urban Health Problem," *Nebraska State Medical Journal* (1969), 54: 677–682; and Owen M. Rennert, Paul Weiner, and John Madden, "Asymptomatic Lead Poisoning in 85 Chicago Children: Some Diagnostic, Therapeutic, Prognostic and Sociologic Considerations," *Clinical Pediatrics* (1970), 9: 9–13.

4. Vincent F. Guinee, "Lead Poisoning in New York City," *Transactions of the New York Academy of Sciences* (1971), 33: 544.

5. Ibid., 539-551. For additional accounts of mass screening in New York City, see "Children at Risk," *Nature* (1970), 228: 1253; Vincent F. Guinee, "Pica and Lead Poisoning," *Nutrition Reviews* (1971), 29: 267–269; Guinee, "Lead Poisoning" (editorial), *American Journal of Medicine* (1972), 52: 283–288; Michael A. Pawel, Christopher N. Frantz, and Ingrid B. Pisetsky, "Screening for Lead Poisoning with the Urinary ALA Test," *HSMHA Health Reports* (1971), 86: 1030–1036; Lloyd A. Thomas, Rita G. Harper, and Dorothy L. Trice, "A Community Centered Approach to the Problem of Lead Poisoning," *Journal of the National Medical Association* (1970), 62: 106–108; and Gary Eidsvold, Anthony Mustalish, and Lloyd F. Novick, "The New York City Department of Health: Lessons in a Lead Poisoning Control Program?" (editorial), *American Journal of Public Health* (1974), 64: 956–962.

6. "In only five patients of 9 percent of those who were asymptomatic on first presentation was mental retardation considered to be a possible sequela. Even in these, however, the reliability of the maternal histories was questionable." Meyer A. Perlstein and Ramzy Attala, "Neurologic Sequelae of Plumbism in Children," *Clinical Pediatrics* (1966), 5: 295.

7. Harriet L. Hardy, "What Is the Status of Knowledge of the Toxic Effect of Lead on Identifiable Groups in the Population?" (editorial), *Clinical Pharmacology and Therapeutics* (1966), 7: 717.

8. Harriet L. Hardy, Richard I. Chamberlin, Clarence C. Maloof, George W. Boylen, Jr., and Mary C. Howell, "Lead as an Environmental Poison" (review article), *Clinical Pharmacology and Therapeutics* (1971), 12: 987.

9. D. Bryce-Smith, "Behavioural Effects of Lead and Other Heavy Metal Pollutants," *Chemistry in Britain* (1972), 8: 242; and Bryce-Smith, "Lead Pollution—A Growing Hazard to Public Health," *Chemistry in Britain* (1971), 7: 54–56. See also D. Barltrop, "Geochemical and Man-Made Sources of Lead and Human Health," *Philosophical Transactions of the Royal Society of London–Series B* (1979), 288: 205–211.

10. Gerald Wiener, "Varying Psychological Sequelae of Lead Ingestion in Children," *Public Health Reports* (1970), 85: 23.

11. Henry A. Schroeder and Isabel H. Tipton, "The Human Body Burden of Lead," *Archives of Environmental Health* (1968), 17: 965.

12. J. Julian Chisholm, Jr., and Eugene Kaplan, "Lead Poisoning in Childhood—Comprehensive Management and Prevention," *Journal of Pediatrics* (1968), 73: 942.

13. Ibid., 942-943.

14. See also Pranab Chatterjee and Judith H. Gettman, "Lead Poisoning: Subculture as a Facilitating Agent?" *American Journal of Clinical Nutrition* (1972), 25: 324–330.

15. Chisholm and Kaplan, "Lead Poisoning in Childhood—Comprehensive Management and Prevention," 943.

16. Ibid., 944.

17. Home visits in Baltimore documented the higher content of lead on outside walls; see J. Julian Chisholm, Jr., and Harold Harrison, "The Exposure of Children to Lead," *Pediatrics* (1956), 18: 943–958.

18. J. Edmund Bradley, "Poverty, Pica, and Poisoning," *Public Health Reports* (1958), 73: 467.

19. National Paint, Varnish, and Lacquer Association, "How to Prevent Lead Poisoning in the Home," and U.S. Department of Health, Education, and Welfare, United States

Public Health Service, Division of Special Services, "The Recognition of Lead Poisoning in the Child," Public Health Service Publication no. 620 (Washington, D.C.: U.S. Department of Health, Education, and Welfare, Public Health Service, 1958), 3.

20. Randolph Byers, discussion, *Journal of Pediatrics* (1959), 55: 111.

21. "In the other five cases with high lead levels, no source of lead was found inside the homes. In each case, however, paint was peeling off the exterior of the houses. Upon questioning, it was found that the children usually played in areas immediately adjacent to the houses." Evelyn E. Hartman, Wilford E. Park, and H. Godfrey Nelson, "The Peeling House Paint Hazard to Children," *Public Health Reports* (1960), 75: 625.

22. "Outdoor paint may still contain a high percentage of lead because of its excellent weather resistance. Thus, flaking outdoor paint may also present a definite hazard if found in a youngster's favored playing corner." Otto P. Preuss, "Childhood Plumbism: Doctor, Would You Think of Lead Poisoning?" *Ohio State Medical Journal* (1962), 58: 666.

23. Emil A. Tiboni, "Control of Childhood Lead Poisoning," *Public Health Reports* (1964), 79: 167.

24. "There is increasing concern over the problem of environmental pollution of all sorts. Much of the controversy with respect to lead was raised by Patterson, who inferred that the body-lead burden in urban dwellers may be 100 times greater than the burden would be under ideal but primitive living conditions." Chisholm and Kaplan, "Lead Poisoning in Childhood—Comprehensive Management and Prevention," 944.

25. Ibid.

26. Ibid., 946.

27. Ibid., 947–948.

28. Jane S. Lin-Fu, *Lead Poisoning in Children*, Children's Bureau Publication no. 452 (Washington, D.C.: U.S. Government Printing Office, 1967).

29. Hearing before the Subcommittee on Health (Senate), *Lead-Based Paint Poisoning* (Washington, D.C.: Government Printing Office, 1970), 188.

30. Jane S. Lin-Fu, "Childhood Lead Poisoning . . . An Eradicable Disease," *Children* (1970), 17: 2–9.

31. Julian Chisholm to Robert Kehoe, July 1969, and Kehoe reply; see correspondence, 1966-1971, Kehoe Papers, Robert A. Kehoe Archives, Cincinnati Medical Heritage Center, University of Cincinnati Medical Center.

32. American Academy of Pediatrics, Subcommittee on Accidental Poisoning, "Prevention, Diagnosis, and Treatment of Lead Poisoning in Childhood," *Pediatrics* (1969), 44: 291.

33. In 1966 the Lead Industries Association surveyed health departments, asking about their criteria for treatment. Most accepted Kehoe's recommendation of 80 micrograms/dl if the patient also had two symptoms attributable to lead poisoning. "Lead Test Criteria Survey," June 29, 1966, Baltimore Health Department (BHD) Archives.

34. American Academy of Pediatrics, Subcommittee on Accidental Poisoning, "Prevention, Diagnosis, and Treatment of Lead Poisoning in Childhood," 291–298.

35. Beginning in the late 1950s, the federal government had distributed educational pamphlets on childhood lead poisoning; see Department of Health, Education, and Welfare, and the National Paint, Varnish, and Lacquer Association, "How to Prevent Lead Poisoning in the Home," 1958; and United States Public Health Service, Division of Special Services, "The Recognition of Lead Poisoning in the Child," Public Health Service Publication no. 620 (Washington, D.C.: U.S. Department of Health, Education, and Welfare, Public Health Service, 1958).

36. "Medical Aspects of Childhood Lead Poisoning," *Pediatrics* (1971), 48: 464.

37. "In some cities, undue exposure to and absorption of lead among children may be so prevalent that an overwhelming number of those screened are found to have blood

lead values of 40 micrograms/dl or more. Under such circumstances, local resources may not permit immediate evaluation of all such children." Ibid., 464.

38. Jane S. Lin-Fu, "Diagnostic and Screening Procedures for Lead Poisoning," *Pediatrics* (1971), 48: 488–489.

39. "The Federal Attack on Childhood Lead Poisoning," *Clinical Pediatrics* (1971), 10: 692–693.

40. Hearings before the Subcommittee on Housing (House of Representatives), *To Provide Federal Assistance for Eliminating the Causes of Lead-Based Paint Poisoning* (Washington, D.C.: Government Printing Office, 1970); and Hearing before the Subcommittee on Health (Senate), *Lead-Based Paint Poisoning* (Washington, D.C.: Government Printing Office, 1970).

41. Thomas Murphy and Martha L. Lepow, "Comparison of Delta-Aminolevulinic Acid Levels in Urine and Blood Lead Levels for Screening Children for Lead Poisoning," *Connecticut Medicine* (1971), 35: 488–492; Lorry A. Blanksma, Henrietta K. Sachs, Edward F. Murray, and Morgan J. O'Connell, "Failure of the Urinary Delta-Aminolevulinic Acid Test to Detect Pediatric Lead Poisoning," *American Journal of Clinical Pathology* (1970), 53: 956–962; Blanksma, "The Resolution on Childhood Lead Poisoning" (letter), *American Journal of Public Health* (1970), 60: 1191–1192; Michael J. Specter, Vincent F. Guinee, and Bernard Davidow, "The Unsuitability of Random Urinary Delta Aminolevulinic Acid Samples as a Screening Test for Lead Poisoning," *Journal of Pediatrics* (1971), 79: 799–804; John L. Clark, "Detection of Lead Toxicity" (letter), *New England Journal of Medicine* (1971), 285: 636; Felix Feldman, Herbert C. Lichtman, Stanley Oransky, Eladia Sta Ana, and Lloyd Reiser, "Serum Delta-Aminolevulinic Acid in Plumbism," *Journal of Pediatrics* (1969), 74: 917–923; William F. Vincent, William W. Ullmann, and Garland L. Weidner, "The Measurement of Urinary Delta-aminolevulinic Acid in Detection of Childhood Lead Poisoning" (letter), *American Journal of Clinical Pathology* (1970), 53: 963–964; Sol Blumenthal, Bernard Davidow, David Harris, and Felicia Oliver-Smith, "A Comparison between Two Diagnostic Tests for Lead Poisoning," *American Journal of Public Health* (1972), 62: 1060–1064.

42. Jane S. Lin-Fu, "Screening for Lead Poisoning" (letter), *Pediatrics* (1970), 45: 720–721.

43. "Mass screening for lead in blood at present is not practical, one reason being that at least 5 ml of blood must be obtained by venipuncture. The sample must be drawn by a physician or other trained professional, and may require the aid of a second person to quiet the child. Furthermore, with potentially exposed children screening tests must be repeated at regular intervals; a child found normal at one time may start ingesting lead immediately afterwards, yet a second blood sample may be much more difficult to obtain since the child with memories of pain may resist." Lester Hankin, Kenneth R. Hanson, Joseph M. Kornfield, and William W. Ullmann, "Simplified Method for Mass Screening for Lead Poisoning Based on Delta-Aminolevulinic Acid in Urine," *Clinical Pediatrics* (1970), 9: 707–712.

44. S. Granick, S. Sassa, J. L. Granick, R. D. Levere, and A. Kappas, "Assays for Porphyrins, Delta-Aminolevulinic Acid Dehydratase, and Porphyrinogen Synthetase in Microliter Samples of Whole Blood: Applications to Metabolic Defects Involving the Heme Pathway," *Proceedings of the National Academy of Science* (1972), 69: 2381–2385.

45. J. Julian Chisholm, Jr., "Screening Techniques for Undue Lead Exposure in Children: Biological and Practical Considerations," *Journal of Pediatrics* (1971), 79: 719–725.

46. Larry P. Kammholz, L. Gilbert Thatcher, Frederic M. Blodgett, and Thomas A. Good, "Rapid Protoporphyrin Quantitation for Detection of Lead Poisoning," *Pediatrics* (1972), 50: 625–631; Sergio Piomelli, Bernard Davidow, Vincent Guinee, Patricia

Young, and Giselle Gay, "The FEP (Free Erythrocyte Porphyrins) Test: A Screening Micromethod for Lead Poisoning," *Pediatrics* (1973), 51: 254–259; "Screening for Lead Poisoning: Measurements and Methodology," (letter), *Pediatrics* (1973), 52: 303–306; Robert D. Fischer, "Lead Poisoning: Status of the FEP and Other Tests" (letter), *Pediatrics* (1973), 52: 467–468; Robert W. Baloh, "Laboratory Diagnosis of Increased Lead Absorption," *Archives of Environmental Health* (1974), 28: 198–208.

47. J. Julian Chisholm, Jr., E. David Mellits, Julian E. Keil, and Maureen B. Barrett, "A Simple Protoporphyrin Assay—Microhematocrit Procedure as a Screening Technique for Increased Lead Absorption in Young Children," *Journal of Pediatrics* (1974), 84: 490–496.

48. Richard E. Cooke, Kathryn L. Glynn, William W. Ullmann, Nicole Lurie, and Martha Lepow, "Comparative Study of a Micro-Scale Test for Lead in Blood, for Use in Mass Screening Programs," *Clinical Chemistry* (1974), 20: 582–585; Douglas G. Mitchell, Kenneth M. Aldous, and Francis J. Ryan, "Mass Screening for Lead Poisoning: Capillary Blood Sampling and Automated Delves-Cup Atomic-Absorption Analysis," *New York State Journal of Medicine* (1974), 74: 1599–1603; Ned V. Schimizzi, "Does Your State Have a Free Lead Testing Program for Children?" *Journal of School Health* (1976), 46: 356–357; Jack Froom, "Lead Screening by Family Physicians," *Journal of Family Practice* (1977), 4: 631–633; Froom, Vincenza Boisseau, and Adele Sherman, "Selective Screening for Lead Poisoning in an Urban Teaching Practice," *Journal of Family Practice* (1979), 9: 65–70; Louis E. Kopito, Michael A. Davis, and Harry Shwachman, "Sources of Error in Determining Lead in Blood by Atomic Absorption Spectrophotometry," *Clinical Chemistry* (1974), 20: 205–211; and Sergio Piomelli and Joseph Graziano, "Laboratory Diagnosis of Lead Poisoning," *Pediatric Clinics of North America* (1980), 27: 843–853.

49. Donald R. Hopkins and Vernon N. Houk, "Federally-Assisted Screening Projects for Childhood Lead Poisoning Control: The First Three Years (July 1972–June 1975)," *American Journal of Public Health* (1976), 66: 485–486. See also Billiamin A. Alli, "Lead Poisoning in Children," *Journal of the National Medical Association* (1977), 69: 797–798. On *Connecticut*, see J. Wister Meigs and Elaine Whitmire, "Epidemiology of Lead Poisoning in New Haven Children—Operational Factors," *Connecticut Medicine* (1971), 35: 363–369; Thomas F. Dolan, Jr., Stephen F. Wang, and A. Meyers, "Treatment of Lead Poisoning at Yale–New Haven Hospital 1970," *Connecticut Medicine* (1971), 35: 482–484; William W. Ullman, "Lead in the Connecticut Environment," *Connecticut Medicine* (1971), 35: 360–362; Mahlon Hale and Martha L. Lepow, "Epidemiology of Increased Lead Exposure among 954 One- to Five-Year-Old Hartford, Connecticut, Children—1970," *Connecticut Medicine* (1971), 35: 492–497; Paul Harris, Alvin H. Novack, and Leonard F. Fichtenbaum, "Lead Poisoning in an Inner City Neighborhood," *Connecticut Medicine* (1971), 35: 485–488. On *Delaware*, see Elizabeth M. Craven, Barbara B. Rose, Vincenta Marquez, and Louis Slyvester, "Lead Poisoning in Wilmington, Delaware," *Delaware Medical Journal* (1973), 45: 1–7; "Lead Poisoning in Children: A Medical Responsibility?" (editorial) *Delaware Medical Journal* (1973), 45: 20. On *Washington, D.C.*, see Robert H. Conn and Dudley Anderson, "D.C. Mounts Unfunded Program of Screening for Lead Poisoning," *HSMHA Health Reports* (1971), 86: 408–413; Raymond L. Standard, "Lead Poisoning in Children," *Medical Annals of the District of Columbia* (1970), 39: 399–400; Stuart Danovitch and Clifton Gruver, "Lead Poisoning," *Medical Annals of the District of Columbia* (1970), 39: 583–584; Raymond L. Standard, "Results of Blood Lead Levels in the Model Cities Area—1971," *Medical Annals of the District of Columbia* (1972), 41: 323–324. On *New Orleans*, see Dan Blumenthal, "Lead Ingestion in New Orleans Children," *Southern Medical Journal* (1971), 64: 364–365. On *Oklahoma*, see Robert Lea Fulwiler and Logan Wright, "Sequelae of Lead Poisoning in Children," *Journal of the Oklahoma State Medical Association* (1972), 65: 372–375. On *New Jersey*, see Ann A. Browder, "Lead

Poisoning in Newark: The Situation Prior to a Case Finding and Intervention Program," *Journal of the Medical Society of New Jersey* (1972), 69: 101–106; D. Gause, W. Chase, J. Foster, and D. B. Louria, "Reduction in Lead Levels among Children in Newark," *Journal of the Medical Society of New Jersey* (1977), 74: 958–960. On *Cincinnati and Norfolk*, see Roger Challop, Edward McCabe, and Robert Reece, "Breaking the Childhood Lead Poisoning Cycle—A Program for Community Casefinding and Self-Help," *American Journal of Public Health* (1972), 62: 655–677. On *Kansas City*, see Vernon A. Green, George W. Wise, and Ned W. Small, "Lead Survey of Selected Children in Kansas City and Some Unusual Cases," *Clinical Toxicology* (1973), 6: 29–37. On *Grand Rapids*, see Robert G. Bulten, John L. Doyle, and Donald G. Young, "Lead Levels in Urban Grand Rapids Children," *Michigan Medicine* (1974), 73: 27–29. On *Milwaukee*, see Ruth Schuh and Ronald C. Backer, "Childhood Lead Poisoning Prevention Program in Milwaukee," *Wisconsin Medical Journal* (1975), 74: S42–S46. On *Charleston, S.C.*, see Norris H. Whitlock, J. Routt Reigart, and Lamar E. Priester, "Lead Poisoning in South Carolina," *Journal of the South Carolina Medical Association* (1977), 73: 378–380; Edward R. Williams and Arthur F. DiSalvo, "Lead Screening in South Carolina," *Journal of the South Carolina Medical Association* (1981), 77: 479–481. On *Wilmington, N.C.*, see Stephen H. Gehlbach, Betty West, Jean Morris, Elizabeth Summey, and Frank R. Reynolds, "Childhood Lead Poisoning in North Carolina: Experience in Wilmington," *North Carolina Medical Journal* (1977), 38: 383–386. On *Arkansas*, see Ruth R. Blackwood, "Childhood Lead Poisoning in Arkansas," *Journal of the Arkansas Medical Society* (1977), 74: 77–78. On *Massachusetts*, see "Lead-Poisoning Prevention in Massachusetts," *New England Journal of Medicine* (1973), 289: 428–429.

50. James M. Simpson, John L. Clark, Roger Challop, and Edward B. McCabe, "Elevated Blood Lead Levels in Children—A 27-City Neighborhood Survey," *Health Services Reports* (1973), 88: 419–422. Cities surveyed were: Chester, Pa.; Des Moines; San Antonio; Trenton; Nashua, N.H.; Denver; Nashville; Pasadena; Toledo; Sacramento; Portland, Ore.; Wilmington, Del.; Spokane; Lexington, Ky.; Indianapolis; Binghamton; Stamford; Salt Lake City; Flint; Wichita; Tulsa; Pensacola; Dayton; Hoboken; Charleston, S.C.; Albuquerque; and Harrisburg.

51. Carol J. Cohen, George N. Bowers, and Martha L. Lepow, "Epidemiology of Lead Poisoning: A Comparison between Urban and Rural Children," *Journal of the American Medical Association* (1973), 226: 1430–1433.

52. "Lead Paint Poisoning Program," *Maryland State Medical Journal* (1974), 23: 29–30.

53. Gerard R. Laurer, Theodore J. Kneip, Roy E. Albert, and Frederick S. Kent, "X-ray Fluorescence: Detection of Lead in Wall Paint," *Science* (1971), 172: 466–468; and "Lead Paint Detectors," *Baltimore Health News* (1971), 47: 33.

54. American Academy of Pediatrics, "News Release," May 20, 1972.

55. Memo, Mary G. Dale (assistant director, Department of Chapters, American Academy of Pediatrics) to Participants in the Eastern Regional Conference on Childhood Lead Poisoning, Conference Program, April 11, 1972, Lead Industries Association (LIA) Archives, housed in the offices of Sullivan, Sullivan, and Nahigian, Boston, Mass.

56. LIA Archives.

57. Raymond L. Tyler, Chief, Accident Control Section, Environmental Health Services, Philadelphia to James C. Roumas, Director of Health and Safety, LIA, October 23, 1969, LIA Archives.

58. American Academy of Pediatrics, Subcommittee on Accidental Poisonings, "Prevention, Diagnosis, and Treatment of Lead Poisoning in Childhood," 296–297.

59. "Medical Aspects of Childhood Lead Poisoning," 466.

60. Lin-Fu, "Childhood Lead Poisoning . . . An Eradicable Disease"; Jean E. Moore, "Community Aspects of Childhood Lead Poisoning," *American Journal of Public Health*

(1970), 60: 1430–1434; Lloyd A. Thomas, Rita G. Harper, and Dorothy L. Trice, "A Community Centered Approach to the Problem of Lead Poisoning," *Journal of the National Medical Association* (1970), 62: 106–108.

61. For examples, see Mark W. Oberle, "Lead Poisoning: A Preventable Childhood Disease of the Slums," *Science* (1969), 165: 991–992; Roger S. Challop, "Lead Poisoning: A Crisis of Conscience," *Medical Annals of the District of Columbia* (1972), 41: 561–563; Edmund O. Rothschild, "Lead Poisoning—The Silent Epidemic" (editorial), *New England Journal of Medicine* (1970), 282: 704–705; Celia S. Deschin, "Knowledge Is Neither Neutral nor Apolitical" (editorial), *American Journal of Orthopsychiatry* (1971), 41: 344–347; J. Julian Chisholm, Jr., "Lead Poisoning," *Scientific American* (1971), 224: 15–23; Jane S. Lin-Fu, "Lead Poisoning in Children—What Price Shall We Pay?" *Children Today* (1979), 8: 9–13; and Robert Klein, "The Pediatrician and the Prevention of Lead Poisoning in Children," *Pediatric Clinics of North America* (1974), 21: 277–290.

62. Moore, "Community Aspects of Childhood Lead Poisoning."

Chapter 14   Air Pollution and an Epidemic Redefined

1. P. B. Hammond, "Lead Poisoning: An Old Problem with a New Dimension," *Essays in Toxicology* (1969), 1: 115–155.

2. United States Working Group on Lead Contamination, *Survey of Lead in the Atmosphere of Three Urban Communities* (Washington, D.C.: U.S. Department of Health, Education, and Welfare, Public Health Service, Government Printing Office, 1965).

3. Ibid., 60.

4. Ibid., 68–75.

5. Ibid., 76–85.

6. Herbert L. Needleman and John Scanlon, "Getting the Lead Out," *New England Journal of Medicine* (1973), 288: 466–467.

7. National Research Council, *Lead: Airborne Lead in Perspective* (Washington, D.C.: National Academy of Sciences, Government Printing Office, 1972).

8. Nevertheless, an investigative reporter from *Science* concluded, "In the overview, there appears to be no evidence that the lead panel's biases, whether real or illusory, were deliberate. More likely, they are an expression of the academy's innate conservatism and the product of a lingering 19th century faith in the virtue of industry and the impartiality of scientists." See Robert Gillette, "Lead in the Air: Industry Weight on Academy Panel Challenged," *Science* (1971), 174: 802.

9. National Research Council, *Lead: Airborne Lead in Perspective*, 12.

10. Ibid., 29–30.

11. Sidney Kaye and Paul Reznikoff, "A Comparative Study of the Lead Content of Street Dirts in New York City in 1924 and 1934," *Journal of Industrial Hygiene and Toxicology* (1947), 29: 178–179.

12. J. Cholak, L. J. Schafer, and R. F. Hoffer, "Results of a Five-Year Investigation of Air Pollution in Cincinnati," *Archives of Industrial Hygiene and Occupational Medicine* (1952), 6: 314–325; and J. Cholak, L. J. Schafer, and T. D. Sterling, "The Lead Content of the Atmosphere," *Journal of the Air Pollution Control Association* (1961), 11: 281–288.

13. Arthur F. W. Peart and Gordon H. Josie, "Planning a Study to Determine the Effects of Air Pollution on Health," *Archives of Industrial Hygiene and Occupational Medicine* (1953), 7: 326–338.

14. National Research Council, *Lead: Airborne Lead in Perspective*, 11.

15. Ibid., 139.

16. Ibid., 159–160.

17. "Recent surveys of children in large cities indicate that many have blood lead con-

centrations in the range of 40–60 micrograms/dl of whole blood. These high blood lead concentrations cannot be ascribed specifically to the inhalation of lead, although that is a possibility. It is also possible that these infants and children eat leaded paint in quantities too small to produce acute poisoning and that at least some of their lead burden comes from the ingestion of lead-bearing street dust and soil, which often attains concentrations in excess of 2000 micrograms/g. Assuming the validity of the relation between daily lead intake and blood lead content, the daily ingestion by a child weighing 10kg of 0.41g of street dust with a lead content of 2000 micrograms/g, would result ultimately in a blood lead concentration compatible with clinical lead poisoning, even without allowing for additional lead acquired by inhalation, from normal dietary sources, or from coincident ingestion of lead paint." Ibid., 210.
18. Barry G. King, "Massive Daily Intake of Lead without Excessive Body Lead-Burden in Children," *American Journal of Diseases of Children* (1971), 122: 337–340. Members of the committee included: Roger Challop, Bureau of Community Environmental Management, Department of Health, Education, and Welfare; J. Julian Chisholm, Jr., Johns Hopkins; Jane Lin-Fu, Maternal and Child Health Service, DHEW; Herbert Stokinger, Bureau of Occupational Safety and Health, DHEW; Lloyd Tepper, Kettering Laboratory; Barry King, Bureau of Community Environmental Management, DHEW.
19. American Academy of Pediatrics, Committee on Environmental Hazards, "Lead Content of Paint Applied to Surfaces Accessible to Children," *Pediatrics* (1972), 49: 918–921.
20. National Research Council, "Report of the Ad Hoc Committee to Evaluate the Hazard of Lead in Paint" (Washington, D.C.: National Academy of Sciences, Government Printing Office, 1973), 5.
21. Hearings before the Subcommittee on Health of the Committee on Labor and Public Welfare (Senate), March 6, 9, 10, 1972.
22. Ibid., 34, 48.
23. Ibid., 58–59, 132–152.
24. Ibid., 164.
25. Ibid., 207.
26. Ibid., 99.
27. Ibid., 20.
28. National Research Council, "Report of the Ad Hoc Committee to Evaluate the Hazard of Lead in Paint."
29. Ibid., 15–17.
30. Ibid., 31–32.
31. Richard O. Simpson, "A Report to Congress in Compliance with Lead-Based Paint Poisoning Prevention Act as Amended (P.L. 93–151)," (Washington, D.C.: U.S. Consumer Product Safety Commission), 1.
32. Hearings before the Subcommittee on Health of the Committee on Labor and Public Welfare (Senate), March 6, 9, 10, 1972, 6–12.
33. Ibid., 39–46.
34. Ibid., 47–50.
35. Subcommittee on Health of the Committee on Labor and Public Welfare, Hearing on Lead-Based Paint Poisoning Prevention Act of 1974, June 6, 1975, 136, 151; for a published account, see Herbert L. Needleman, "Lead-Paint Poisoning Prevention: An Opportunity Forfeited" (editorial), *New England Journal of Medicine* (1975), 292: 588–589.
36. National Research Council, Committee on Toxicology, "Recommendations for the Prevention of Lead Poisoning in Children" (Washington, D.C.: National Academy of Sciences, Government Printing Office, 1976); for a published summary of the report, see "Recommendations for the Prevention of Lead Poisoning in Children," *Nutrition Reviews* (1976), 34: 321–327.

37. F. W. Alexander, Barbara E. Clayton, and H. T. Delves, "Mineral and Trace-Metal Balances in Children Receiving Normal and Synthetic Diets," _Quarterly Journal of Medicine_ (1974), 43: 89–111; F. W. Alexander, "The Uptake of Lead by Children in Differing Environments," _Environmental Health Perspectives_ (1974), 7: 155–159; and Ekhard E. Ziegler, Barbara B. Edwards, Robert L. Jensen, Kathryn R. Mahaffey, and Samuel J. Fomon, "Absorption and Retention of Lead by Infants," _Pediatric Research_ (1978,) 12: 29–34.

38. Center for Disease Control, "Increased Lead Absorption and Lead Poisoning in Young Children: A Statement by the Center for Disease Control," _Journal of Pediatrics_ (1975), 87: 824–830. The biggest change from the Public Health Service statement in 1970 was a lowering of the blood lead level for "undue or increased lead absorption" to 30–79 micrograms/dl.

39. National Research Council, Committee on Toxicology, "Recommendations for the Prevention of Lead Poisoning in Children," app. F.

40. Consumer Product Safety Commission, "Final Environmental Impact Statement on Lead Content of Paint," May 27, 1977, XI-2.

41. U.S. Department of Health, Education, and Welfare, 37 Fed. Reg. 4915-6 (March 7, 1972); U.S. Department of Housing and Urban Development, 37 Fed. Reg. 16,872-3 (August 22, 1972); and HUD 37 Fed. Reg. 22,732-3 (October 21, 1972).

42. U.S. Food and Drug Administration, 37 Fed. Reg. 5,229-31 (March 11, 1972); and U.S. Consumer Product Safety Commission, 42 Fed. Reg. 44,199-201 (September 1, 1977).

43. Consumer Product Safety Commission, "Final Environmental Impact Statement on Lead Content of Paint," May 27, 1977, III-22-23; the original petition came in response to an FDA regulation in 1972 which defined lead-based paints as hazardous substances; National Paint and Coatings Association (NPCA) to Commissioner of Food and Drug Administration, October 24, 1972.

44. NPCA to Commissioner of Food and Drug Administration, October 24, 1972, 13–14.

45. Mark Silbergeld (attorney, Washington, D.C., office, Consumers Union) to Sadye Dunn (secretary, CPSC), March 16, 1977.

46. J. Julian Chisholm, Jr. (Baltimore City Hospital) to Sadye Dunn (secretary, CPSC), March 9, 1977; and Lewis D. Polk (acting health commissioner, Philadelphia) to CPSC, March 11, 1977.

47. U.S. Food and Drug Administration, 37 Fed. Reg. 5,229-31 (March 11, 1972); and FDA, 37 Fed. Reg. 16, 078-9 (August 10, 1972).

48. Harriet L. Hardy, Richard I. Chamberlin, Clarence C. Maloof, George W. Boylen, Jr., and Mary C. Howell, "Lead as an Environmental Poison," _Clinical Pharmacology and Therapeutics_ (1971), 12: 982–1002.

49. For a summary of state and municipal ordinances, see National Research Council, _Lead: Airborne Lead in Perspective_, 77. See also the ordinances of Minneapolis and Massachusetts: (Minneapolis) "Housing Maintenance Code: Maintenance by Owners Relating to Lead Poisoning in Paint," Minneapolis Code of Ordinances Chapter 72, July 15, 1969; (Massachusetts) "An Act Providing for a Comprehensive Program of Lead Paint Poisoning Prevention and Control," General Laws of Massachusetts, Chapter 1081, Sections 190–199, Nov. 15, 1971.

50. Robert G. Oliver, "Lead and the Legislature–1971," _Connecticut Medicine_ (1971), 35: 498–500. Years when legislation passed: New York State, 1970 ("Public Health—Lead Poisoning," Laws of New York, Chapter 338, Title 10, Sections 1370–1376, May 1, 1970); New Orleans, 1971 (see Dan Blumenthal, "Lead Ingestion in New Orleans Children," _Southern Medical Journal_ [1971], 64: 364–365); Maryland, 1971 ("Prohibit the Use of Lead-Based Paint in Dwellings in Order to Protect Children," Annotated

Code of Maryland, Chapter 495, Article 13, Section 117A, May 17, 1971); New Jersey, 1971 ("An Act Prohibiting the Use of Lead Paint under Certain Circumstances," New Jersey Revised Statutes, Chapter 366, Title 24A1-12, Dec. 28, 1971); Chicago, 1972 ("Prohibit Use of Lead or Toxic Based Substances on Exposed Surfaces," Municipal Code of Chicago, Chapter 78, Section 17.2, Feb. 23, 1972); Kentucky, 1972 ("Restrictions on Sale and Use of Paint Containing Lead; Labeling," KY ST § 217.801, June 16, 1972); Louisiana, 1973 ("Sale and Use of Lead-Based Paint," Louisiana Revised Statutes 40: 1299. 26(a), Jan. 1, 1973).

51. Consumer Product Safety Commission, "Final Environmental Impact Statement on Lead Content of Paint," May 27, 1977, I-A-11.

52. Irwin Harold Billick and V. Eugene Gray, *Lead-Based Paint Poisoning Research: Review and Evaluation, 1971–1977* (Washington, D.C.: U.S. Department of Housing and Urban Development, Office of Policy Development and Research, Government Printing Office, 1978).

53. Irwin H. Billick, Anita S. Curran, and Douglas R. Shier, "Analysis of Pediatric Blood Lead Levels in New York City for 1970–1976," *Environmental Health Perspectives* (1979), 31: 183–190.

54. D. Gause, W. Chase, J. Foster, and D. B. Louria, "Reduction in Lead Levels among Children in Newark," *Journal of the Medical Society of New Jersey* (1977), 74: 958–960; Henrietta K. Sachs, "Effect of a Screening Program on Changing Patterns of Lead Poisoning," *Environmental Health Perspectives* (1974), 7: 41–45.

55. Billick and Gray, *Lead Based Paint Poisoning Research*, table 6, 4, 80.

56. Ibid., executive summary.

57. Ibid., 70. For a cost-benefit analysis of childhood lead programs, see David W. Broudy, and J. Michael Swint, and David R. Lairson, "Prospective Economic Evaluation of Lead Poisoning Prevention Programs, *Journal of Community Health* (1979), 4: 291–301.

58. Billick and Gray, *Lead Based Paint Poisoning Research: Review and Evaluation, 1971–1977*, chap 2.

59. Center for Disease Control, "Preventing Lead Poisoning in Young Children: A Statement by the Center for Disease Control," *Journal of Pediatrics* (1978), 93: 710.

60. Ibid.

61. Ibid., 717.

62. Ibid.

63. Ibid., 718.

64. Massachusetts, "An Act Providing," 1971; New Jersey, "An Act Prohibiting," 1971. For an analysis of the abatement program in Newark, New Jersey, see James D. Foster, Donald B. Louria, and Lydia Stinson, "Influence of Documented Lead Poisoning on Environmental Modification Programs in Newark, New Jersey," *Archives of Environmental Health* (1979), 34: 368–371. See also Chicago, "Prohibit Use of Lead," 1972.

65. U.S. Department of Housing and Urban Development, 41 Fed. Reg. 28,876-81 (July 13, 1976).

Chapter 15 **Dust, Dirt, and Mouthing in 1980**

1. F. W. Alexander, Barbara E. Clayton, and H. T. Delves, "Mineral and Trace-Metal Balances in Children Receiving Normal and Synthetic Diets," *Quarterly Journal of Medicine* (1974), 43: 89–111; and Ekhard E. Ziegler, Barbara B. Edwards, Robert L. Jensen, Kathryn R. Mahaffey, and Samuel J. Fomon, "Absorption and Retention of Lead by Infants," *Pediatric Research* (1978), 12: 29–34.

2. Alan J. Clark and George W. Hallett, "Lead Poisoning Survey—Portland, Maine, July–August, 1970," *Journal of the Maine Medical Association* (1971), 62: 6–7.

3. Bart Barnes, "Lead Poisoning in Remodeling of Old Homes," *Children Today* (1973),

2: 7–9; Muriel D. Wolf, "Lead Poisoning from Restoration of Old Homes," *Journal of the American Medical Association* (1973), 225: 175–176.

4. Evan Charney, "Lead Poisoning in Children: The Case against Household Lead Dust," *Lead Absorption in Children: Management, Clinical, and Environmental Aspects*, ed. J. Julian Chisholm, Jr., and David M. O'Hara (Baltimore: Urban and Schwarzenberg, 1982), 79–88. Despite the title, Charney argues that dust and dirt became the major new source of household lead.

5. J. Julian Chisholm, Jr., "Screening for Lead Poisoning in Children," *Pediatrics* (1973), 51: 281–282. Cleveland researchers were not able to discover an elevated urinary CPP-III in children playing in dirt outside the home, see Robert C. Griggs, Irving Sunshine, Vaun A. Newill, Burritt W. Newton, Stuart Buchanan, and Cleo A. Rasch, "Environmental Factors in Childhood Lead Poisoning," *Journal of the American Medical Association* (1964), 187: 706. Clair Patterson estimated the amount of lead in soil in 1965; see Patterson, "Contaminated and Natural Lead Environments of Man," *Archives of Environmental Health* (1965), 11: 353.

6. Herbert L. Needleman and John Scanlon, "Getting the Lead Out," *New England Journal of Medicine* (1973), 288: 466; and R. M. Hicks, "Air-Borne Lead as an Environmental Toxin," *Chemico-Biological Interactions* (1972), 5: 367.

7. James W. Sayre, Evan Charney, Jaroslav Vostal, and I. Barry Pless, "House and Hand Dust as a Potential Source of Childhood Lead Exposure," *American Journal of Diseases of Children* (1974), 127: 167–170.

8. Jane S. Lin-Fu, "Vulnerability of Children to Lead Exposure and Toxicity, part 2," *New England Journal of Medicine* (1973), 289: 1289. This article was actually published before the Rochester study (see note 7) but cited its conclusions. See also Michael C. Klein, James W. Sayre, and David Kotok, "Lead Poisoning: Current Status of the Problem Facing Pediatricians," *American Journal of Diseases of Children* (1974), 127: 805; Donald Barltrop, "Children and Lead," *American Journal of Diseases of Children* (1974), 127: 165; and Dennis Malcolm, "Environmental Lead Pollution," *Proceedings of the Royal Society of Medicine* (1974), 67: 167–168.

9. Jaroslav J. Vostal, Ellen Taves, James W. Sayre, and Evan Charney, "Lead Analysis of House Dust: A Method for the Detection of Another Source of Lead Exposure in Inner City Children," *Environmental Health Perspectives* (1974), 7: 96.

10. Martha L. Lepow, Leonard Bruckman, Marybeth Gillette, Steven Markowitz, Robert Robino, and Janet Kapish, "Investigations into Sources of Lead in the Environment of Urban Children," *Environmental Research* (1975), 10: 419.

11. Kathryn R. Mahaffey, "Quantities of Lead Producing Health Effects in Humans: Sources and Bioavailability," *Environmental Health Perspectives* (1977), 19: 285–295.

12. F. Strait Fairey and John W. Gray III, "Soil Lead and Pediatric Lead Poisoning in Charleston, S.C.," *Journal of the South Carolina Medical Association* (1970), 66: 79–82.

13. Gary Ter Haar and Regine Aronow, "Tracer Studies of Ingestion of Dust by Urban Children," *Environmental Quality and Safety* (1975), suppl. 2: 197–201.

14. Lepow et al., "Investigations into Sources of Lead in the Environment of Urban Children."

15. Carol R. Angle, Matilda S. McIntire, and Gary Vest, "Blood Lead of Omaha School Children—Topographic Correlation with Industry, Traffic, and Housing," *Nebraska Medical Journal* (1975), 60: 97–102.

16. James W. Sayre and Monica Katzel, "Household Surface Lead Dust: Its Accumulation in Vacant Homes," *Environmental Health Perspectives* (1979), 29: 179–182; Bruce P. Lanphear, T. D. Matte, J. Rogers, R. P. Clickner, B. Dietz, R. L. Bornschein, P. Succop, K. R. Mahaffey, S. Dixon, W. Galke, M. Rabinowitz, M. Farfel, C. Rohde, J. Schwartz, P. Ashley, and D. E. Jacobs, "The Contribution of Lead-Contaminated House Dust and Residential Soil to Children's Blood Lead Levels: A Pooled Analy-

sis of 12 Epidemiologic Studies," *Environmental Research* (1998), 79: 51–68.

17. S. D. Walter, A. J. Yankel, and I. H. von Lindern, "Age-Specific Risk Factors for Lead Absorption in Children," *Archives of Environmental Health* (1980), 35: 53–58.

18. Donald Barltrop, "The Prevalence of Pica," *American Journal of Diseases of Children* (1966), 112: 116–123.

19. Martha F. Leonard, "The Significance of Pica in Children," *Connecticut Medicine* (1971), 35: 479–482; Reginald S. Lourie, "Prevention of Lead Paint—or Prevention of Pica," *Pediatrics* (1971), 48: 490–491; Lourie, "Pica and Poisoning," *American Journal of Orthopsychiatry* (1971), 41: 697–699; James M. Oleske, "Not All Children Are Magpies," *Pediatrics* (1975), 55: 297–298; Siegfried M. Pueschel, Susan M. Cullen, Rosanne B. Howard, and Marie M. Cullinane, "Pathogenetic Considerations of Pica in Lead Poisoning," *International Journal of Psychiatry in Medicine* (1977–78), 8: 13–24; Steven M. Marcus, Rhodora Damaso-Diaz, and Robert Ziering, "Mouthing Activities and Their Relationship to Lead Poisoning," *Journal of the Medical Society of New Jersey* (1978), 75: 837–838; Nancy A. Madden, Dennis C. Russo, and Michael F. Cataldo, "Environmental Influences on Mouthing in Children with Lead Intoxication," *Journal of Pediatric Psychology* (1980), 5: 207–216; Edward B. McCabe, "Age and Sensitivity to Lead Toxicity: A Review," *Environmental Health Perspectives* (1979), 29: 29–33; Brigitte de la Burdé and Betty Reames, "Prevention of Pica, the Major Cause of Lead Poisoning in Children," *American Journal of Public Health* (1973), 63: 737–743.

20. Evan Charney, Barry Kessler, Mark Farfel, and David Jackson, "Childhood Lead Poisoning: A Controlled Trial of the Effect of Dust-Control Measures on Blood Lead Levels," *New England Journal of Medicine* (1983), 309: 1089–1093.

21. Michael C. Klein, James W. Sayre, and David Kotok, "Lead Poisoning: Current Status of the Problem Facing Pediatricians," *American Journal of Diseases of Children* (1974), 127: 805.

22. Jane S. Lin-Fu, "Vulnerability of Children to Lead Exposure and Toxicity: Part 1," *New England Journal of Medicine* (1973), 289: 1229–1233.

23. Hugo Dunlap Smith, Robert L. Baehner, Thomas Carney, and William Joseph Majors, "The Sequelae of Pica with and without Lead Poisoning," *American Journal of Diseases of Children* (1963), 105: 609–616.

24. Meyer A. Perlstein and Ramzy Attala, "Neurological Sequelae of Plumbism in Children," *Clinical Pediatrics* (1966), 5: 292–298.

25. Emil A. Tiboni and Raymond L. Tyler, "Childhood Lead Poisoning in Philadelphia," *Philadelphia Medicine* (1960), 56: 668–669.

26. "Lead-Based Paint Poisoning," hearing before the Subcommittee on Health of the Committee on Labor and Public Welfare, United States Congress, Senate (Washington, D.C.: Government Printing Office, 1970), 203.

27. American Academy of Pediatrics, Subcommittee on Accidental Poisoning, "Prevention, Diagnosis, and Treatment of Lead Poisoning in Childhood," *Pediatrics* (1969), 44: 291–298.

28. "Medical Aspects of Childhood Lead Poisoning," *Pediatrics* (1971), 48: 464–468.

29. Siegfried M. Pueschel, Louis Kopito, and Harry Schwachman, "Children with Increased Lead Burden: A Screening and Follow-up Study," *Journal of the American Medical Association* (1972), 222: 462–466.

30. Siegfried M. Pueschel, "Neurological and Psychomotor Functions in Children with an Increased Lead Burden," *Environmental Health Perspectives* (1974), 7: 13–16.

31. Brigitte de la Burdé and McLin S. Choate, Jr., "Does Asymptomatic Lead Exposure in Children Have Latent Sequelae?" *Journal of Pediatrics* (1972), 81: 1088–1091; and de la Burdé and William E. Laupus, "Subclinical Lead Poisoning in a Group of Children," *Virginia Medical Monthly* (1973), 100: 623–628.

32. Brigitte de la Burdé and McLin S. Choate, Jr., "Early Asymptomatic Lead Exposure

and Development at School Age," *Journal of Pediatrics* (1975), 87: 638–642. See comment, Evan Charney, "Lead in Teeth as a Determinant of Long-Term Exposure to Lead" (letter), *Journal of Pediatrics* (1976), 89: 1040–1041.

33. David Kotok, "Development of Children with Elevated Blood Lead Levels: A Controlled Study," *Journal of Pediatrics* (1972), 80: 57–61.

34. Phillip Nieburg, David Kotock, and J. J. Chisholm, Jr., "Development of Children with Elevated Blood Lead Levels" (letter), *Journal of Pediatrics* (1972), 81: 627–628; and Keith R. Powell, U. T. Rolfe, and D. Kotock, "Development of Children with Elevated Blood Lead Levels" (letter), *Journal of Pediatrics* (1972), 81: 628–630.

35. Nieburg, Kotock, and Chisholm, "Development of Children with Elevated Blood Lead Levels."

36. R. E. Albert, R. E. Shore, A. J. Sayres, C. Strehlow, T. J. Kneip, B. S. Pasterack, A. J. Friedhoff, F. Covan, and J. A. Cimino, "Follow-Up of Children Overexposed to Lead," *Environmental Health Perspectives* (1974), 7: 33–39.

37. Ralph Barocas and Bernard Weiss, "Behavioral Assessment of Lead Intoxication in Children," *Environmental Health Perspectives* (1974), 7: 47–52.

38. Philip J. Landrigan, Randolph H. Whitworth, Robert W. Baloh, Norman W. Staehling, William F. Barthel, and Bernard F. Rosenblum, "Neuropsychological Dysfunction in Children with Chronic Low-Level Lead Absorption," *Lancet* (1975), 1: 708–712.

39. Oliver J. David, "Association between Lower Level Lead Concentrations and Hyperactivity," *Environmental Health Perspectives* (1974), 7: 17–25; David, Stanley P. Hoffman, and Jeffrey Sverd, "The Role of Lead in Hyperactivity," *Psychopharmacology Bulletin* (1976), 12: 11–13; David, Hoffman, Sverd, Julian Clark, and Kytja Voeller, "Lead and Hyperactivity: Behavioral Response to Chelation: A Pilot Study," *American Journal of Psychiatry* (1976), 133: 1155–1158; and David, Clark, and Hoffman, "Childhood Lead Poisoning: A Re-Evaluation," *Archives of Environmental Health* (1979), 34: 106–111.

40. Robert Baloh, Randall Sturm, Bonnie Green, and Goldine Gleser, "Neuropsychological Effects of Chronic Asymptomatic Increased Lead Absorption: A Controlled Study," *Archives of Neurology* (1975), 32: 326–330.

41. Donald Barltrop, "Sub-Clinical Lead Poisoning in Children," *Journal of Child Psychology and Psychiatry* (1976), 17: 225–227.

42. J. Julian Chisholm, Jr., "Management of Increased Lead Absorption and Lead Poisoning in Children," *New England Journal of Medicine* (1973), 289: 1016–1018.

43. Herbert L. Needleman and Irving M. Shapiro, "Dentine Lead Levels in Asymptomatic Philadelphia School Children: Subclinical Exposure in High and Low Risk Groups," *Environmental Health Perspectives* (1974), 7: 27–31.

44. Richard W. Moriarty, "Screening to Prevent Lead Poisoning," *Pediatrics* (1974), 54: 626–628.

45. "Lead and Mental Handicap" (editorial), *Lancet* (1978), 1: 365–367; "Child Health and Environmental Lead" (editorial), *British Medical Journal* (1977), 1: 255–256.

46. Center for Disease Control, "Increased Lead Absorption and Lead Poisoning in Young Children: A Statement by the Center for Disease Control," *Journal of Pediatrics* (1975), 87: 1152–1160.

47. Herbert L. Needleman, Charles Gunnoe, Alan Leviton, Robert Reed, Henry Peresie, Cornelius Maher, and Peter Barret, "Deficits in Psychologic and Classroom Performance of Children with Elevated Dentine Lead Levels," *New England Journal of Medicine* (1979), 300: 689–695. For earlier work, see Irving M. Shapiro, Bruce Dobkin, Orphan C. Tuncay, and Herbert L. Needleman, "Lead Levels in Dentine and Circumpulpal Dentine of Deciduous Teeth of Normal and Lead Poisoned Children," *Clinica Chimica Acta* (1973), 46: 119–123; Needleman, "Lead Poisoning in Children: Neurologic Implications of Widespread Subclinical Intoxication," *Seminars in Psy-

chiatry (1973), 5: 47–54; and Herbert L. Needleman, Isobel Davidson, Edward M. Sewell, and Irving M. Shapiro, "Subclinical Lead Exposure in Philadelphia School Children: Identification by Dentine Lead Analysis," *New England Journal of Medicine* (1974), 290: 245–248.

48. Michael Rutter, "Raised Lead Levels and Impaired Cognitive/Behavioural Functioning: A Review of the Evidence," *Developmental Medicine and Child Neurology* (1980), suppl. 42: 1–36.

49. James R. Varga, "More on Long-Term Sequelae of Exposure to Lead" (letter), *Journal of Pediatrics* (1979), 94: 680–681; and Philip Graham, "Research into Lead Pollution" (letter), *Lancet* (1979), 1: 1024–1025. For Needleman's reply to Graham, see Herbert L. Needleman and Alan Leviton, "Lead Deficit in Children" (letter), *Lancet* (1979), 2: 104.

50. R. Lansdown, "Moderately Raised Blood Lead Levels in Children," *Proceedings of the Royal Society of London, Series B: Biological Sciences* (1979), 205: 145–161.

51. Henrietta K. Sachs, Donald A. McCaughran, Vita Krall, Irving H. Rozenfeld, and Nillawan Yongsmith, "Lead Poisoning without Encephalopathy: Effect of Early Diagnosis on Neurologic and Psychologic Salvage," *American Journal of Diseases of Children* (1979), 133: 786–790.

52. Herbert L. Needleman and Alan Leviton, "Neurologic Effects of Exposure to Lead" (letter), *Journal of Pediatrics* (1979), 94: 505–506.

53. Phillip J. Landrigan, "Neurologic Effects of Exposure to Lead" (letter), *Journal of Pediatrics* (1979), 94: 504–505.

54. Judith Horn Rummo, Donald K. Routh, Nicholas J. Rummo, and James F. Brown, "Behavioral and Neurological Effects of Symptomatic and Asymptomatic Lead Exposure in Children," *Archives of Environmental Health* (1979), 34: 120–124.

55. Michael Rutter, "Raised Lead Levels and Impaired Cognitive/Behavioural Functioning."

56. Robert Bornschein, Douglas Pearson, and Lawrence Reiter, "Behavioral Effects of Moderate Lead Exposure in Children and Animal Models: Part 1, Clinical Studies," *CRC Critical Reviews in Toxicology* (1980), 8: 43–99.

57. M. R. Moore, "Exposure to Lead in Childhood: The Persisting Effects," *Nature* (1980), 283: 334–335; "Children and Lead: Some Remaining Doubts" (editorial), *Archives of Diseases of Childhood* (1980), 55: 497–499.

58. J. Julian Chisholm, Jr., and Donald Barltrop, "Recognition and Management of Children with Increased Lead Absorption," *Archives of Diseases of Childhood* (1979), 54: 258–259. In Britain the debate over the long-range effects of lead poisoning often queried whether lead was responsible for children institutionalized with mental handicaps. For opinions regarding the relationship between mental retardation and lead poisoning, see B. E. Oliver, "Aspects of Lead Absorption in Hospitalized Psychotic Children," *Journal of Mental Deficiency Research* (1967), 11: 132–142; Sheila L. M. Gibson, C. N. Lam, W. M. McCrea, and A. Goldberg, "Blood Lead Levels in Normal and Mentally Deficient Children," *Archives of Diseases of Childhood* (1967), 42: 573–578; Joan Bicknell, Barbara E. Clayton, and H. T. Delves, "Lead in Mentally Retarded Children," *Journal of Mental Deficiency Research* (1968), 12: 282–293; A. D. Beattie, M. R. Moore, A. Goldberg, Margaret J. W. Finlayson, Janet F. Graham, Elizabeth M. Mackie, Joan C. Main, D. A. McLaren, K. M. Murdoch, and G. T. Steward, "Role of Chronic Low-Level Lead Exposure in the Aetiology of Mental Retardation," *Lancet* (1975), 1: 589–592; and "Lead and Mental Handicap" (editorial), *Lancet* (1978), 1: 365–367.

59. CDC, "Preventing Lead Poisoning in Young Children."

60. A. D. Beattie, "The Use of D-Penicillamine for Lead Poisoning," *Proceedings of the Royal Society of Medicine* (1977), 78 (suppl. 3): 43–45; C. S. Bartsocas, J. A. Grunt, G. W. Boylen, Jr., and I. K. Brandt, "Oral D-Penicillamine and Intramuscular BAL + EDTA in the Treatment of Lead Accumulation," *Acta Paediatrica Scandinavica*

(1971), 60: 553–558; Leonard F. Vitale, Amy Rosalinas-Bailon, Dave Folland, J. F. Brennan, and Beryl McCormick, "Oral Penicillamine Therapy for Chronic Lead Poisoning in Children," *Journal of Pediatrics* (1973), 83: 1041–1045; J. Julian Chisholm, Jr., "Treatment of Acute Lead Intoxication—Choice of Chelating Agents and Supportive Therapeutic Measures," *Clinical Toxicology* (1970), 3: 527–540; Chisholm, "Childhood Lead Intoxication: Diagnosis, Management, and Prevention," *Medical Times* (1970), 98: 92–105; Chisholm, "Chelation Therapy in Children with Subclinical Plumbism," *Pediatrics* (1974), 53: 441–443; Chisholm, "Management of Increased Lead Absorption and Lead Poisoning in Children," *New England Journal of Medicine* (1973), 289: 1016–1018; and Michael C. Klein and Mary Schlageter, "Non-Treatment of Screened Children with Intermediate Blood Lead Levels," *Pediatrics* (1975), 56: 298–302.

Epilogue

1. The CDC had an additional category of "lead toxicity," which was defined in terms of free erythrocyte protoporphyrin of greater than 50 micrograms/dl, which corresponded to a blood lead of 30 micrograms/dl. So "lead toxicity" and "elevated lead level" were equivalent categories. Many health departments did not have ready access to blood lead measurements. Center for Disease Control, "Preventing Lead Poisoning in Young Children: A Statement by the Center for Disease Control," *Journal of Pediatrics* (1978), 93: 709–720.
2. Ibid., 710.
3. Ibid., 715.
4. Ibid., 710.
5. "The Nature and Extent of Lead Poisoning in Children in the United States: A Report to Congress," U.S. Department of Health and Human Services, Agency for Toxic Substances and Disease Registry, July 1988, V-32.
6. "Update: Blood Lead Levels—United States, 1991–1994," *Morbidity and Mortality Weekly Report* (1997), 46: 141–146.
7. Centers for Disease Control, "Preventing Lead Poisoning in Young Children," U.S. Department of Health and Human Services, Public Health Service, October 1991, 65.

Index

The following typographical conventions are used in the index: *f* identifies a figure; *t* identifies a table.

AAP. *See* American Academy of Pediatrics

abatement, of lead: American Academy of Pediatrics and, 161–162; Centers for Disease Control and, 172, 183; in factory dust, 30, 33, 35, 44, 47, 51; HUD funding for, 171–172; U.S. Public Health Service and, 162; in urban housing, 133–134, 168; using whitewash for, xiii, 101

abdominal pain, as lead poisoning symptom, xi, 8, 15, 18, 63, 65, 77

abortifacient, lead as, 44, 45

Abrahams, R., 12–13

absorption, of lead, 35–36; adult vs. infant, 173; hyperactivity and, 177–178, 179; neurological system damage from, 93, 175–176, 178, 179 (*see also* encephalopathy); psychological functioning and, 177–179. *See also* lead poisoning; sources, of lead

Abt, Isaac, 61, 62

African American children: blood lead levels of, 182*t*; lead attack rate for, 92–93, 97; lead poisoning in, xiii–xiv, 97,

108, 133, 134–135; pica among, 111

age, of children: afflicted with lead poisoning, 65, 67, 85–86, 92, 220n32; blood lead level by, 182*t*

air: lead content of, 1–2; as lead source, 164, 172, 173, 230n24. *See also* air pollution

air pollution, 140. *See also* air; dirt, as lead source; dust, as lead source; tetraethyl lead workers

ALA. *See* delta-aminolevulinic acid

Albert, R. E., 177

aldehyde, 53

Altshuller, Lillis, 118

AMA. *See* American Medical Association

American Academy of Pediatrics (AAP), 97, 123, 125, 127; accidental poisoning subcommittee of, 141–142; large-scale screening programs and, 157–158; lead abatement and, 161–162; and prevention/diagnosis/treatment of lead poisoning, 176; role in undue lead absorption program, 155; safe lead levels for paint recommended by, 169–170

American College of Physicians, 87

American Hospital Association, 125

American Medical Association (AMA), 96, 125, 126

About the Author

PETER C. ENGLISH is a professor of pediatrics and a professor of history at Duke University. He has published on the histories of surgical shock, child abuse, pneumonia, diphtheria, and rheumatic fever.

CPSIA information can be obtained at www.ICGtesting.com
Printed in the USA
BVOW010452300513

321866BV00008B/87/A